Obsessive-Compulsive Disorder Spectrum

Pathogenesis, Diagnosis, and Treatment

Obsessive-Compulsive Disorder Spectrum
Pathogenesis, Diagnosis, and Treatment

José A. Yaryura-Tobias, M.D., F.A.C.P.M.
Medical Director
Institute for Bio-Behavioral Therapy and Research
Great Neck, New York
Professor of Psychiatry
National University of Cuyo
Mendoza, Argentina

and

Fugen A. Neziroglu, Ph.D., A.B.B.P., A.B.P.P.
Clinical Director
Institute for Bio-Behavioral Therapy and Research
Great Neck, New York
Associate Professor
Hofstra University
Hempstead, New York

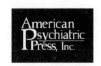

Washington, DC
London, England

Note: The authors have worked to ensure that all information in this book concerning drug dosages, schedules, and routes of administration is accurate as of the time of publication and consistent with standards set by the U.S. Food and Drug Administration and the general medical community. As medical research and practice advance, however, therapeutic standards may change. For this reason and because human and mechanical errors sometimes occur, we recommend that readers follow the advice of a physician who is directly involved in their care or the care of a member of their family.

Books published by the American Psychiatric Press, Inc., represent the views and opinions of the individual authors and do not necessarily represent the policies and opinions of the Press or the American Psychiatric Association.

Copyright © 1997 American Psychiatric Press, Inc.
ALL RIGHTS RESERVED
Manufactured in the United States of America on acid-free paper
00 99 98 97   4 3 2 1

American Psychiatric Press, Inc.
1400 K Street, N.W., Washington, DC   20005

Library of Congress Cataloging-in-Publication Data
Yaryura-Tobias, José A., 1934–
    Obsessive-compulsive disorder spectrum : pathogenesis, diagnosis,
and treatment / José A. Yaryura-Tobias, Fugen A. Neziroglu.
        p.   cm.
    Includes bibliographical references and index.
    ISBN 0-88048-707-0 (cloth : alk. paper)
    1. Obsessive-compulsive disorder.   I. Neziroglu, Fugen A., 1951–
II. Title.
    [DNLM: 1. Obsessive-Compulsive Disorder.   2. Mental Disorders.
WM 176 Y29o 1997]
RC533.Y369   1997
616.86'227—dc20
DNLM/DLC
for Library of Congress   96-26096
                                                                      CIP

British Library Cataloguing in Publication Data
A CIP record is available from the British Library.

Contents

Section II: Neuropsychiatric Disorders Associated With OCD

Chapter 5: Obsessive-Compulsive Disorder

Section III: Research Issues

Prologue

O bsessive-compulsive disorder (OCD) is a neurobehavioral process characterized by a strong desire to control the outer environment; to engage in forceful, unwanted, repetitive thoughts; and to perform irresistible mental or motor activities, all within a substratum of doubting.

Historically, OCD symptoms remain unchanged. This observation indicates the distinctness of permanent symptoms unmodifiable by biopsychosocial variables that could emerge in time. However, as OCD's nucleus stays solidly uniform, parallel morbidity may overlap it to conform to a set of clinical entities that are self-incorporated with OCD's mainstream pathophysiology.

Some of these entities are major neuropsychiatric disorders that thus far, under the influence of undetermined factors, trade symptoms with OCD (i.e., schizophrenia, neurological disorders, affective disorders). Recently an increased interest in studying other OCD-related conditions has been observed. These include body dysmorphic disorder, hypochondriasis, eating disorders, self-mutilative syndromes, mental retardation, and Tourette's syndrome.

Hereafter, these conditions will be considered part of the *spectrum,* or the conditions that might overlap with OCD. *Comorbidity* is the coexistence of two conditions in the cerebral structure.

A comorbid condition adopts the phenomenological profile of the previously established disorders. Consequently, a new nosography emerges. This novel entity assembles new pathophysiological parameters that may modify symptom prevalence, disorder course, and treatment response.

The book is organized in three parts, the first comprising four chapters, the second comprising eight chapters, and the third comprising one chapter. The first four chapters relate to OCD. Chapter 1 looks at the disorder's natural history. Important factors such as magic, religion, and semantics are explored. These influence the OCD dynamic and primary symptom meaning. Cultural aspects signal OCD's worldwide prevalence, where the disorder's social acceptance might be questioned.

OCD symptoms' significance and their division into primary and secondary symptoms offers a better grouping for prioritizing treatment goals. In addition, a grasp of OCD symptomatology helps establish a differential diagnosis. Current epidemiological surveys are a good introduction to studying OCD comorbidity. The emphasis placed on childhood and adolescent onset of OCD enables its early detection. Furthermore, observing late OCD onset may suggest a structural lesion, and this may require additional testing.

Chapter 2 is dedicated to biological and psychological therapies; this chapter emphasizes OCD drug therapy, and monopharmacy versus polypharmacy is discussed. Special notes are made on side effects, notably the importance of explaining them to an apprehensive patient population. This chapter reviews benzodiazepines and antipsychotic medications, drugs that are becoming important for treating certain comorbid conditions. Treatment outcome and prognosis also are discussed.

Behavior therapy appears to be the most effective psychological therapy. In fact, a combination of drug and behavior therapy seems to be the treatment of choice. We added to this chapter a discussion of self-help group therapy as an additional tool to better the patient's recovery. We consider it important to approach the mental patient in an integral manner.

Chapter 3 discusses childhood OCD. Overall, it is similar to its adult counterpart and is treated as such. Chapter 4 covers many medical and psychological tools. Rapid advances in medical technology, mainly in cerebral imagery, literally puts the brain in a new light. The capacity to visualize the brain and study its metabolism may help us understand OCD pathology, resulting in new therapeutic techniques. Currently OCD psychological assessment instruments are valid and reliable; they confirm diagnosis and measure symptom changes systematically. The standardization of psychological instruments helps communicate worldwide research results.

Section II is divided into eight chapters on disorders that might present interconnections with OCD or have a clear comorbid presentation. Chapter 5 looks into schizophrenia and OCD. The association between both disorders is about 100 years old. Not only are both conditions major psychiatric disorders, but also they present a vast pathology that seems to overlap in certain groups of patients with OCD or schizophrenia. As a result, their comorbidity evolves into what seems to be a new nosological profile. If this is correct, new treatment provisions should be made.

Chapter 6 focuses on the association between OCD and major affective disorders. Some schools of thought have included OCD as part of the affective disorders, notably depression. This concept was substantiated by the presence of strong depressive symptomatology in patients with OCD and by the therapeutic efficacy of antidepressants in OCD. These ideas are currently disputed. Not every patient with OCD has endogenous depression, and some antidepressant agents are antiobsessive compulsive agents as well. Finally, the interface of OCD with manic depressive symptomatology calls for the need to outline a therapeutic regimen able to control the symptoms of both conditions.

Chapter 7 reviews the interactions between OCD and alcohol and drug abuse. The presence of insertion or comorbidity, although scarcely researched, has been documented. The major problem concerns how to treat conditions with induced biochemical pathology and its action on the putative biochemistry of OCD and drug abuse mechanisms.

Chapter 8 presents a variety of disorders that share OCD features as variant forms. The main disorder in this chapter is hypochondriasis, an illness described by Galen that has remained enigmatic throughout the centuries. Currently it is classified as a somatization disorder. Nonetheless, it has many aspects that seem related to OCD.

Chapter 9 discusses body dysmorphic disorder (BDD). This condition was discovered by Morselli during the 19th century and named *dysmorphophobia*. Currently there is strong evidence to consider it a comorbid condition with OCD. However, the complexity of its symptoms and thought pathology deem it necessary to reconceptualize BDD.

Chapter 10 discusses the eating disorders, which manifest many obsessions and compulsions in their symptomatology. Specific mention should be made of primary anorexia nervosa, which may be considered a comorbid condition. Chapter 11 concerns self-mutilation syndromes. These syndromes, notably related to mental retardation, constitute another group of disorders that present obsessional and compulsive symptomatology.

Chapter 12 introduces us to the communion of psychiatry and neurology. We believe these two disciplines, each with a clear cerebral origin, should be closely investigated. Starting with the encephalitic process that shows OCD symptomatology and continuing with Tourette's syndrome, a number of neurological conditions seem to interconnect with OCD.

Chapter 13, dedicated to clinical and experimental research, is a bridge between OCD and the comorbid conditions. In this chapter we present OCD's historical course. There also is a description of OCD models that might shed light on the genesis of comorbidity. In addition, we examine the various biological challenges, or markers, used to expand our knowledge of OCD's pathogenesis. In synthesis, this chapter speaks of OCD pathology's advancement.

We would like to thank Jonathan Hoffman and Theresa Campisi for their valuable suggestions in the preparation of this book. We would also like to thank the two anonymous reviewers of the American Psychiatric Press whose useful comments have been fundamental for the completion of the book. We also would like to thank Deborah DiRaimo, library assistant of the Nassau Academy of Medicine who obtained journal articles that were difficult to find, as well as some out-of-print books. We also appreciate the technical assistance provided by Fran Noone and Allen Pabo.

Section I

Primary Obsessive-Compulsive Disorder

Section I comprises four chapters dedicated to primary obsessive-compulsive disorder (OCD). The first aim of these chapters is to introduce the reader to OCD study. The second aim is to acquaint the reader with OCD and to facilitate an understanding of it. The third aim is to become familiarized with OCD biobehavioral treatment, a fundamental part of the bio-psychosocial model.

Overall, Section I provides suitable information to diagnose and treat OCD. Chapter 1 is the stepping stone to move into the world of the OCD spectrum.

Chapter 1
History, Culture, and Clinical Aspects of OCD

Historical Background

Magic and Religion

Primitivism, the Middle Ages, and contemporary times narrate the interactions among magic, religion, and psychiatry (Rosen 1969). In ancient times, mental illness or madness was attributed to magic and religion, for psychiatry was in an embryonic stage. Ignorance and uncertainty were two factors affecting the behavior of ancient humans, two factors that unfortunately remain in the modern world. Consequently, humans experienced the fear of the unknown, pain, death, losses, and catastrophes. To compensate for all those fears, humans need to believe in others and in hope. These two vital needs keep humans in equilibrium. Otherwise, a loss of balance disrupts the thinking process and the behavior required to function. This loss of balance is currently interpreted as mental illness or emotional disorder caused by biopsychosocial factors, whereas in primitive societies, it was interpreted as the consequence of a supernatural act. Therefore, in ancient times the path to follow was to conjure the spirits to ease fears and restore health. Currently, psychiatry could be defined as the science and art of studying both the body and the mind in the human biopsychosocial milieu.

Perhaps the history of obsessive-compulsive disorder (OCD) can be traced to humanity's beginning. As will be seen later, OCD encompasses many symptoms closely related to magic and religion. Magic entails using means, having supernatural powers, or causing a supernatural being to produce or prevent a particular result (e.g., healing). Magic thinking and avoidance are two well-known mechanisms used in OCD and phobias.

Religion (from the Latin word *religare*, to tie back) is a personal commitment to and serving a god. This commitment includes a belief system, a moral code to live by, and a degree of faith. Because reasoning cannot explain religious dogma, the believer uses faith to accept it. In the case of patients who have OCD with an obsessional content of religious scrupulosity, faith becomes an important characteristic of the patient's moral values. Thus, the therapist must consider not only the obsessionality, but also the concomitant faith intensifying the belief. Gradually psychiatry emerged as an independent entity, although it still shows vestiges of its past, rooted in magic and religion. In OCD, these vestiges include ceremony performance; avoidance behaviors; superstitious beliefs; certain obsessional religious contents (e.g., fear of going to hell); and scrupulosity, obsessional belief, and the degree of attached scrupulosity.

In magic and religion's psychology, ceremonies decrease the anxiety and fear elicited by inexplicable natural phenomena. A ceremony, or *ritual*, is a careful act that pays great attention to form and detail and is performed to emphasize hygiene rules, celebrate past events, prevent catastrophes, or worship a god. A ritual can be witnessed in both the hand washing performed to purify and the hand washing performed by a patient who just touched a contaminated object.

An example of religion and psychiatry's relationship is the analogy between taboo and obsessional neurosis (Freud 1913/1953). Both insist on rigid adherence to rules and prohibitions. When a rule is broken, a ceremony or ritual must be performed. In psychiatric anthropology these acts were described as part of controlling taboo beliefs by the Northeastern Argentinean Indians many centuries ago (Perez De Nucci 1988).

Scrupulosity's obsessional content closely relates to morality and the "right-and-wrong" paradigm. In fact, scrupulosity also may be known as *moral hypertrophy*. Some patients who have scrupulosity might be religious individuals. When this occurs, OCD and religiosity may blend, worsening the disorder. OCD and theology seem to share common interests regarding religiosity and scrupulosity. Theology establishes the difference between compulsion and temptation concepts. In compulsions, the moral issue is not raised, whereas in temptation, an intense, painful desire to perform an unacceptable or immoral act is described. Nonetheless, for a scrupulous patient the moral issue is raised. Moreover, religious patients may regard temptation and compulsion equally. This brings serious guilt and sinful feelings every time a patient engages in sinful obsessionality. If need be, we request pastors to intervene to discuss matters with our severe scrupulosity patients, hoping to decrease guilt intensity.

Another classic connection between OCD and religion is found in demonology treatises (Oesterreich 1974; Spranger and Kramer 1486/1975). Individuals possessed by demons demonstrate behaviors characterized by repetitive acts—yelling, trembling, cursing, sinful obsessionality, and involuntary movements, similar to symptoms seen in OCD, Tourette's syndrome, conversion hysteria, manic-depressive illness, and epilepsy. Charcot, Richer, Janet, Tourette, and Meige made important contributions to studying demonic possession's psychiatric aspect. They tried to explain how many of these thoughts and behaviors were illness symptoms rather than devil manifestations. These beliefs and behaviors are not ascribed only to those in the Western world. In Burma, China, Indochina, Africa, Japan, and Egypt, possession may involve animals instead of the devil.

One aspect related to magic and religion is superstitious beliefs. Superstition is a fixed unreasonable belief based in ignorance, in spite of contrary evidence. A superstitious individual performs brief rituals to prevent harm from occurring. Superstition and magic also contribute to founding OCD dynamics. In OCD, magic thinking and morbid obsessionality are two important clinical symptoms.

Finally, the higher incidence of paranoid symptoms in Caribbean patients might be caused by the presence of both magic and superstition (Meyer 1968). Later we will see the similarities between the obsessional and schizophrenic thought process where magic thinking seems prevalent.

Cultural Factors

The social concepts and ensuing traditions regarding mental illness vary among cultures. These concepts are determined by religious and superstitious beliefs, moral codes, cultural knowledge, and economic factors. There is no worldwide agreement on the definition of mental illnesses or a common understanding of how to classify and diagnose it. A consensus exists among Western countries to agree on an official nosological nomenclature. However, some cultures still accept attitudes and behaviors that are otherwise rejected as abnormal elsewhere. For instance, cultural idiosyncratic values in Germany, Japan, and Switzerland foster promptness, order, organization, and cleanliness—clear reminders of OCD qualities.

One question requiring attention is: how do cultural factors influence psychiatry generally, and OCD in particular? Is OCD accepted or rejected socially? What are OCD's phenomenological aspects and cultural patterns? What is the influence of religion on OCD's content?

Leighton and Murphy (1965) reported that Yorubans' psychiatric disorder conception overlaps with that of Westerners. Interestingly, Yorubans base their concept of handicap on the degree to which a person's symptoms interfere with his or her ability to relate to his or her immediate family and earn a living.

Carothers (1948) believed compulsive symptoms appear in the "guilt culture." In these cultures ritual performance controls guilt, just as in the Shaman culture. He stated that obsessive neurosis is rare in Africa, because it is tied to cultural factors as well as religious and magic beliefs (Carothers 1953).

Only one compulsive act case was found among Sudanese Arab children (Cederblad 1968). The author believed the reason obsessive-compulsive symptoms are not elicited in these cultures is a result of misunderstanding the question's implication. Pfeiffer (1962) found no obsessional illness cases in a hospital population in West Java. The author explained the negative findings by indicating that the population usually consults with faith healers.

Religion helps develop obsessive-compulsive patterns in OCD patients. These patterns are expressed by either religious obsessionality or ritualistic behavior, related to religious belief or practice, respectively. Among the factors identified, guilt and doubting are prominent (Higgins et al. 1992; Mahgoub and Abdel-Hafeiz 1991; Steketee et al. 1991; Wallace 1983). In three African cases, faith healing and religious ceremonies are performed to dispose of religious obsessions, hatred contents, and demon possession (Lambo 1962). In Moslem countries religious topics are more important than cleanliness compulsions because such compulsions may seem to be an exaggeration of the normative, daily cleanliness ritual (Okasha et al. 1968). In the Jewish population consulting with us, religious scholars affected by OCD exaggerate and overanalyze obsessions with religious content.

Religion's influence also is observed in countries where researchers perform fieldwork. Gaitonde's (1958) obsessional population in Bombay was all Catholic. In a larger study ($N = 412$), also in India, the obsessive-compulsive sample's predominant religion was Hinduism ($n = 347$) (Khanna et al. 1986). In Israel patients with strong religious backgrounds had high scrupulosity (Greenberg et al. 1987). In 157 patients with OCD from our institute in Long Island, no significant differences were found among Catholic, Protestant, and Jewish patients. However, when the OCD sample was compared with a non-OCD psychiatric patient sample ($n = 157$), a significant difference was found between atheistic and agnostic OCD patients (Neziroglu et al. 1994).

In conclusion, magic and religion affect the obsessional content and ritualistic behavior of OCD patients. This historical remnant should concern those practicing psychotherapy and those interested in psychiatric anthropology. OCD exists worldwide, and although one may suspect a strong sociocultural influence in content and form, this may not be the case. For some investigators, OCD cultural variation may be more apparent than real (Greenberg and Witztum 1994).

Semantics

Semantics studies word meanings, signs, or forms relating to a referent. Semantic changes may indicate a linguistic development. The process of semantic evolution stems from new ways of thinking or from knowledge acquisition resulting in connotation changes. These changes indicate a new understanding or a referential modification. Presently there is an excessive tendency to change word meanings. These new connotations incorporate words with a different referential. Consequently, misunderstandings can arise on certain issues.

Considering that OCD was described in the 17th century, it would be expected to undergo semantic changes in its nosological concepts and signs. What is an obsession? What is a compulsion? How should OCD be defined? These are some classic questions subject to change. One main interest in OCD semantics focuses on describing and understanding the meanings of the words *obsession, compulsion,* and *doubting.*

In 1638 Younge spoke about the obsessional ruminator's indecisiveness, and in 1757 Woodard described an obsessional delusion (both cited in Hunter and Macalpine 1963). However, the scientific study of obsessions and compulsions belongs to the French and German schools. In 1799 Wartburg coined "obsession's" actual, or current, meaning (cited by Monserrat-Esteve 1971). In 1838 Esquirol described the *delire du toucher* (compulsion to touch) and the *monomanie raissonnante* (obsession).

In 1856 Morel considered obsessions an emotional delusion. Falret (1866) described *la folie du doute,* and in 1875 Legrand du Saulle (1875; cited by Bourgeois 1975) described *la folie du doute avec delire du toucher.* Obsessions as fixed ideas were described by Buccola (1880) and Tamburini (1883). In 1872 Westphal coined the term *zwang* to imply obsession; in popular German this term means to obligate, coerce, or compel. This word, which also denotes violence and force, was accepted as a medical term. A description of obsessions and compulsions should also be attributed to Luys (1883), who wrote, "les malhereux patient expériment avec douleur les obsessions qui les dominent, les pensées penibles qui les poursuivent, les impulsions à faire des gestes, à faire des grimaces, à grimper sur les meubles,

à courir malgré eux, comme s'ils etaient possédé par de forces aveugles. . . ."
[the unfortunate patients painfully experience the imposing obsessions that
dominate them, the painful thoughts that follow them, the urges to gesticu-
late, to grimace, to jump on the furniture, or to run in spite of, as if they
were possessed by blind forces. . .] (pp. 20–21).

In England, Tuke (1894) called obsessions *imperative ideas.* Three years
later Donath (1897) used the term *anancasmus* (from the Greek *ananke*, meaning destiny or fatality) to express obsessions without phobias. Thus the
anancastic personality is described, and at times confused, with an obsessive personality or obsessive neurosis.

The term *compulsion,* usually interchanged with *impulse,* is a classic example of clinical misunderstandings. Compulsion denotes the act of compel-
ling; a state of being compelled; or a strong, irresistible urge to act. However,
a compulsion can be reasoned and, with training, resisted and controlled.
However, an impulse is the spontaneous and uncontrollable act of driving
forward with sudden force, almost without previous reasoning.

Currently a compulsion is viewed as an irresistible desire that goes
against one's will, whereas an impulse is accepted by the will. An impulse also differs from a compulsion because it is usually punishable by
society and goes against the person's conscience or moral values. The
differences between compulsions and impulses should be addressed with
patients. Patients usually consider a compulsion an impulse; hence they
fear acting on them. This common belief is primarily observed in patients
afflicted by fear of harming others.

Doubt is the uncertainty of a belief or opinion. In doubting, judgment is held
when facing a statement's truth or an event's reality. Chronic doubting, as in
OCD, is masked by the presence of iterative questioning or double checking.
At times doubting elicits the inability to make decisions. Although some clinicians use the term as a synonym for being unable to make decisions, they are
not synonymous.

In conclusion, semantics occupies an important place in OCD's evolution.
Its presence reflects an active dynamic force driven and challenged by research advancements in OCD phenomenology, comorbidity, and pathogenesis. An understanding of OCD semantics benefits an understanding of the
disorder and interpretation of the symptoms. Semantics assists professionals
internationally to communicate and discuss OCD and its spectrum by enabling them to share the same scientific language.

Clinical Aspects

Definitions

Westphal (1872) described obsessions as parasitic ideas in an intact intellect that intrude into normal thought processes or ideation against the will. Schneider (1930) defined obsessions as "contents of consciousness which, when they occur, are accompanied by the experience of subjective compulsions, and which cannot be gotten rid of, though, on quiet reflection they are recognized as senseless." Lewis (1936) found Schneider's definition practical and acceptable. However, Lewis believed the OCD patient needed to resist the obsession. Schneider's and Lewis's definitions were encompassed by Pollitt (1957), who described the obsession as "thought, images, feelings, impulses, recurring or persistent movements, that are accompanied by immediate sensation of subjective compulsion, and a desire to oppose it" (p. 95). Although many other contributory definitions have been proposed to foster an understanding of OCD (Freud 1917; Green 1965; Janet 1903; Kanner 1948; Kringlen 1965; Tuke 1894), Westphal's definition still stands on solid ground.

A compulsion is a strong ideational or motor urge that, although against one's will, must be satisfied by performance of the compulsion or by a repetitive act fulfilling the compulsion's emotional and intellectual component. If the act is not performed, anxiety develops and stays until the urge is carried out.

Our experience indicates the obsessive-compulsive process is an experiential set of objects and actions containing sensorial activity translated into understanding and behavior. The OCD thought process does not follow the law of logic (i.e., linear logic). Instead, it follows a spiral-like logic with back-and-forth motions. In OCD sensorial activity no longer makes sense. Patients complain of obsessions represented by images or melodies that keep coming back and cannot be repelled. Are these melodies and images pure obsessional material, or do they combine a dysperception at first, becoming an obsession at the end? Reality remains intact but questionable and, as Janet (1903) observed, might be weakened.

Doubting, with its checking companion, rounds out the process. Doubting affects decision making and performance. The patient reports losing evidence ("Has it really occurred?"), losing meaning ("Is it worth doing?"), and losing control ("Can I continue to run my life?"). The patient is rigid, demanding, and self-centered. Clinicians wonder whether patients can resist obsessions or compulsions. Generally patients consider it necessary to resist obsessions and compulsions, although in one study only 32% of 45 patients manifested a high degree of resistance (Stern and Cobb 1978).

OCD's basic dynamic includes obsessions, compulsions, doubting, hypervigilance, and a need to control the world. All these symptoms, as isolated emergents, might be observed in other neuropsychiatric disorders. Nonetheless, doubting seems exclusive to OCD. This may explain why the French knew OCD as the "folie du doute."

Symptomatology

The first and most comprehensive obsession and compulsion study was done by Janet (1903). Important clinical observations also were done by those in the psychoanalytical school, such as Freud. These colleagues took the time to interview and listen to their patients and gathered a wealth of useful information.

Obsessive-compulsive symptoms are protean and vast in extension. They emerge with numerous symptoms classified as secondary symptoms or blend with other nosology symptoms that are part of a comorbid process. Sufficient time is needed for a complete examination of the patient. It is impossible to clinically assess an OCD patient in one interview. Listening to patients tell their stories is fundamental, because there are no diseases, merely patients, and each is a distinct entity. During interviews patients are usually anxious, speech content is circumstantial, and patients tend to get off track. Symptom quality exploration will assist the practitioner to obtain a better evaluation of the patient. This wealth of information is applicable to the use of cognitive-behavioral techniques (Table 1–1).

Sometimes it is rewarding to invite a family member, with the patient's authorization, to sit in during the diagnostic evaluation. This serves to 1) help patients focus on their condition, 2) explain the disorder to patients and their families, and 3) obtain family support as part of the therapeutic strategy. Asking for the chronological history of the illness, hospitalizations, and treatment received helps in developing a treatment outline.

Primary Symptoms

Obsessions.   An obsessive thought appears in an intrusive, invasive manner. It cannot be stopped and may stay for long periods. At the beginning the

Table 1–1. Symptoms in obsessive-compulsive patients

Thought	Mood
Doubtful	Anxious-depressed-cyclothymic
Intrusive	
Obstinate	**Motor**
Magical	Repetitive
Behavior	**Social**
Ritualistic	Inability to function
Iterative	Family disturbance
Bizarre	
Aggressive	
Vigilant	

obsessive thought can be justified, but later the patient realizes these thoughts are parasites—purposeless and impractical. The thoughts have an iterative quality, and the patient may not be able to switch off obsessive thoughts. Although the patient tries to resist, the thought persists and cannot be erased from the mind.

We find contamination, religious, sexual, and morbid thought contents to be the most common; this agrees with observations by Khanna and Channabasavanna (1987). Morbid thoughts seem to differ from other obsessions in that thought content is usually sinful and unacceptable. Most morbid thoughts are sexual or aggressive. In the sexual form, patients report thoughts or images of having sex, mostly with their own or other children, parents, or animals. In aggressive thoughts, knives, scissors, or other sharp objects evoke thoughts of stabbing their children, family members, or themselves. Although aggressive thoughts are common, follow-up studies report no evidence that obsessive behavior predisposes to homicide or other criminal behavior (Goodwin et al. 1969).

Obsessive thinking might be magical in that patients believe they can undo or change events just by the thought process. These thoughts may relate to superstition or religious practices and are reminiscent of ceremonial compulsions, where magical thinking or superstitious beliefs are common. However, patients manifesting magical thinking do not have to be religious, and magical thinking may be associated with delusional beliefs. When that occurs, a psychotic process must be ruled out.

During the examination clinicians may be exposed to three types of thinking: obsessional beliefs, delusional beliefs, and overvalued ideas.

The obsessional belief is basically real, the delusional belief is fixed and unquestionable, and the overvalued idea is fixed but questionable under pressure. Our experience indicates that reality is weakened when obsessionality is intense. At such moments an obsession may appear delusional or overvalued.

Another important symptom is the moral issue, characterized by scrupulosity and the right-and-wrong criterion. These symptoms are usually elicited in people with religious and ethic obsessionality. When moral issues are intense, *moral hypertrophy* is present. This symptomatology may accompany seizure disorders (notably those with a temporal lobe location) with or without OCD.

St. Ignatius Loyola was concerned with obsessions as a thought disorder or affect. For him, obsessions represented the chronic interrogation of life. In fact, OCD patients question life incessantly. Patients perceive the world as a threat; hence, they take precautions to avoid harm and therefore become hypervigilant. This belief and attitude remind us of the paranoid patient.

In some patients obsessions closely relate to body image and focus on one anatomical area. Sometimes patients become extremely concerned and obsessed with their heart rate, breathing, or bowel activity.

One important aspect of the obsession is conflicting doubt. Patients believe, and yet do not believe, in their obsessions. If asked whether the thought is logical, patients hesitate to answer. In time, such doubtfulness incapacitates patients, preventing them from functioning. As noted by Tamarin (1977), patients are trapped in the hypothetical premise that their thoughts turn into a circular perpetual mobility; their incompatibilities and prohibitions lead them to social isolation.

Compulsions.   Compulsions can be divided into 1) ideational or mental and 2) motor. An ideational compulsion is an urge to perform an act in one's mind (e.g., arithmomania, onomatomania). A motor compulsion is an urge to perform an act by muscular participation.

Ideational compulsions are more discreet because they are invisible. Patients use them to avoid having witnesses of their condition. After all, OCD should be "kept in the closet," because many symptoms' bizarreness cause embarrassment. Many patients double-check visually; others count objects, possessions, coins, or stamps. Some configure letters, words, or even complete sentences in their mind. Arithmomania, a common form, causes patients to engage in addition, division, subtraction, and multiplication endlessly.

Motor compulsions are subdivided into aggressive, physiological, bodily movement, and ceremonial. Aggressive compulsions are urges to act out verbally, as in coprolalia, or physically, as in self-mutilation. Self-mutilation varies and includes hair pulling, eyebrow plucking, slashing, head banging, self-punching, self-slapping, self-biting, picking, and digging. Aggressive compulsions should not be confused with anger, a mood state.

Physiological compulsions include defecation, urination, eating, drinking, smoking, swallowing, and performing sex acts endlessly. In a way, in these types compulsive physiological satiation is impaired. This compulsive activity seems to result from obsessions pertaining to bodily physiology. These physiological modifications affect the biopsychosocial profile of the patient (Table 1–2).

Bodily movement compulsions consist of touching, tics, clapping, sneezing, jumping, stretching, throat clearing, rocking, rubbing, stereotyped movements, echokinesis, and exercising. Ceremonial compulsions relate to purification and decontamination rituals. They include cleanliness forms, hand washing, and showering, as well as clothing and house cleaning.

Other compulsions include ordering, arranging, collecting, list making, echolalia, retracing, rereading, and rewriting. Compulsions may be performed repetitively, without purpose, or to undo some anticipated disastrous consequence. Finally, the two major compulsions are washing and double-checking.

Secondary Symptoms

Many authors touch on secondary OCD symptoms such as sexual anxiety disturbances, anger, depression, and phobias (Beech 1971; Cammer 1973; Kendell and Discipio 1970; Yaryura-Tobias 1977; Yaryura-Tobias and

Table 1–2. OCD physiological changes

Characteristic	How affected
Reproduction/cohabitation	Decreased
Eating habits	Normal to abnormal
Thirst	Normal to increased
Death	Nonsuicidal
Flight/fight	Flight
Life coping mechanisms	Poor
Urination	Normal to pollakiuria
Defecation	Abnormal patterns
Sleep	Normal, unless severe hypervigilance
Sexual activity	Decreased copulation
	Masturbation

Neziroglu 1978; Yaryura-Tobias et al. 1979; Walker and Beech 1969). Here we discuss what we consider essential aspects of secondary symptoms that may require treatment modification. Finally, secondary symptoms may overlap OCD spectrum phenomenology. This requires close attention for differential diagnosis purposes and consequent therapeutic strategies (Table 1–3).

Phobias.   About 50% of OCD patients suffer from phobias. The presence of phobias in the obsessive-compulsive phenomenology modifies the patient's attitude toward handling the illness. Patients use avoidance behavior and may ritualize to undo fear. There is a close affinity between phobias and compulsions: both involve avoidance behaviors and anxiety as a response to a feared object. The difference is, the phobic individual usually avoids anxiety-provoking situations more readily than the compulsive individual, because in the compulsive individual, the fears are all-pervasive. The compulsive individual has to engage in rituals to undo the fear.

Rachman and Hodgson (1980) suggested that compulsive cleaners engage in more passive avoidance than compulsive checkers. *Passive avoidance*, as seen in patients with simple phobias, refers to directly avoiding a feared situation. *Active avoidance*, as seen in individuals with compulsions, refers to engaging in behaviors to undo the fear. Rachman and Hodgson (1980)

Table 1–3.   Incidence of secondary symptoms in 100 OCD patients

Symptom	%
Depression	94
Anxiety	90
Aggression	65
Dysperception	60
Phobias	58
Checking	55
Other rituals	54
Washing	41
Sleep disorders	49
Family disturbance	45
Sexual dysfunction	34
Appetite disorder	33
Meticulosity	27
Self-mutilation	16
Tics	1

suggested that compulsive cleaners are more similar to phobia patients and can avoid situations, whereas compulsive checkers need to undo their fears. Consequently, it was hypothesized that compulsive cleaners are more likely to have concurrent phobias or a history of earlier phobias. Theoretically, this assumption may be sound, but practically, most compulsive cleaners engage in active avoidance (cleaning). Further research is needed to determine the accuracy of this hypothesis.

Sexual disturbances. Sexual disturbances in OCD patients include an increase or decrease in libido, frigidity, impotence, and delayed or premature ejaculation. These may be caused by the patient's strict religious or moral views, depression, or anxiety. Obsessional phobia patients who manifest fear of contamination regarding semen, vaginal secretion, and urine also may avoid sexual contact.

Patient attitudes toward sexual practices result in careful analysis and organization by the patient about how to perform the sex act or whether it should be performed. Consequently, spontaneity is lost, and anxiety and tension build up. Patients who have sexual disturbances and are treated with tricyclic or heterocyclic agents should be informed of the possibilities of sexual side effects (e.g., loss of libido, anorgasmia, impotence, delayed ejaculation).

Anger. Anger is a common secondary symptom. Its pathogenesis might relate to psychological and biochemical components. OCD causes frustration because of the inability to function and to socialize. Frustration can then be channeled into outer or inner anger. Outer anger is basically verbally manifested, whereas inner anger becomes depression. We make a clear distinction between anger and the compulsive aggression that afflicts many OCD patients. The anger's biochemical basis might be associated with serotonin metabolism. Low brain serotonin levels seem to trigger anger; this has been seen in animal experiments and in indirect observations in humans.

Speech pattern. OCD linguistic patterns can be examined as expressive behavior (Lorenz 1955), yielding clues for diagnostic and prognostic purposes. The speech is usually iterative, stuttering, stammering, circumstantial, circular, or redundant and can be fast or slow. Tone and its modulation vary from high to low pitch. Speech quality is characterized by preciseness and good diction. Patients usually express themselves carefully; their words often contain a lot of information. With the use of first-person pronouns and past tense, speech becomes reflexive.

Noting the speech pattern might help for differential diagnosis. For instance, speech is altered in relation to the thought stream, as seen in patients with accelerated thinking who are unable to synchronize thought and speech speed (e.g., patients with a manic disorder). Schilder (1938) indicated that OCD patients' speech is characterized by verborrhagia and propulsive features. The difference between obsessive and hysteroid speech is that, in the latter, interruptions by the listener are less welcome, and an anxious overtone is noticeable throughout.

Weintraub and Aronson (1974) compared 17 compulsive patients' verbal behavior with a control group and demonstrated significant differences between both. Compared with control subjects, compulsive patients did more explaining and used more negatives, retractors, and evaluators. They also used fewer nonpersonal references and more expressions of feeling, but not significantly.

Perceptual disturbances. du Saulle (cited in Bourgeois 1975) described changes of taste and smell in OCD. Neziroglu (1983) observed that some patients complained of visual disturbances, such as "floaters" or transient spots in front of their eyes. At times patients report the passing or falling of objects, perceived by their lateral vision (e.g., books falling from a shelf). This may force the patient to check once, but does not relate to double-checking. Research has indicated the presence of dysperception in OCD patients, similar to schizophrenic patients (Yaryura-Tobias et al. 1995). Dysperceptions also are observed in the OCD spectrum (see Chapters 5 and 8–10).

Other characteristics. Seriously ill patients present four major characteristics: strong dependence needs, social isolation, school failure, and job loss. This psychosocial sequence in OCD's evolution is crucial to determining an unfavorable prognosis. Therefore, we shall review these factors to have a better understanding of patient needs.

Disturbances in the family constellation are common and expected. Why do they occur? Living with an OCD patient is difficult. OCD patients are self-centered, demanding, and ungrateful, and their mood changes and anger aggravate matters.

Families are partially to blame for their condition. They become an anchor for patients, keeping them in contact with the social milieu; they also provide food and medicine. With the current drastic changes in health care, OCD patients feel abandoned and, hence, unprotected. Because of their inability to make decisions and doubtfulness involving their actions, they develop a strong dependency on family. An overprotective parent, spouse, relative, or friend, responding to the patient's uncertainty, will make decisions for him or her.

If a family member living with the patient has OCD or an obsessive-compulsive personality, the patient's behavior may be reinforced. Therefore, treating family disturbances to achieve a better prognosis is imperative. One important factor is that patients or families sometimes need to sabotage treatment for secondary gains. Patients who remain ill can be taken care of, and families with an ill member may fulfill a purpose in life. The therapist should look into the possible gains for both patients and families to maintain the status quo.

Patients have serious difficulties interacting socially. Several factors influencing socialization can be isolated: low self-esteem, fear of ridicule, thought rigidity, inability to accept others' values systems, inflexible moral codes, and a need to control others' behaviors and ways of thinking. The presence of social phobias in many patients should not be overlooked.

Children, adolescents, and adults have many problems performing in school or academic settings. Intense and lasting obsessions prevent them from listening in class and studying. Long hours spent in ritualization activities make it difficult to do homework or get sufficient sleep. All this interference leads to school or college failure.

The condition also may affect the ability to work or maintain a job. Although many successful people have obsessive-compulsive characteristics, OCD is not conducive to success. Continuous obsession causes distractions and prevents the patient from performing; perfectionism, double-checking, and doubting reduce productivity.

Conclusions

Overall, OCD symptomatology remains unchanged. Cross-cultural studies have shown uniform symptomatology. However, the obsessional content may vary among patients because of the patient's intellectual profile, values, or cultural factors. In our experience, secondary symptoms are usually eliminated by merely treating the obsessions and compulsions; however, in case of failure, specific therapeutic modalities should be used in treating secondary symptoms (see Table 1–3).

After examining many patients who have chronic OCD, we find they have a quality of catastrophe and chronic indecisiveness. When explored further, the person seems to be an "unfinished product." This might be a philosophical reflection of his or her inability to complete a task. The challenge is to return the patient to the mainstream.

Epidemiology

Gradually the international scientific community is acknowledging OCD's presence, as acknowledged in mental health surveys done in Hong Kong (Chen et al. 1993), Benin (Bertschy and Ahyi 1991), Australia (Hafner and Miller 1990), Egypt (Okasha et al. 1968), and Italy (Ronchi et al. 1992) and in Afro-Americans (Horwath et al. 1993) and Mexican Americans (Karno et al. 1989), among others. OCD comorbidity was reported in Japan (Hayashi 1992; Takahashi et al. 1987), and OCD and anxiety disorders were reported in Italy (Faravelli et al. 1989).

Prevalence

Historically, prevalence in the general white population has ranged from 0.05% (Woodruff and Pitts 1964) to 0.32% (Nica Udangiu 1977). More recently, a 2.5% lifetime prevalence rate was reported (Reiger et al. 1988), which is 25 to 60 times greater than previous estimates (Karno et al. 1989).

Incidence

The incidence of obsessional illness symptoms in inpatient or outpatient populations varies from 0.99% to 3.0% (Chakraborty and Banerji 1975; Costa Molinari 1971a; Goodwin et al. 1969; Ingram 1961b; Judd 1965; Kringlen 1965; Leitenberg 1976; Okasha et al. 1968; Pollitt 1957). We feel the percentage is probably higher because obsessive-compulsive patients are secretive about their symptoms.

Sex Ratio

The male-to-female ratio is about 1:1 (Costa Molinari 1971a; Judd 1965; Kayton and Borge 1967; Kringlen 1965; Muller 1957; Neziroglu et al. 1994; Okasha et al. 1968; Pacella 1944; Pollitt 1957; Pujol and Savy 1968; Rosenberg 1968; Rudin 1953).

Age at Onset

Illness onset seems unrelated to cultural patterns and remains unmodified over the years. It usually starts between ages 10 and 30 (Chakraborty and

Banerji 1975; Ingram 1961a; Khanna et al. 1986; Kringlen 1965; Neziroglu et al. 1994; Okasha et al. 1968; Pollitt 1960; Taschev 1970; Thyer et al. 1985).

First Consultation

For several authors, first consultation takes place between ages 25 and 35 (Chakraborty and Banerji 1975; Costa Molinari 1971a; Taschev 1970; Yaryura-Tobias et al. 1979). Between illness onset and first consultation, a 7.5-year lapse may occur (Pollitt 1957; Pujol and Savy 1968). According to Dowson (1977), the mean age at hospital admission was 31.6 years, and 68% of the sample were women.

Marital Status

Most authors find a celibacy incidence of 48% (Ingram 1961a; Lo 1967; Neziroglu et al. 1994; Okasha et al. 1968; Rudin 1953). Generally, if the illness is severe before marriage, the chance of marrying decreases, and if it is severe during marriage, marital disturbances are reported in half of cases (Neziroglu et al. 1994).

Socioeconomic Level

In a study by Ballus (1971), 1.59% of patients belonged to the upper class, 23.81% to the upper middle class, and 53.97% to the middle class. A higher incidence among the upper socioeconomic level was reported by Chakraborty and Banerji (1975), Ingram (1961a), and Lo (1967). However, in pre-Allende metropolitan Santiago de Chile, lower class groups experienced more obsessive-compulsive tendencies (Williamson 1976). However, Kringlen (1965) found, in a comparison with a control group, that obsessive-compulsive patients existed in all social classes. These findings are similar to ours. Socioeconomic strata do not seem to be an important variable in understanding the illness's pathology but are important in treatment outcome, because upper class patients can better afford treatment.

Scholarship and Working Adaptability

Empirical evidence indicates that most patients who come for consultation cannot work or study. If they can, it is only at a rudimentary level. In one study, compared with a general population, 26% could not work (Neziroglu et al. 1994).

Intelligence Quotient

Ballus (1971) found a high intelligence quotient (IQ) in 28.53% of the OCD population, and Skoog (1959) found feeblemindedness in 12%. We agree

with Ingram (1961a) and Lo (1967) that obsessive-compulsive patients have
a high verbal IQ.

Premorbid Personality

Premorbid personality types were found in 66% of the cases reported by
Pollitt (1960), in 25.5% reported by Chakraborty and Banerji (1975), in 47%
reported by Lo (1967), and in 72% reported by Kringlen (1965).

Genetic Factors

In evaluating the origin of OCDs, both genetic and social learning factors
should be considered. Arguments for a genetic component were presented by
Inouye (1965), Marks et al. (1969), Parker (1964), and Woodruff and Pitts
(1964). They all indicated a high concordance rate for monozygotic twins. In
contrast, Black (1974), and Rachman and Hodgson (1980) expressed concern about these findings' validity based on methodological considerations.
However, they did not present data supporting their assumptions.

Studies of the illness' family incidence may provide important information
about how symptoms are transmitted through learning. It is difficult to ascer-
tain from the studies whether the reported obsessionality refers to obsessive-
compulsive symptoms or personality traits.

Since 1930 systematic observations on the presence of obsessive-compulsive
traits in blood relatives have been reported in 20%–40% of studied cases
(Chakraborty and Banerji 1975; Costa Molinari 1971a; Kringlen 1965; Lewis
1936; Neziroglu et al. 1994; Storring 1930). Studies have shown
an 18% incidence of psychiatric illness in OCD patients' parents, as follows:
OCD, 7.5%; obsessive-compulsive pesonality, 3%; alcoholism, 5.5%; psychosis
and affective disorders, 2% (Neziroglu et al. 1994).

Brown (1942) stated that 7.5% of parents ($n = 40$) and 7.1% of siblings
($n = 56$) demonstrated obsessive traits. Likewise, Lo (1967) reported that
8.6% of parents ($n = 186$) and 4.6% of siblings ($n = 309$) exhibited pro-
nounced obsessive traits.

Nonpsychiatric pathophysiological family members' background indicates
a high incidence of tubercular meningitis (DeBoor 1949), migraine, epilepsy
(Alberca Lorente 1953), arteriosclerosis, and myxedema (Lewis 1936).
Whether this background contributes to the illness' genesis is unknown.
In this regard, Bustamante (1934) did not find common abnormal factors in
blood relatives. So far, there are no current studies on family members' general pathology, except psychiatric history.

Birth and Birth Order

According to Kayton and Borge (1967), 31 of 40 patients were firstborn or only children. Capstick and Seldrup (1977) examined the theory of a positive relationship between physical abnormalities occurring at birth and subsequent development of obsessional states. They found that separating children and mothers because of an abnormality was more relevant than the abnormality per se. Compared with the general population, there was no difference in the percentage of birth abnormalities in OCD populations (Neziroglu et al. 1994).

Fertility Rate

(Ingram 1961a), found that the fertility rate for obsessive-compulsive patients is one child per marriage for both sexes; according to Lo (1967), three children; and according to Chakraborty and Banerji (1975), 0–2 children. A low fertility rate was reported by Hare et al. (1972). A nonsignificant number of premature children was reported in a 392-case sample. In the same sample, an analysis of family size indicated that smaller ones had more prematurely born Slater's index cases (Khanna and Channabasavanna 1987).

Suicide

Although suicide is uncommon among obsessive-compulsive patients—perhaps because of their inability to make decisions—it was reported in three compulsive narcissist cases (Bach 1977).

Classification

Modern nosology history begins with Sydenham's work (1682). Describing a variety of symptoms pertaining to individual cases produces the need to group and classify. Linnaeus's botanical classification was applied to medicine by Boissier de Savages de la Croix and Cullen. Nonetheless, Cullen followed the nervous disease concept introduced by Willis (1672) and Sydenham.

Thereafter, Pinel (1802) and Cullen, ascribing to the concept of madness as a medical illness, opened the door for a new psychiatry perspective. Cullen introduced the terms *hypochondriasis* and *hysteria* with the meanings that we currently know. However, Pinel left the study of "neurosis" to general medicine.

Gradually, with hesitation, a nosological composite took place while clinicians witnessed nosology's semantic evolution, the grouping process, and the emergence of new clinical conditions.

Luys (1883) advanced the most important OCD classification by dividing obsessions in three groups: 1) intellectual, 2) emotional, and 3) psychomotor. These divisions represent various OCD phases, suggesting the presence of parallel conditions. These conditions now would be considered comorbidities. Following this line of thought, other classifications have been proposed by Blanc (1956), Coullaut Mendigutia (1960), Ingram (1961a), and Seva Diaz (1964). In 1971 Costa Molinari (1971a) introduced an OCD classification comprising psychiatric and neurological elements.

Classificatory activity demands scientific testing (interdisciplinary, predictive, retrodictive, and statistical). One needs to consider clinical, therapeutic, and philosophical issues. These issues have socioeconomic and political ramifications, including professional interest and popular cultural needs. Wallace (1994) has presented an interesting philosophical retrospective study of psychiatry and its nosology.

The current OCD classification is based on two major symptoms: obsessions and compulsions. This narrowly limits classification by excluding other accompanying symptoms, notably doubting. However, 100 years ago, doubting was considered an important symptom, to the point that the French called OCD "the disease of the doubt." At that time European psychiatrists tended to accept doubting as a determinant OCD core component. Other symptoms pertain to the motor area and are fundamental because they produce phenomenological variations conducive to "organic" comorbidity.

Traditionally, the major mental illness divisions are neurosis, affective disorders, psychosis, and character disorders, with OCD included in the neurosis group. This view of OCD remains unchanged in DSM-IV (American Psychiatric Association 1994). This edition classifies OCD as an anxiety disorder form, stating ". . . Obsessive-Compulsive Disorder is characterized by obsessions (which cause marked anxiety or distress) and/or by compulsions (which serve to neutralize anxiety) (p. 393)." This argument uses the posteffect of obsessive-compulsive symptoms (e.g., anxiogenic effect), rather than causative factors, to classify OCD as an anxiety disorder.

Usually OCD is classified by blending phenomenology, dynamics, evolution, pathology, etiology, and treatment response. This approach further confuses OCD's complexity. Classifying it in various categories for clearer understanding and promoting communication among those dedicated to researching this condition is advantageous. Hence, we proposed a modified classification (Yaryura-Tobias 1986).

Our classification is flexible and considers the various disciplines focusing their interest on segments of OCD and removing it from its total concept for easier access and interpretation. The first classification is based on clinical findings grouped in symptom clusters, reflecting the syndrome or disease concept (Table 1–4). The second classification is geared toward the student of the OCD phenomenon and its spectrum. This classification is more ambitious because it looks into causes and mechanisms that in many instances are still disputable (Table 1–5).

In concluding, psychiatric nosography is not sacred and undergoes periodic revision. Consequently, classifications still keeping a Kraepelinian and Krestchmerian frame of reference continue to change.

Differential Diagnosis

The differential diagnosis between OCD and other psychiatric disorders should be carefully done. Because the symptomatology of OCD is protean, its symptoms may easily be mistaken for similar symptoms of other conditions. The first task is to identify the fundamental symptoms of OCD: obsessions, compulsions, and doubting. This task is followed by the listing of secondary symptoms, notably anxiety, depression, and anger. At this point clinicians should proceed to assess the characteristics and qualities of the symptoms. This basic guideline may help to evaluate the patient.

Overall, the aim is to identify the OCD core and isolate it from other symptoms. These symptoms may belong to diseases considered as part of the OCD spectrum or to diseases without any nosological connection with OCD. Consider, for instance, attempting to distinguish among an obsession, an overvalued idea, or a delusion. This symptom may be present in OCD, schizophrenia, hypochondriasis, or body dysmorphic disorder, but it must be connected with the specific condition. A symptom on its own does not constitute a syndrome or a disease.

When obsession and compulsion symptoms are masked by intense anxiety, depression, disturbed thoughts, or bizarre behavior, clinicians may miss the OCD diagnosis and erroneously diagnose the patient as having general anxiety disorder, major depression, or psychosis. Anxiety symptoms, when intense and disabling, lead the patient to consult with a physician. The

Table 1–4.   OCD clinical classification

Complex forms
   Body dysmorphic disorder
   Compulsive orectic mutilative syndrome
   Tourette's syndrome
   Hypochondriasis
   Eating disorders
With related disorders
   Choreas
   Encephalitis
   Extrapyramidalism
   Parkinson's
   Seizure
With compulsive self-mutilation
   Cornelia de Lange syndrome
   Lesch-Nyhan syndrome
   Prader-Willi syndrome
With major psychiatric disorders
   Affective disorders
   Schizophrenia
   Phobias

Table 1–5.   Putative etiopathological classification

Biological
   Biochemical (neurotransmitters, coenzymes, hormones)
   Infectious (viral, microbial)
   Traumatic (cerebrovascular disorders, brain trauma, tumors)
   Iatrogenic (psychotropic medication, neurosurgery)
   Degenerative (brain atrophy, cerebral arteriosclerosis)
   Genetic (traits)
Psychological
   Analytical (fixations, defense mechanisms)
   Behavioral (classic conditioning, negative reinforcement)
Social
   Environmental (ecological, cultural, idiosyncracies)

practitioner might be misdirected by the prominent, anxious picture masking an underlying OCD. A long depression, making the patient dysfunctional, also may disguise an underlying OCD process. Finally, an odd obsession, accompanied by bizarre behavior, may lead to a schizophrenia diagnosis.

Our OCD experience shows a considerable number of misdiagnoses, mostly with major depression and schizophrenia. Currently, access to a wealth of information pertaining to the diagnosis and treatment of OCD improves the diagnostician's skills. Renewed interest in OCD variants and comorbidities also will help improve diagnostic techniques.

Walker (1973) described four main characteristics distinguishing an obsessional ritual from other psychiatric symptoms and from healthy behavior:

1. It is a purposeful action, rather than a series of movements. In other words, the washing or checking activity is not only a series of body movements, but also coordinated actions performed to reduce anxiety, thus becoming purposeful acts.
2. It is performed according to rules. Usually there are a certain number of times one must wash or check, and in a particular order, to feel satisfied.
3. It is not an end in itself but is designed to cause or prevent some future state of affairs. The washing is usually performed to prevent further contamination.
4. The activity does not bring about the state of affairs it was designed to produce. In other words, patients may wash their hands to remove visible dirt, and this is normal. However, when they wash their hands 100 times to remove nonexistent dirt, the behavior is considered bizarre.

We offer two more important characteristics of an obsessional ritual:

1. The activity or thought is considered illogical or ridiculous but cannot be resisted. There is a subjective urge to think or perform an act, even though the patient knows it is unreasonable.
2. The probability that the action's consequences will occur is overestimated. OCD patients are usually obsessed with improbable ensuing actions or disasters. The relevance of these actions is difficult for others to understand. For example, patients may keep rechecking a faucet to prevent dripping. They may believe the drip will produce a flood, wet the electrical sockets, and start a fire.

References

Alberca Lorente R: Las bases del analisis existencial. Rev Psiq y Psicol Med Barcelona 1:31–107, 1953

American Psychiatric Association: Diagnostic and Statistical Manual of Mental Disorders, 4th Edition. Washington, DC, American Psychiatric Association, 1994

Bach GR: Narzismus und Gruppentherapie: Uberlegungen zu drei Misserfolgen. Gruppenpsychotherapie Gruppendynamen 12:100–107, 1977

Ballus C: Eiologia y patogenia, in Patologia Obsesiva. Edited by Monserrat-Esteve S, Costa Molinari JM, Ballus C. Malaga, Graficasa, 1971, pp 81–114

Beech HR: Ritualistic activity in patients. J Psychosom Res 15:417–422, 1971

Bertschy G, Ahyi RG: Obsessive-compulsive disorders in Benin: five case reports. Psychopathology 4:398–401, 1991

Black A: The natural history of obsessional neurosis, in Obsessional States. Edited by Beech HR. London, Methuen, 1974, pp 19–54

Blanc M: Neurose obsessionelle et syndromes obsessionelles. Rev Prat 6:935–947, 1956

Bassier de Savages de la Croix F: Nosologie methodique dans laquelle les maladies sont rangeos par classe suivant le systeme de Sydenham et pordre des botanistes. Lyon, 1770

Bourgeois M: Apropos d'un centenaire: la folie du doute (avec delire du toucher), Legrand du Saulle (1875). Ann Med Psychol (Paris) 2:937–956, 1975

Brown FW: Heredity in the psychoneurotic. Proc R Soc Med 35:785–790, 1942

Buccola G: Les idees fixes et leurs conditions physiopathol. Revista Sperimentallede Freniatria 6:155–181, 1880

Bustamante M: Historiales clinicos de neurosis obsesiva. Arch Neurobiol 14:927–978, 1934

Cammer L: Antidepressants as a prophylaxis against depression in the obsessive-compulsive person. Psychosomatics 14:201–206, 1973

Capstick N, Seldrup JA: Study in the relationship between abnormalities occurring at the time of birth and the subsequent development of obsessional symptoms. Acta Psychiatr Scand 56:427–431, 1977

Carothers JC: A study of mental derangement in Africans, and an attempt to explain its peculiarities, more especially in relation to the African attitude to life. Psychiatry 11:47–86, 1948

Carothers JC: The African mind in health and disease (World Health Organization monograph, series 17). Geneva, Switzerland, World Health Organization, 1953

Cederblad M: A child psychiatric study on Sudanese Arab children. Acta Psychiatr Scand 200(44):1–230, 1968

Chakraborty A, Banerji G: Ritual, a culture specific neurosis, and obsessional states in Bengali culture. Indian Journal of Psychiatry 17:273–283, 1975

Chen CN, Wong J, Lee N, et al: The Shatin community mental health survey in Hong Kong II: major findings. Arch Gen Psychiatry 50:125–33, 1993

Costa Molinari JM: Clasificacíon, clínica, evolucíon y diagnóstico, in Patología Obsesiva. Edited by Monserrat-Esteve S, Costa Molinari JM, Ballús C. Málaga, Graficasa, 1971a, pp 159–191

Costa Molinari JM: Semiología clinica, in Patalogia Obsesiva. Edited by Monserrat-Esteve S, Costa Molinari JM, Ballús C. Málaga, Graficasa, 1971b, pp 49–62

Coullaut Mendigutia R: El uso Asociado de Ipronizida y Alcaloides de la Rawolfia Serpentina en Enfermos Mentales. Act Luso-Esp de Neurol y Psiquiat 19: 130–133, 1960

Cullen W: Apparatus and Nosologiam Methodicam, seu Synopsis Nosologiae Methodicae in Usum Studiosorum. Edinburgh, Creech, 1769.

DeBoor W: Die Lehre von Zwang. Sammelbericht uber die Jahre 1918 bis 1947. Fortschr Neurol Psychiatr 17:49–85, 1949

Donath J: Zur Kenntnis des Anankasmus (Psychicheszwangzustade). Arch Fortschr Psych u Nervenkrankh 1897:29–39, 1897

Dowson JW: The phenomenology of severe obsessive-compulsive neurosis. Br J Psychiatry 131:75–78, 1977

Esquirol JEE: Des maladies mentales considerées sous le rapport medical, hygienique et medico-legal (Paris 1838), cited in Oesterreich TK, Possession and Exorcism. New York, Causeway Books, 1974, p 191

Falret J: De la folie raisonnante ou folie morale. Ann Med Psychol 7:382–386, 1866

Faravelli C, Guerrini Degl'Innocenti B, Giardinelli L: Epidemiology of anxiety disorders in Florence. Acta Psychiatr Scand 79:308–312, 1989

Freud S: The Standard Edition of the Complete Psychological Works of Sigmund Freud, Vol 16. Translated and edited by Strachey J. London, Hogarth Press, 1917, pp 258–259

Freud S: Totem y Tabu (1913). Buenos Aires, Brazil, Santiago Rueda, 1953, p 37

Gaitonde MR: Cross-cultural study of the psychiatric syndromes in outpatient clinics in Bombay, India and Topeka, Kansas. Int J Soc Psychiatry 3: 98–104, 1958

Goodwin DW, Guze SB, Robins E: Follow-up studies in obsessional neurosis. Arch Gen Psychiatry 20:182–187, 1969

Green A: Obsess et psychoneur obsess. Encyclopedie Medico-Chirurgicale Psychiatrie, 1965

Greenberg D, Witztum E: Cultural aspects of obsessive-compulsive disorder, in Obsessive Compulsive Disorder. Edited by Hollander E, Zohar J, Marazziti D, Olivier B. London, Wiley, 1994, pp 11–21

Greenberg D, Witztum E, Pisante J: Scrupulosity: religious attitudes and clinical presentations. Br J Med Psychol 60:29–37, 1987

Hafner RJ, Miller RJ: Obsessive-compulsive disorder: an exploration of some unresolved clinical issues. Aust N Z J Psychiatry 24:480–485, 1990

Hare E, Price J, Slate E: Fertility in obsessional neurosis. Br J Psychiatry 121: 197–205, 1972

Hayashi N: Neurotic symptoms of borderline patients: a case review study. Seishin Shinkeigaku Zasshi 94:648–681, 1992

Higgins NC, Pollard CA, Mekel WT: Relationship between religion-related factors and obsessive-compulsive disorder. Current Psychology Research and Reviews 11:79–85, 1992

Horwath E, Johnson J, Hornig CD: Epidemiology of panic disorder in African-Americans. Am J Psychiatry 150:465–469, 1993

Hunter R, Macalpine I: Three Hundred Years of Psychiatry. London, University Press, 1963

Ingram IM: La personalite obsessive et la maladie obsessive. (The obsessional personality and obsessional illness). Am J Psychiatry 117:1016–1019, 1961a

Ingram IM: Obsessional illness in mental hospital patients. Journal of Mental Science 107:382–396, 1961b

Inouye E: Similar and dissimilar manifestations of obsessive-compulsive neurosis in monozygotic twins. Am J Psychiatry 121:1171–1175, 1965

Janet P: Les Obsessions et la Psychastenie, Vol 1. Paris, France, Alcan, 1903

Judd LL: Obsessive-compulsive neurosis in children. Arch Gen Psychiatry 12:136–143, 1965

Kanner L: Child Psychiatry, 2nd Edition. Oxford, England, Blackwell, 1948

Karno M, Golding JM, Burnam MA, et al: Anxiety disorders among Mexican Americans and non-Hispanic whites in Los Angeles. J Nerv Ment Dis 177:202–209, 1989

Kayton L, Borge C: Birth order and the obsessive-compulsive character. Arch Gen Psychiatry 17:751–755, 1967

Kendell RE, Discipio WJ: Obsessional symptoms and obsessional personality traits in patients with depressive illness. Psychol Med 1:65–72, 1970

Khanna S, Channabasavanna SM: Birth order in obsessive-compulsive disorder. Psychiatr Res 21:349–354, 1987

Khanna S, Rajendra PN, Channabasavanna SM: Sociodemographic variables in obsessive-compulsive neurosis in India. Int J Soc Psychiatry 32:47–54, 1986

Kringlen E: Obsessional neurotics. Br J Psychiatry 111:709–772, 1965

Lambo TA: The importance of cultural factors in treatment. Acta Psychiatr Scand 38:176–181, 1962

Leighton AJ, Murphy JM: The problem of cultural distortion. Milbank Mem Fund Q 43:189–198, 1965

Leitenberg J: Behavioral approaches to treatment of neuroses, in Handbook of Behavior Modification and Behavior Therapy. Edited by Leitenberg H. Englewood Cliffs, NJ, Prentice-Hall, 1976

Lewis A: Problems of obsessional illness. Proc R Soc Med 29:325–336, 1936

Lo WH: A follow-up study of obsessional neurotics in Hong Kong Chinese. Br J Psychiatry 113:823–832, 1967

Lorenz M: Expressive behavior and language patterns. Psychiatry 18:353–366, 1955

Luys M: Des obsessions pathologiques dans leurs rapports avec l'activite automatique des elements nerveus. Encephale 3:20–61, 1883

Mahgoub OM, Abdel-Hafeiz HB: Pattern of obsessive-compulsive disorder in Eastern Saudi Arabia. Br J Psychiatry 158:840–842, 1991

Marks IM, Crow J, Drewe E, et al: Obsessive-compulsive neurosis in identical twins. Br J Psychiatry 115:991–998, 1969

Meyer A: Superstition and magic in the Caribbean: some psychiatric consequences. Psychiatria, Neurologia, Neurochirurgia 71:421–434, 1968

Monserrat-Esteve S: In Patologia Obsesiva. Edited by Monserrat-Esteve S, Costa Molinari JM, Ballus C. Malaga, Graficasa, 1971, pp 12–29

Morel M: Du delire emotif: neurose et systeme nerveux ganglionnaire visceral. Archives General de Medicine 1:385–402, 1856

Muller C: Weitere Beobachtungen zum Verlauf der Zwangskrankheit. Psychiatr Neurol (Basel) 133:80–94, 1957

Neziroglu FA: Symptomatology and symptoms, in Obsessive-Compulsive Disorders: Pathogenesis, Diagnosis, Treatment. Edited by Yaryura-Tobias JA, Neziroglu FA. New York, Marcel Dekker, 1983, pp 7–17

Neziroglu FA, Yaryura-Tobias JA, Lemli JM, et al: Estudio demografico del trastorno obseso-compulsivo. Acta Psiquiatr Psicol Am Lat 40:217–223, 1994

Nica Udangiu S: Epidemiology of psychic disorders of neurotic intensity in old age. Rev Roumanian Med Ser Neurol Psychiat 15:167–176, 1977

Oesterreich TK: Possession and Exorcism. New York, Causeway Books, 1974

Okasha A, Kamel M, Hassan AH: Preliminary psychiatric observations in Egypt. Br J Psychiatry 114:949–955, 1968

Pacella B: Clinical and electroencephalographic studies of obsessive-compulsive states. Am J Psychiatry 100:830–838, 1944

Parker N: Close identification in twins discordant for obsessional neurosis. Br J Psychiatry 110:496–504, 1964

Perez De Nucci AM: La Medicina Tradicional del Nordeste Argentino. Buenos Aires, Brazil, Ediciones del Sol, 1988, pp 49–60

Pfeiffer WM: Geistige Storungen bei den Sudanesen. Psychiatr Neurol (Basel) 143:315–333, 1962

Pinel P: A Treatise on Insanity. Translated by Davis D. Sheffield, England,W Todd, 1802

Pollitt J: Natural history of obsessional states: a study of 150 cases. BMJ 1:194–198, 1957

Pollitt J: Natural history studies in mental illness. Journal of Mental Science 106: 93–113, 1960

Pujol R, Savy L: Le Devenir de l'Obsede. Paris, France, Masson et Cie, 1968

Rachman S, Hodgson R: Obsessions and Compulsions. Englewood Cliffs, NJ, Prentice-Hall, 1980

Reiger DA, Boyd HH, Burke JD, et al: One month prevalence of mental disorders in the United States. Arch Gen Psychiatry 45:977–978, 1988

Ronchi P, Abbruzzese M, Erzegovesi S, et al: The epidemiology of obsessive-compulsive disorder in an Italian population. European Psychiatry 7:53–59, 1992

Rosen P: The historical sociology of mental illness, in Madness in Society. New York, Harper & Row, 1969

Rosenberg CM: Complications of obsessional neurosis. Br J Psychiatry 114: 477–482, 1968

Rudin E: Ein Beitrag zur Frage der Zwang Krankheit, insbesondere ihrer hereditaren Beziel ungen. Arch Psychiatr Nervenkr 191:14–54, 1953

Schilder P: The organic background of obsessions and compulsions. Am J Psychiatry 94:1397–1416, 1938

Schneider K: Psychologie der Schizophrenen. Leipzig, Germany, Thieme, 1930

Seva Diaz A: Investigaciones en torno al fenomento obsesivo. Actas-Luso-Esp. Neurobiol y Psiquiat 23:260271, 1964

Skoog G: The anancastic syndrome and its relation to personality attitudes. Acta Psychiatr Scand 134:205–207, 1959

Spranger J, Kramer H: Malleus maleficarum. London, Pushkin Press, 1951

Spranger J, Kramer H: Maleus Maleficarum (1486). Buenos Aires, Brazil, Ediciones Orion, 1975

Steketee G, Quay S, White K: Religion and guilt in obsessive-compulsive disorder patients. Journal of Anxiety Disorders 5:359–367, 1991

Stern RS, Cobb JP: Phenomenology of obsessive-compulsive neurosis. Br J Psychiatry 132:233–239, 1978

Storring GE: Uber Zwangsdeken bei Blickrampfen. Arch Psychiatr Nervenkr 89:836–840, 1930

Takahashi S, Nakamura M, Iida H, et al: Prevalence of panic disorder and other subtypes of anxiety disorder and their background. Jpn J Psychiatry Neurol 41:9–18, 1987

Tamarin GR: Some formal logical and social specificities of the obsessive and paranoid life style and though organization. Isr Ann Psychiatry Relat Discip 15:1–11, 1977

Tamburini A: Sur la folie du doute and sur les idees fixes impulsives. Revista Esperimental di Freniatria 9:75–97, 1883

Taschev T: Zur Klinik der Zwangszustande. Fortschr Neurol Psychiatr 38:89–110, 1970

Thyer B, Parrish RT, Curtis GC, et al: Ages of onset of DSM-III anxiety disorders. Compr Psychiatry 26:113–122, 1985

Tuke DH: Imperative ideas. Brain 2:179, 1894

Walker VJ: Explanation in obsessional neurosis. Br J Psychiatry 123:675–680, 1973

Walker VJ, Beech HR: Mood state and the ritualistic behavior of obsessional patients. Br J Psychiatry 115:1261–1263, 1969

Wallace ER: Reflections on the relationship between psychoanalysis and Christianity. Pastoral-Psychology 31:215–243, 1983

Wallace ER: Psychiatry and its nosology: a historico-philosophical overview, in Philosophical Perspectives on Psychiatric Diagnostic Classification. Edited by Sadler JZ, Wiggins OP, Schwartz MA. Baltimore, MD, The John Hopkins University Press, 1994, pp 16–86

Weintraub W, Aronson J: Verbal behavior analysis and psychological defense mechanisms. Arch Gen Psychiatry 30:297–300, 1974

Westphal C: Ueber Zwangsvorstellungen. Berliner Klinischen Wochenschrift 3:390–397, 1872

Williamson RC: Socialization, mental health, and social class: a Santiago sample. Soc Psychiatry 11:69–74, 1976

Willis T: De Anima Brutorum. London, R. Davis, 1672.

Woodruff R, Pitts FN: Monozygotic twins with obsessional illness. Am J Psychiatry 120:1075–1080, 1964

Yaryura-Tobias JA: Obsessive-compulsive disorders: a serotonergic hypothesis. Journal of Orthomolecular Psychiatry 6:317–326, 1977

Yaryura-Tobias JA: Symptoms and classification of obsessive-compulsive disorder. Biol Psychiatry 1:521–523, 1986

Yaryura-Tobias JA, Neziroglu F: Compulsions, aggression, and self-mutilation: a hypothalamic disorder? Journal of Orthomolecular Psychiatry 7:114–117, 1978

Yaryura-Tobias JA, Neziroglu F, Fuller B: An integral approach in the management of the obsessive-compulsive patient. Pharmaceutical Medicine 2:155–167, 1979

Yaryura-Tobias JA, Campisi T, McKay D: Schizophrenia and obsessive-compulsive disorder: shared aspects of pathology. Neurology, Psychiatry and Brain Research 3:143–148, 1995

Chapter 2
Biological and Behavior Therapies

C urrent treatment of obsessive-compulsive disorder (OCD) is multi-disciplinary. The introduction of anti–obsessive-compulsive agents; improvement in behavioral techniques; and the addition of cognitive formulation, family therapy, and self-help groups constitute an integrative direction for treatment.

Biological and behavior treatment is basically symptom oriented, because no etiopathogenetic factors have been isolated. Therefore, the aim of therapy is to 1) decrease symptom intensity and frequency, 2) suppress some of the symptoms, 3) facilitate indifference toward the symptoms, and 4) eradicate the illness.

The protean nature of the symptoms complicates treatment strategies. Therefore, it is convenient to divide symptoms into two groups: primary and secondary. Primary symptoms include the core of OCD: obsessions, compulsions, and doubting. Secondary symptoms include those primarily manifesting an altered affect. This division allows the therapist to select medications whose actions are known to affect a given group of symptoms (e.g., an anti–obsessive-compulsive agent for the primary symptoms and an anxiolytic drug for anxiety). Current medications given to patients with OCD have multiple actions that act not only on the primary symptoms, but also on the patient's affect. The use of antipsychotic medication has been displaced by the introduction of the more specific anti–obsessive-compulsive agents. However, the coexistence of OCD with schizophrenia, schizoaffective disorders, overvalued ideas, or paranoid symptoms may require a new therapeutic approach.

The behaviorist will treat the patient using techniques to basically modify the presence of obsessions, compulsions, and anxiety. In addition, cognitive therapy is used to change false beliefs. The therapist should not overlook the dynamic aspects of the condition. Awareness of past events, childhood development, and phobic components, among others, may facilitate a better response to the standard procedures. Family intervention and participation are key elements for successful treatment. Because patients are usually dependent, family involvement is helpful in limiting this dependency.

Our experience indicates that the treatment strategy has to be tailored to the patient. The concept that there are no diseases, just patients, is applicable here. Before starting the chosen treatment, an integral assessment of the patient must be made. Knowing the patient as much as possible will enhance the treatment response. We find that a gradual approach to treatment is useful. Launching a fast, "all-the-way" therapeutic program might be erroneous, because patients with OCD are fearful and have a need to be in control. Also, a hasty treatment approach, immediately applying standard therapies, may lead to overlooking important components of the particular patient's illness. Each patient is unique, with special needs and his or her own history. Time will allow the therapist to know the patient, and vice versa.

Finally, a nonpsychiatric medical history, a physical examination, blood tests and urinalysis, an electrocardiogram, and an electroencephalogram should be obtained. Baseline measurements are useful, because therapy alters one's biology and often must be modified accordingly.

Psychopharmacotherapy

For many centuries drugs were widely used for the treatment of patients, without specific targets. In 1845 in France Moreau de Tours—for the first time—used a drug to induce and treat mental symptoms. The drug was cannabis, and that event marked the onset of psychopharmacology. At the beginning, drug treatment of mental illness lacked objectives. However, current psychopharmacology drugs are more specific and selective to reach certain targets.

The treatment of OCD also has suffered from the lack of specificity in treating the symptoms in particular and the illness in general. This lack of specificity was compounded by the confusion surrounding its symptomatology and phenomenology. For example, mistakenly diagnosing OCD for another mental disorder, or vice versa, was a common occurrence.

Since 1970 a great variety of psychostimulants, neuroleptics, antidepressants, anxiolytics, anticonvulsants, vitamins, minerals, and amino acids have been tried to treat OCD. Currently clinicians have a greater choice of drugs that are more specific, and therefore more target oriented, than those in the past.

Before discussing the pharmacotherapy of OCD, it is important to set some guidelines as to the role of the psychiatrist who is ready to prescribe medicines. There are three major issues to consider: diagnosis, treatment tailoring, and coexistent nonpsychiatric medical illnesses. The following are the guidelines that we implement:

1. Perform the following:
   a. Physical examination
   b. Psychiatric and medical history
   c. Laboratory testing
2. Discuss with the patient:
   a. Treatment outcome, with and without medication
   b. Choices between medical and psychological treatment
   c. Medication choice and dosage
   d. Drug action and side effects
   e. Interaction with other medications the patient is taking
   f. Drug action with other acute or chronic medical illnesses
   g. Treatment duration
   h. Overdosing
   i. Dietary and beverage restrictions
   j. The use of illegal drugs
   k. Warnings regarding operating machinery or driving a vehicle
   l. Discontinuation of therapy and withdrawal side effects

Psychotomimetics and Psychostimulants

Cocaine is given by iontophoresis, via a transfrontal or pernasal mode. Cocaine's beneficial effects are 1) diminishing the concern for harming oneself or others by reducing moral rigidity, and 2) eliciting indifference similar to that seen in presenile dementia (Rojo Sierra 1954, 1959). One patient reported that psychedelic drugs (i.e., LSD and psilocin) reduced his severe OCD symptoms' intensity (Leonard and Rapoport 1987). Patients who chronically used hashish and marijuana reported a decrease in anxiety, which helped control obsessive-compulsive symptoms. Other substances, such as amphetamine-like substances, were administered with equivocal results (Giberti and Gregoreti 1957). It is believed that these compounds make symptoms tolerable by elevating the mood, impairing memory (which facilitates transient forgetfulness of the obsessional content), and giving a false sense of self-assurance.

Acetylcholine

Administration of acetylcholine also was proposed for treating OCD and produced good results (Lopez Ibor 1952).

Neuroleptic Medication

In 1967 Dally reported using perphenazine in low doses to treat obsessive-compulsive patients. Patients with severe obsessive-compulsive syndromes were treated with L-promazine, 50% of the cases improved (Baruk et al. 1959). Properiazine, an antipsychotic with antiaggressive action, was given in oral doses of 500 mg daily by Lanfranchi (1968), who considered aggressiveness the etiopathological factor in obsessions.

Tapia (1969) indicated that haloperidol seemed to be effective against whatever mechanism sets off obsessive-compulsive or ruminative concerns that bring about tics, Tourette's syndrome, obsessive-compulsive thoughts, and perhaps some forms of stuttering (Tapia 1969). However, haloperidol was sometimes reported to be inefficacious (Hussain and Ahad 1970).

Lambertet et al. (1966) treated a youngster experiencing an encephalopathic syndrome characterized by athetotic movements, urges to scream and touch, and self-mutilation obsessions. High L-mepromazine (also known as methotrimeprazine) doses with poor results were followed by a thioproperazine trial (average dose, 300 mg/day) and trihexyphenidyl (10 mg/day) with good results. Crying impulses and self-harm urges disappeared. The authors suggested that the mesodiencephalic region participated in the case's etiology.

From 1972 to 1978 we saw more than 500 OCD patients, many of whom were at different stages of their illnesses, under neuroleptic medication. Thioridazine, chlorpromazine, trifluoperazine, and perphenazine were the most often used agents. One severely obsessive-compulsive patient received 3,000 mg of chlorpromazine daily over a 6-month period, to no avail. We also observed several cases of haloperidol therapy using 100 mg/day doses. Patients treated with high neuroleptic doses developed extrapyramidal symptoms, tardive dyskinesia, or psychomotor rituals.

Neuroleptic medications are not acceptable treatment for primary OCD. They may help secondary OCD symptoms, such as aggressive behavior or insomnia, but their side effects outweigh the therapeutic gains. Furthermore, neuroleptics may induce obsessive-compulsive symptoms such as iterative thinking, compulsions, and movement disorders.

Anxiolytic Medication

Historically, anxiolytics have been widely used to treat OCD, based on the idea that obsessions and compulsions result from anxiety. Several uncontrolled studies using different benzadiazepines, in small or large doses, showed an improvement in anxiety symptoms but not in obsessive-compulsive symptoms (Bethune 1964; Breitner 1960; Burrell et al. 1974; Hussain and Ahad 1970; Okuma et al. 1971; Orvin 1967; Venkoba Roa 1964).

Alprazolam, an anxiolytic medication with a strong antipanic effect, was tried in a few patients, resulting in moderate to marked improvement (Tesar and Jenike 1984; Tollefson 1985). A comparative double-blind study between alprazolam and imipramine showed negative results for both drugs (Yaryura-Tobias et al., unpublished data). Clonazepam, a benzodiazepine with action in serotonergic neural transmission, was tried in the treatment of OCD, with satisfactory results (Hewlett et al. 1990). Buspirone, a serotonergic agonist, when used to treat OCD as a coadjuvant drug in combination with fluoxetine in an open-label trial, was effective (Markovitz et al. 1990). However, when used with fluvoxamine, its effects were similar to those of placebo (McDougle et al. 1993). When buspirone was compared with clomipramine, both produced clinical "improvement" in half the patients ($N = 18$) (Pato et al. 1991). In another study, which involved augmentation of a potent serotonin reuptake inhibitor with either placebo or buspirone in a double-blind controlled trial, only 29% of the patients ($N = 14$) had a 25% reduction in OCD symptoms. This led to the conclusion that there was not a significant difference between placebo and buspirone in terms of augmentation (Pigott et al. 1992a).

Antidepressant Medication

Various authors (Brown 1942; Lewis 1957; Sakai 1967) have found a genetic relationship between manic-depressive illness and obsessive-compulsive neurosis, suggesting a link between the two. Gittelson (1966a, 1966b, 1966c, 1966d), in a series of publications, reported that 52 of 388 depressed patients showed frank, obsessional symptoms before the onset of depressive illness. Similarly, Kendell and Discipio (1970) not only confirmed these findings, but also indicated that obsessional symptoms correlated with depression depth and continued through the duration of depression. These findings were conducive to viewing OCD as a psychoaffective illness. Therefore, a trial of antidepressant medication was the logical next step taken by psychiatrists.

Tricyclic antidepressants. Tricyclic antidepressants may be helpful in the treatment of OCD, even when depressive symptoms are absent.

Imipramine is used extensively because of its thymoleptic properties (Baruk et al. 1959; Borenstein and Dabbah 1959; Guyotat et al. 1960; Navarro 1960; Tellenbach 1963; Trabucci et al. 1959; Vidal and Vidal 1965). Some of these data were reviewed by Angst and Theobald (1970), who found that most studies used small samples, and the results varied.

Protriptyline was used in psychasthenic patients (Malik and Chainia 1968) and amitriptyline in obsessional and psychasthenic patients (Carles Egea 1963). A report was published by Needleman and Waber (1977) on five women diagnosed with anorexia nervosa who had concomitant parkinsonian syndrome-like symptoms and obsessive-compulsive pathology. These patients responded well to hospitalization and amitriptyline therapy in doses ranging from 75 to 150 mg/day.

Doxepin, a dibenzoxazepine compound that is closely related structurally to the tricyclic antidepressants, helped by defusing symptoms rather than suppressing them (Ananth et al. 1975).

Nontricyclic antidepressants. A trial with nisoxetine, a nontricyclic antidepressant with selective blocking action on norepinephrine uptake, did not improve symptoms in a group of 18 OCD patients (Yaryura-Tobias and Neziroglu 1983).

Phenethylhydrazine (phenelzine), a monoamine oxidase inhibitor (MAOI), was successful in treating patients with OCD, phobia, or both (Annesley 1969; Izikowitz 1960; Jain et al. 1970). Phenelzine given to a 52-year-old female with poor response to imipramine improved her condition dramatically (Isberg 1981). Other MAOIs, such as tranylcypromine, nialamide, isocarboxazid, and iproniazid, had unpredictable results (Dally 1967; Yaryura-Tobias and Neziroglu 1979). MAOIs produced good results in four of eight OCD patients (Jenike 1982). Trazodone was effective in a few patients (Baxter 1985; Hermesh et al. 1990) but ineffective in a double-blind placebo-controlled trial involving 21 OCD patients (Pigott et al. 1992b).

Anti–Obsessive-Compulsive Agents

Clomipramine was the first drug to show therapeutic efficacy in OCD (Capstick 1971; Fernández de Córdoba and López Ibor 1967; Van Reynynghe De Voxurie 1968; Yaryura-Tobias and Neziroglu 1975). In 1976 the first double-blind, placebo-controlled study of clomipramine showed significant improvement in obsession and compulsion symptoms (Yaryura-Tobias et al. 1976).

Since that time, many studies of clomipramine have been conducted, and currently its efficacy in the treatment of OCD is widely accepted (Clomipramine Collaborative Study Group 1991; Jenike et al. 1989). The average dose is 200 mg daily. To prevent the onset of some untoward effects, it is advisable to titrate medication gradually in steps of 25 mg over 3 weeks. To prevent nausea, the drug should be given immediately after a meal. It is usually administered orally or intravenously, with the intravenous route chosen for severe obsessive-compulsive syndrome cases (López Ibor Alino and López Ibor Alino 1973; Porta Biosca and Vallejo Ruiloba 1971; Rego et al. 1970) or cases refractory to oral administration (Fallon et al. 1992; Thakur et al. 1991; Warneke 1984). Marshall and Micev's (1973) comprehensive intravenous clomipramine study showed good results in a 118-patient sample. Clomipramine's efficacy was best reflected in patients lacking hysterical symptoms and those with predominant obsessive-compulsive symptoms.

The clinical clomipramine response is unrelated to depression, but depression appears to be a predictor of poor outcome in patients with a long history of illness (DeVeaugh-Geiss et al. 1990). Plasma levels required for therapeutic efficacy range from 100 to 250 ng/ml for clomipramine and from 230 to 550 ng/ml for N-desmethylclomipramine (Stern et al. 1980). Plasma levels of clomipramine, but not of N-desmethylclomipramine, correlate significantly with posttreatment outcome measures, with responders having significantly higher clomipramine levels (Mavissakalian et al. 1990). The maintenance clomipramine dose is 75–100 mg (Pato et al. 1990; Yaryura-Tobias et al. 1976).

The side effects of clomipramine are similar to those of tricyclic antidepressants. Perhaps the two most important clomipramine side effects are weight gain and sexual disorders (loss of libido, delayed ejaculation, anorgasmia). Anorgasmia is seen in both male and female patients (Monteiro et al. 1987). An anecdotal report described the successful treatment of anorgasmia with yohimbine (Price and Grunhaus 1990).

Clomipramine has been compared with tricyclic antidepressants, MAOIs, and selective serotonin reuptake inhibitors in the treatment of OCD. In a double-blind placebo-controlled trial conducted with clomipramine and nortriptyline, clomipramine was superior to placebo, whereas nortriptyline was not (Thoren et al. 1980). A comparative study between clomipramine and doxepin indicated that clomipramine reduced phobic and obsessive-compulsive symptoms, whereas doxepin only alleviated the interference of obsessive symptoms (Ananth and Van Den Steen 1977). Another study showed that clomipramine had better therapeutic effects and fewer side effects than amitriptyline (Zhao 1991).

When compared with imipramine, clomipramine more effectively reduced the symptoms of OCD and depression (Volavka et al. 1985).

In another study, clomipramine and phenelzine yielded the same therapeutic efficacy (Vallejo et al. 1992).

Comparative studies suggest that fluoxetine is a viable alternative to clomipramine in the treatment of OCD (Jenike et al. 1990a; Pigott et al. 1990). Comparative trials that included clomipramine, clonazepam, clonidine, and diphenhydramine indicated that clonazepam is a useful alternative treatment for OCD patients (Hewlett et al. 1992). Systematic comparison of clomipramine and fluvoxamine showed that the two are equally effective (Tamini et al. 1991)

Clomipramine also was administered to children experiencing phobias, obsessions, and anorexia nervosa. Good phobic anxiety remission and amelioration of obsession, anorexia nervosa, and depression were reported (Dugas and Velin 1972).

Furthermore, clomipramine may facilitate behavior therapy involving relaxation practice and thought stopping (Symonds 1973). We also found that clomipramine administration, before exposure and response prevention, helped patients resist their rituals by decreasing the urges' intensity.

Selective Serotonin Reuptake Inhibitors

Sertraline successfully controlled obsessive-compulsive symptoms in several double-blind placebo-controlled trials (Chouinard 1992; Chouinard et al. 1990; Jenike et al. 1990b).

Fluvoxamine also significantly improved OCD treatment (Mallya et al. 1992). In a comparative trial with desipramine, fluvoxamine reduced OCD symptoms, whereas desipramine did not (Goodman et al. 1990). In another study, fluvoxamine and clomipramine were compared in 12 OCD patients, with equal improvement reported for both drugs (Smeraldi et al. 1992).

In one long-term study, fluoxetine was successful in OCD patients (Frenkel et al. 1990). In a double-blind crossover study of 13 OCD patients treated with fluoxetine, buspirone, or placebo, there were no significant differences between buspirone and placebo (Grady et al. 1993).

In a sample of six OCD patients, a comparative sequential trial of fluoxetine, phenelzine, and tranylcypromine did not improve obsessive-compulsive symptoms. Lack of efficacy, short-term study duration, and intolerable side effects are possible reasons for the negative results (Modell et al. 1989).

Zimeldine was given to six patients with OCD accompanied by cognitive deficits and hyperactive thinking. Their hyperactive thinking normalized, and the obsessive-compulsive symptoms decreased (Kahn et al. 1984).

Coadjuvant Drugs

Fenfluramine. Fenfluramine, an amphetamine analogue, acts as a serotonin releasing agent and reuptake inhibitor. Administering it as an augmentation agent moderately reduces obsessive-compulsive symptoms (Hollander et al. 1990; Judd et al. 1991).

Lithium. Lithium alone is ineffective in the treatment of OCD (Geisler and Schou 1969; Hesso and Thorell 1969). However, in patients with OCD and the manic-depressive subset, a combination of lithium and clomipramine, lithium alone, and a combination of lithium and L-tryptophan all showed efficacy (Yaryura-Tobias 1981). Lithium is used as an adjuvant in treating OCD, with a positive therapeutic outcome resulting when lithium is combined with clomipramine (Pigott et al. 1991), fluoxetine (Ruegg et al. 1992), or desipramine (Eisenberg and Asnis 1985). A controlled trial of lithium augmentation in patients with fluvoxamine-refractory OCD indicated a lack of efficacy (McDougle et al. 1991). Our experience indicates that lithium is helpful in patients with OCD with a manic subset or patients with "racing of the mind."

Anticonvulsants

The relationship between epilepsy and obsessive-compulsive symptoms, and the presence of abnormal electroencephalograms as well as findings of cerebral abnormality in such patients calls for trials with anticonvulsant medication to treat OCD.

According to Haward (1970), 150 mg of phenytoin significantly improved concentration in anancastic patients compared with a placebo group. Compulsive eating was treated in 10 patients, 9 of whom had abnormal electroencephalograms. These nine patients were successfully treated with 300–400 mg/day of phenytoin (Green and Rau 1974).

Tryptophan

According to our hypothesis, OCD is an organic disorder and relates to a central disturbance in serotonin metabolism. We conducted an open study of oral L-tryptophan (3,000–9,000 mg) along with divided doses of nicotinic acid (2,000 mg) and pyridoxine hydrochloride (200 mg). Results were satisfactory (Yaryura-Tobias 1981; Yaryura-Tobias and Bhagavan 1977).

L-Tryptophan and trazodone were inefficacious in 12 OCD patients. However, considerable side effects, including complaints of dizziness, sedation, or feeling "spaced out," forced patients to take trazodone ($n = 6$) or withdraw from the trial ($n = 5$), thus invalidating the results reported (Mattes 1986). Lithium or L-tryptophan, combined with clomipramine in patients refractory to clomipramine therapy alone, improved obsessive-compulsive symptoms (Rasmussen 1984).

Miscellaneous

Anecdotal reports have been published regarding the use of intranasal oxytocin to improve OCD symptoms, but severe memory disturbances discourage its use (Ansseau et al. 1987). Milnacipran (300 mg/day) used for 10 months resulted in partial control of obsessive and compulsive symptoms (Papart and Ansseau 1990). Clonidine did not improve OCD symptoms in a 10-patient sample (Lee et al. 1990).

Seasonal OCD, which occurs in autumn or winter, has been treated by administering full-spectrum bright light concurrently with 125 mg of amitriptyline daily for 12 days; this regimen was followed by complete recovery (Hoflich et al. 1992). In contrast, six patients with a history of OCD and seasonal variations did not respond to light therapy (Yoney et al. 1991).

To test the involvement of endogenous opiates in OCD, two patients were treated with naloxone; however, both patients experienced exacerbated obsessional doubting (Insel and Pickar 1983).

Polypharmacy

Practitioners frequently combine psychopharmacological agents. Based on experimental and clinical evidence, one drug usually produces side effects that require an additional one. For instance, chlorpromazine, prescribed for a psychotic episode, may cause depression, which has to be treated with an antidepressant that may in turn aggravate the psychosis. Thus, it is important to tailor drug treatment to patient needs. As a result, a combined therapeutic approach to OCD has become part of clinical practice.

In a long-term treatment program, the combination of iproniazid and reserpine in daily doses of 150 and 30–45 mg, respectively, was ineffective (Coullaut Mendigutia 1960).

Combination treatments, such as chlordiazepoxide with an antidepressant drug, can be useful in OCD patients (Dally 1967). In a double-blind clinical trial, coadministration of doxepin and amitriptyline was beneficial (Bauer and Novack 1969).

In one study, a 28-year-old man with mysophilia, an abnormal attraction to filth, presented the clinical picture of urolagnia and the compulsive behavior of a toucheur, a voyeur, a compulsive listener, and a sniffer. He was treated with diethylstilbestrol, chlordiazepoxide, and supportive psychotherapy for 2 years, with apparent success (Rousal and Brichoin 1971). The attraction to filth is common among patients refractory to improvement. The compulsion to touch, "peep," listen, and smell constitutes a group of somatosensory compulsions we are investigating. Our preliminary findings indicate that only on questioning do patients respond in the affirmative.

In one study, clomipramine and sulpiride used to treat obsessive-compulsive neurosis improved obsessive ideation, anancasmus, and phobias in about 2 weeks; depression and anxiety improved almost immediately (Amabile et al. 1973).

After reviewing pharmacological treatment of obsessive neurosis, López Ibor Alino and López Ibor Alino (1973) preferred a combination of clomipramine and propericiazine. They also considered infusion of clomipramine superior to oral administration. Moreover, they believed clomipramine should be administered at its highest dose (López Ibor Alino and López Ibor Alino 1974).

Vitamins and Minerals

There is no evidence that vitamins have direct anti–obsessive-compulsive action. However, as coenzymes, they may act as coadjuvants in treatment programs. For instance, using niacin as a tryptophan by-product and pyridoxine as an essential coenzyme in monoamine metabolism may help to mediate the availability of L-tryptophan.

Because OCD is a stressful condition, it might produce a subclinical vitamin dependency or a clinical vitamin depletion. For instance, one report indicated thiamine and folic acid deficiency in a group of 30 patients with OCD (Hermesh et al. 1988). We have conducted a vitamin analysis (vitamins A, C, and B complex) in 180 patients with OCD, with equivocal results (Yaryura-Tobias and Neziroglu, unpublished data, October 1985). The assumption that OCD produces a vitamin deficiency may hold validity when dietary habits or food availability is improper or insufficient. Also, the administration of psychotropic substances may cause vitamin depletion.

Diet

Nutrition is important when treating any medical illness; therefore, diets are prepared for organs affected by different ailments. It is medically unsound to treat a cardiac insufficiency, liver dysfunction, nephrosis, or diabetic condition without a proper dietetic regimen. However, the brain seems spared from nutritional considerations, although ancient medicine books recommended foods, herbs, and even wine as part of the psychiatric armamentarium. For OCD patients, the presence of an appetite disturbance is a common event precipitated by depression, anger, or the concurrent presence of eating disorders. Therefore, poor nutrition leading to a subclinical metabolic imbalance might be expected to affect the illness's therapeutic outcome. One example is the presence of a glucose disturbance in many OCD patients. Postprandial hypoglycemia (Berlin et al. 1994) and abnormal oral glucose tolerance tests (Yaryura-Tobias 1988) have been reported in patients with OCD. Furthermore, in one anecdotal report, two patients with obsessionality and ruminations secondary to functional hypoglycemia seemed to improve after dietary control (Rippere 1984).

It is beneficial for the clinician to prescribe a diet high in complex carbohydrates and low in processed sugar. Patients who abstain from using substances known to cause reactive hypoglycemia (e.g., chocolate, alcohol, acetylsalicylic acid, caffeine, and marijuana) also may benefit.

Stimulant foods, such as those containing tyramine (e.g., aged cheese, wine, and liver), should be avoided. Furthermore, alcohol is generally incompatible with the use of antidepressants because it may produce anxiety, agitation, depression, or aggressive behavior toward oneself or others. Also, alcohol produces hyposerotoninemia. Caffeine may inhibit the action of psychotropics because it depletes potassium and produces weight loss, irritability, hyperactivity, and insomnia. Both alcohol and caffeine may cause functional hypoglycemia (see Chapter 13). Following the preceding guidelines may decrease anxiety, irritability, and depression.

Constipation is common in obsessive-compulsive patients with intense symptoms of depression or anorexia. Constipation is one of the vegetative symptoms in depression and may be caused or aggravated by antidepressants. In anorexia, constipation stems from the lack of food and liquid intake. The use of laxatives may deplete nutrients by affecting the intestinal absorption of food. In such cases, a corrective diet and abdominal exercises may help.

In conclusion, it should be remembered that psychotropic medication may alter plasma glucose levels in psychiatric patients (Yaryura-Tobias and Neziroglu 1975).

Physical Exercise

Bruxism and muscular tension in the neck, back, and sural muscles are common complaints of OCD patients. Relaxation exercises comprising different techniques, such as yoga, may be beneficial. Swimming (a natural form of hydrotherapy) is known to control anxiety. Aerobic exercises stimulate circulation in general as well as circulation for particular organs such as the liver, which metabolizes many drugs used for treating OCD.

Sleep Therapy

Cheng et al. (1968) used sleep therapy for patients with compulsive water drinking and had good results. Minkowski and Citrome (1953) reported that one patient with advanced obsessive neurosis superimposed on a schizophrenoid background improved with sleep therapy. The literature on sleep therapy and OCD is practically nonexistent.

Electroconvulsive Therapy

Most authors concur on the poor therapeutic response of patients with OCD to electroconvulsive therapy, although temporary improvement may be observed in patients with severe depressive symptoms. The use of electroconvulsive therapy was common before psychotropic agents were introduced.

Electroconvulsive therapy was successful as part of a conditioning technique that included acting out obsessions and compulsions. Four patients with compulsive self-mutilation improved considerably using this technique (Rubin 1976). In another study, a 60-year-old man with refractory OCD and tardive dyskinesia was successfully treated with electroconvulsive therapy (Mellman and Gorman 1984).

In a review of the use of electroconvulsive therapy, Salzman (1978) found that electroconvulsive therapy for OCD may even be contraindicated.

Behavior Therapy and OCD

Given the scope of this book, it is impossible to review the entire psychological treatment history of OCD. Both the psychodynamic and behavioral literature have been reviewed elsewhere (Yaryura-Tobias and Neziroglu 1983). Although the psychodynamic school provided an excellent clinical description of the disorder, it contributed little to the treatment of OCD. In fact, before the advent of behavior therapy, patients with OCD had a poor prognosis, especially those with severe symptoms. In 1966 Meyer introduced exposure and response prevention, a behavioral approach subsequently found to be effective (Boersma et al. 1976; Boulougouris and Bassiakos 1973; Catts and McConaghy 1975; Emmelkamp and Kraanen 1977; Foa and Goldstein 1978; Marks et al. 1975; Meyer et al. 1974; Rabavilas et al. 1976; Roper et al. 1975). In this approach, Meyer (1966) exposed patients to anxiety-evoking stimuli and constant staff supervision to prevent compulsions.

Before this formal application of exposure and response prevention, Janet (1903) had described exposure therapy. The resulting procedures were derived from animal experimental studies conducted by Maier (1949) and Baum (1966). Exposure and response prevention exposes patients to their feared stimuli and then prevents them from engaging in compulsions. Another term for exposure is *flooding*. For example, patients who obsess about germs may be asked to expose themselves to floors, hospitals, and related objects (e.g., handrails, telephones, excrement, and so forth) and then are prevented from washing their hands. Patients who obsess about fires starting when they are away from home may be asked to leave appliances plugged in before leaving the house; put the stove on and walk out of the kitchen; not pick up cigarette butts; and then not double-check the stove, appliances, or ground.

These examples illustrate the two components of this treatment: first, exposure and second, response prevention. The question of whether both components are necessary was answered in a study conducted by Foa et al. (1980). They found that exposure reduced anxiety to contaminants more than it affected washing behavior, whereas the reverse was true for response prevention. Therefore, it seems both components are needed to treat OCD.

Success Rate

Exposure and response prevention treatment success rates of 60%–85% (median, 75%) have been reported. (For a review, see Foa and Steketee

[1979] and Yaryura-Tobias and Neziroglu [1983].) "Success" in most studies means an improvement rate of 50% or more; "failure" means an improvement rate of less than 30%. The various studies used different lengths of treatment, both in total duration and time dedicated within sessions. Our experience with motivated patients who engaged in 90-minute intensive behavior therapy sessions three to six times a week for a mean duration of 6 weeks indicated a 75% reduction in symptoms. Of course, not every patient engages in intensive treatment. The number of weekly sessions may range from one to six, and the total number of weeks of intensive treatment may range from four to eight, depending on symptom severity and the patient's prior level of functioning.

Although behavior therapy success rates are high, in clinical practice the outcome may not be as encouraging. For clinicians who have treated many patients with OCD, a failure rate of 25% seems low. Patients included in published studies are motivated and compliant and tend to complete treatment. In addition, studies are usually conducted in centers specializing in OCD. Therefore, these patients would have a better than average chance of improving, because most studies do not report on patients who refuse treatment, do not fit the entrance criteria, or drop out of therapy early. In clinical practice, therapists encounter patients who have severe symptoms, do not respond or respond only minimally to medications, are discouraged by previous failures, have one or more comorbid conditions, feel defeated and are minimally motivated, have personality disorders, are depressed, or have highly overvalued ideas. If we take into consideration the entire population of OCD patients, the percentage who improve is considerably lower.

Behavior Therapy, Medications, and the Combined Approach

Only a few studies have compared behavior therapy, medications, and a combination of both. Marks et al. (1980) examined the effects of clomipramine with and without exposure and response prevention. Both psychological treatments—exposure and response prevention and relaxation therapy—consisted of 45-minute sessions, 5 days a week. After 4 weeks of receiving either placebo or clomipramine, patients began one of the psychological therapies. At week 7, there was a significant reduction in rituals among patients who had received both clomipramine and exposure and response prevention than among patients who had received only one of these treatments. By week 10, all patients had received exposure and response prevention so the effect of the two treatments could no longer be differentiated. Marks et al. (1980) concluded that at week 7 the combined approach's superiority reflected the additive influence of two effective treatments given together, rather than one treatment strengthening the other.

Mavissakalian et al. (1985) concluded that a combination of both pharmacological and behavioral intervention is optimal. However, 20% of patients treated with the combined approach failed to improve.

Solyom and Sookman (1977) compared 6 weeks of clomipramine treatment with 6 months of exposure and response prevention conducted twice weekly. They concluded that there were no differences between the two in reduction of depression and obsessive-compulsive symptoms. However, at a 3-year follow-up, patients who had behavior therapy continued to improve; those on drugs did not.

Clomipramine may reduce compulsions enough for patients to have behavior therapy. In one study, clomipramine administered for 4 weeks reduced symptoms by 60% (Neziroglu 1979). Afterward, exposure and response prevention treatment commenced for 10 weekly sessions, yielding a further reduction of 18.7% in symptoms. After 6 months, gains were maintained, and at 1 year, 9 of 10 patients were symptom free (Neziroglu and Yaryura-Tobias 1980). A meta-analysis based on 38 trials of a variety of effective treatments (i.e., clomipramine, exposure and response prevention, and psychosurgery) indicated that clomipramine and exposure and response prevention did not significantly differ from each other in terms of the results produced. However, both were significantly superior to nonspecific treatment programs (Christensen et al. 1987).

Most comparative studies investigated the efficacy of clomipramine. However, one study looked at the efficacy of fluvoxamine with antiexposure instructions, fluvoxamine with exposure, or placebo with exposure in 60 patients for 24 weeks (Cottraux et al. 1990). Most patients did not comply with antiexposure instructions. All three groups improved in rituals and depression from week 0 to week 24 and at 48-week follow-up, with a slight but nonsignificant superiority of the combined approach at week 24.

Despite nearly 30 years of behavior therapy research and more than 20 years in psychopharmacological outcome studies, little is known about the additive or interactive effects of these approaches. Also, no data are available on whether medications should be used before behavioral treatment, as suggested by Foa and Steketee (1984), or if tricyclic medication is a treatment worthy of a direct empirical comparison with behavior therapy (Christensen et al. 1987). Our experience of more than 20 years using both medications and exposure and response prevention leads us to believe that for the majority of patients, the combined treatment approach is most effective. Economically, it shortens the duration of treatment. After many years these clinical observations are being experimentally tested. The crucial questions may be: Who responds to which medications? Who responds to behavior therapy? Who needs the combined approach, and for how long?

Long-Term Effects of Behavior Therapy

Some follow-up data are available on behavior therapy's long-term efficacy. (For a review, see Baer and Minichiello [1990], Neziroglu and Yaryura-Tobias [1994], and Yaryura-Tobias and Neziroglu [1983].) In one study, 34 chronic OCD patients were followed up 6 years after receiving exposure and response prevention for either 3 or 6 weeks, along with clomipramine or placebo for 36 weeks (O'Sullivan et al. 1991). Patients remained significantly improved on obsessive-compulsive symptoms, work or social adjustment, and depression at the end of 6 years. However, they had returned to pretreatment levels of general anxiety. The best predictor of long-term outcome was improvement at posttreatment. Those taking clomipramine or other antidepressants 6 years later were no more improved than those who had stopped such treatment long before. Patients who had received 6 weeks of behavior therapy were doing better than those who had received 3 weeks of behavior therapy.

The long-term effects of exposure in vivo have been reported to last 2 years (Emmelkamp and Rabbie 1981; Kasviskis and Marks 1988; Marks et al. 1975; Mawson et al. 1982), 3.5 years (Visser et al. 1991), 5 years (Marks 1990), and 6 years (O'Sullivan et al. 1991). However, 20%–30% of patients fail to maintain treatment gains at 1 year follow-up (Kirk 1983; Steketee et al. 1982).

Patients who receive more intensive behavior therapy for longer periods of time do better than those in short-term behavior therapy. We recommend, for the average patient, 6 weeks of intensive treatment (90-minute sessions, three to six times a week), and then weekly sessions for 6 months to 1 year. What constitutes an "average patient"? For us, an average patient is one who is either obsessing or engaging in compulsions for 3 hours or more each day, who is distressed about his or her symptoms, and who demonstrates dysfunctionality in at least one of the following areas: work, school, interpersonal relations, household responsibilities, leisure or social activities, and sex.

The nature of the patient population from the early 1970s to the present has changed as many more patients have sought treatment. In the 1970s, patients who had severe symptoms and were incapacitated by the illness sought treatment. The average duration from onset to first consultation was approximately 7 years. By the late 1980s, patients had become more familiar with the symptoms, and the general acceptance of OCD as a "chemical imbalance" took away some of the stigma. The Obsessive Compulsive Foundation was instrumental in destigmatizing the disorder and disseminating information to the public via the media. Patients with various degrees of symptom severity began to seek help. As a consequence, researchers in the field began to see similarities between OCD and other disorders, and studies evolved investigating the continuum, the spectrum, and comorbid conditions. In Section II, these disorders will be discussed in depth. In addition, interest was aroused in refractory cases. To deal with this new set of disorders and cases, new pharmacological agents and cognitive therapy were introduced. Up to this point, behavior therapy referred only to exposure and response prevention and not to cognitive therapy and exposure and response prevention treatment.

Cognitive Therapy

Cognitive therapy is another form of behavior therapy. This approach is based on modifying the anxiety component of OCD by altering patients' faulty beliefs, which are rooted in their appraisal of threat and their ability to cope with it. Although many obsessions and compulsions are mediated cognitively, some are not (e.g., tapping, counting, and touching). For those cognitively mediated compulsions, cognitive therapy may be helpful.

Carr (1974) suggested that patients with OCD overestimate the probability of danger occurring. Expanding on this, McFall and Wollershein (1979) formulated a cognitive-behavioral model of OCD. They stated that after the "primary appraisal" of danger, a "secondary appraisal" occurs, and the individual believes he or she is unable to cope with it. Thus, anxiety results from these faulty appraisals and the individual engages in obsessive-compulsive behaviors to reduce or avoid anxiety.

Few studies have tested the efficacy of a cognitive-behavioral approach. This is surprising, given the number of patients unresponsive to exposure and response prevention; at least 25% refuse to enter behavioral treatment and 12% drop out after starting (Emmelkamp et al. 1980). It has been suggested that patients who have difficulty with exposure and response prevention are depressed, have pure obsessions, and refuse or drop out of treatment (Foa et al. 1983b; Rachman 1983). Although it is obvious that those who refuse or drop out cannot benefit from treatment, current research demonstrates that depressed and purely obsessional patients do respond to behavior therapy (Foa et al. 1992; Neziroglu and Neuman 1990; Salkovskis and

Westbrook 1989). We believe that the major reason patients refuse, drop out, or are treatment refractory is because of highly overvalued ideas. Cognitive therapy may be expected to modify the fixity of beliefs (overvalued ideas), thus shortening the duration of exposure and response prevention.

The first attempt to use cognitive therapy on OCD was by Emmelkamp et al. (1980), and the first to put forth a cognitive-behavioral formulation of obsessions was Salkovskis (1985). Emmelkamp et al. (1980) found that modifying cognition via self-instructional training does not enhance exposure effectiveness in vivo. However, self-instructional training is questionable because it does not target obsessive-compulsive symptoms; therefore, in another study rational emotive therapy was used. In this study, cognitive therapy proved to be as effective as exposure in vivo (Emmelkamp et al. 1988). This finding is further substantiated in another study that found no differences on obsessive-compulsive measures between cognitive therapy and exposure and response prevention nor between cognitive therapy administered before exposure and response prevention compared with exposure and response prevention alone (Emmelkamp and Beens 1991). However, on irrational belief measures, patients who received the combination of cognitive therapy and exposure and response prevention were more improved than patients who received exposure and response prevention alone, thus attesting to cognitive therapy's construct validity. At 6-month follow-up, both groups had maintained their gains. This result suggests that cognitive therapy does not add anything to exposure treatment, even though it modifies patients' faulty cognitions. However, we believe it is important to correctly identify faulty cognitions for therapy to be effective (see "Faulty Cognitions Seen in OCD"). It is unclear from this study what irrational beliefs were challenged.

The cognitive-behavioral formulation states that obsessions are cognitive intrusions, the content of which patients interpret or appraise as harmful to themselves or others, and for which they are responsible to prevent from occurring (Salkovskis 1985; Salkovskis and Warwick 1985). To diminish the possibility of harm, and their sense of responsibility, patients neutralize their thoughts, images, or impulses (Salkovskis and Westbrook 1989). By neutralizing their thoughts via covert rituals or reassurance seeking, they prevent reappraisal of the true risks and amplify preexisting beliefs about responsibility. Cognitive therapy focuses on 1) preventing neutralization, thus increasing exposure to the obsessions; 2) modifying attitudes toward responsibility; 3) modifying the appraisal of intrusive thoughts; and 4) increasing exposure to responsibility by exposure in vivo and stopping reassurance seeking. Neziroglu

(1994) provided case examples and illustrated how to apply behavior and cognitive therapy in OCD. For a review of the application of cognitive therapy to pure obsessions, see "Behavior Therapy Myths."

Faulty Cognitions Seen in OCD

It is important to challenge the proper cognitions to obtain maximum improvement. The most common clinician's mistake is directly challenging the faulty beliefs (e.g., "Where is the evidence that you have AIDS?"). Staying at this level of disputation does not lead to generalization and permanent change.

Below is a list of faulty cognitions we have identified:

- I must have guarantees.
- I cannot stand the anxiety/discomfort.
- I must not make mistakes.
- I am responsible for causing harm.
- I am responsible for not preventing harm to others.
- Thinking is the same as acting.
- It is terrible to make the wrong decision.
- There is a right and a wrong in every situation.
- I must have complete control over everything at all times.
- I am in continuous danger.
- I am responsible for others.
- I must be perfect.
- I alone am responsible for the outcome of events (there is no diffusion of responsibility).

Challenging these core cognitions in OCD are clinically effective in reducing highly overvalued ideas and producing more rapid shifts in cognition during exposure and response prevention treatment. Controlled studies are needed to further test the efficacy of cognitive therapy.

Few studies assess how patients process information. Areas that have been investigated include reduced cognitive inhibition (Enright and Beech 1993); attention failure (Gordon 1985); deficits in cognitive shifting (Head et al. 1989); and cognitive deficit in the form of complex, overly specific, concept formation for obsessional/fear items (Pearson and Foa 1984).

Behavior Therapy Myths

Despite behavior therapy's history of experimentation, there are still erroneous beliefs about it. This may be because psychology's history is rooted in philosophy and psychoanalysis. A discussion of some of these faulty beliefs follows.

All types of behavior therapy work with OCD. Behavior therapy is a psychological treatment based on experimentally derived theories about maladaptation. Many forms of behavior therapy are ineffective in treating core symptoms of OCD. These include systematic desensitization, thought stopping, assertion training, social skills training, paradoxical intention, aversion therapy, behavior modification, and mass practice. These behavior therapies may be necessary for other problems OCD patients may have, such as social skill deficits, unassertiveness, lack of motivation, and family problems. However, these therapies are ineffective in treating obsessions and compulsions. Only exposure and response prevention and cognitive therapy yield positive outcome.

Depressed patients do not respond to treatment. In general, patients with OCD are not depressed. However, those who are exhibit depression secondary to their OCD. They are upset by their lifestyle and their inability to function as a consequence of their disorder. Some patients have depression as a comorbid condition to OCD. If their depression is severe and they are unable to engage in behavior therapy, the depression may have to be treated first with antidepressants.

Foa et al. (1979) suggested treating depression with imipramine before starting behavior therapy for OCD treatment. In a later study, they found no differences between highly depressed and mildly depressed patients with regard to obsessive-compulsive symptoms and their responses to behavior therapy (Foa et al. 1992). In addition, those patients who received imipramine before behavior therapy had the same response as those who received placebo. Essentially, imipramine does not potentiate the effects of behavior therapy. Marks et al. (1980) noted that clomipramine, by reducing depression, increased compliance with behavior therapy. It is not clear whether it is clomipramine's antidepressive or antiobsessive properties that help increase compliance.

In a meta-analysis of 38 trials, exposure and response prevention produced a significant change on depression measures, similar to the change produced by clomipramine (Christensen et al. 1987). This is contrast to Foa and Goldstein's (1978) initial observation that depressed patients do not respond successfully to behavior therapy.

Use of drugs is necessary. Medications may be used in conjunction with behavior therapy. Once patients reduce their obsessions and compulsions, they may be gradually taken off their medications. This may be 6 months to 1 year later. In these cases, the medications reduce the urge to give into compulsions, thus making behavior therapy more "user-friendly."

Antidepressants reduce patients' depression. Depressed OCD patients do not habituate as well as OCD patients who are not depressed (Foa 1979). Once again, it is important to differentiate between patients with secondary depression and those with comorbid depression.

Medications are not always necessary. However, medication with behavior therapy yields the best results for most patients. Many more studies are needed to determine which patients need medication and for what duration of time.

Obsessions (ruminations) do not respond to behavior therapy. The percentage of patients reported to have only obsessions varies. Dowson (1977) reported 15%; Akhtar et al. (1975), 24%; Kirk (1983), 44%; and Hoogduin et al. (1987), 17%. Although Kirk's findings seem high in comparison, approximately 20% of OCD patients have only obsessions.

Studies investigating the efficacy of behavior therapy for obsessions have demonstrated at least a 50% reduction in about 46% of patients (Emmelkamp and Giesselbach 1981; Emmelkamp and Kwee 1977; Emmelkamp and Van der Heyden 1980; Likiermein and Rachman 1982). In these studies, behavior therapy took the form of thought stopping versus imaginal exposure, exposure to obsessions versus exposure to irrelevant fear-provoking scenes, assertiveness training versus thought stopping, and thought stopping versus habituation. Two other studies reported that 73% (Hoogduin et al. 1987) and 81% (Kirk 1983) of obsessional patients responded to exposure and response prevention, with the majority maintaining their gains at follow-up. Even if these two studies are averaged with the others, 50% to 60% of patients with obsessions benefit from behavior therapy.

Although a 50% reduction in obsessions in 50% to 60% of patients with pure obsessions is far from excellent, this result is not less than that obtained with medications (Clomipramine Collaborative Study Group 1991; Jenike 1990). In addition, as Salkovskis and Westbrook (1989) have pointed out, the poor results with obsessions may be a result of ineffective implementation of treatment (e.g., patients with compulsions are included with insufficient response prevention, and the number of sessions are severely limited). Thus, the somewhat discouraging outcome may be from "technical failures" (incorrect methodology) rather than "serious failures" (poor response) (Rachman 1983).

If obsessions are divided into anxiety-elevating obsessions (pure obsessions or ruminations) and anxiety-reducing obsessions (cognitive rituals), as Wolpe (1958) has suggested, behavior therapy results may be different. *Cognitive rituals* are compulsions performed with the intellect rather than the body, as happens in *overt compulsions*. With cognitive rituals, patients engage in active avoidance and essentially try to neutralize, or undo, the anxiety. With *ruminations,* patients engage in passive avoidance by trying to avoid contact with triggering stimuli (e.g., churches/synagogues that elicit religious obsessions, children or magazines that elicit sexual obsessions, or sharp objects that elicit aggressive obsessions).

Both cognitive rituals and ruminations respond to exposure and response prevention. The only obsessions more difficult to treat with behavior therapy are 1) repetitive melodies or sentences and 2) counting. We categorize these types as "obsessions without a theme." Most patients with ruminations have an image or thought, as if they perceive or think the end result but not how they arrive at it. For example, a patient with an aggressive obsession has an image of stabbing her husband; however, she does not know how she obtained that image. Through deductive reasoning, the patient and therapist explore the specific detailed steps to achieve the stabbing outcome. Exposure in imagination and, when possible, in vivo (e.g., having the patient hold a knife in the presence of her husband), leads to habituation. Patients are then asked to prevent passive avoidance of the triggering stimuli (e.g., not shopping in aisles with sharp objects), active avoidance (e.g., putting away all knives in drawers), or both. In a study comparing exposure, rational emotive therapy, and thought stopping in patients with obsessions (ruminations) only, both exposure and rational emotive therapy reduced obsessions (Neziroglu and Neuman 1990).

When this form of exposure does not work, a revised habituation technique may be implemented. Several single-case studies have demonstrated the efficacy of audiotaped exposure (Headland and MacDonald 1987; Salkovskis 1985; Salkovskis and Westbrook 1989; Thyer 1985). Audiotaped exposure uses loop cassette tapes (duration: 6 seconds to 16 minutes) to record patients speaking their obsessional thoughts. These thoughts are played back over headphones; patients hear their voices, and obsessing follows unless active attempts prevent it. Patients are encouraged not to neutralize or prevent covert rituals by distracting themselves, or they are instructed to use thought stopping to disrupt covert rituals.

Cognitive therapy is ineffective. Cognitive therapy effectively treats pure obsessions (see preceding section) and may also treat obsessive-compulsive symptoms (see discussion of cognitive therapy).

Symptom substitution occurs. Behaviorists are frequently accused of leaving room for symptom substitution by superficially treating problems. However, in almost every study, symptom substitution is absent. The emergence of other fears during treatment is not common among obsessive-compulsive patients (Foa and Steketee 1987). When and if such emergence occurs, it is not symptom substitution but instead is caused by the possible existence of high anxiety-evoking stimuli not dealt with during exposure treatment. Careful behavior analysis and exposure to the most salient cues impedes emergence of new fears.

Prognostic Indicators

Probable causes of failure of behavior therapy include the following:

1. *Overvalued ideas.* The stronger the patient's belief in the reality basis of his or her fear, the more difficult it is to treat the obsession/compulsion (Foa 1979; Lelliott et al. 1988, Neziroglu and Yaryura-Tobias 1995). Although patients with OCD doubt whether their fears will come true, some doubt it less than others.
2. *Personality factors.* Patients with certain personalities, such as schizotypal, histrionic, dependent, passive-aggressive, and borderline, tend to be poorer responders to both drug and behavior therapy than those without personality disorders (Baer and Jenike 1990; Jenike et al. 1986; McKay et al. 1996; Minichiello et al. 1987; Steketee 1988).
3. *Other concomitant psychiatric disorders.* Patients with comorbid disorders usually need treatment for both and thus require more time for therapy. For example, a patient with a comorbid condition of depression may lack energy and ability to resist compulsions, and agoraphobic patients may experience difficulty coming for treatment (Foa et al. 1983a; Marks et al. 1980). Some concomitant OCD disorders are eating disorders, body dysmorphic disorder, and Tourette's syndrome. Determining which disorder to treat first may be difficult, yet treating both simultaneously may hinder OCD symptom habituation.
4. *Prior level of functioning.* Patients who attain a relatively high level of functioning before the disorder's onset seem to respond better to treat-

ment. Once again, it is important to question patients about their prior functioning level in school, work, leisure, and daily routine activities, as well as in interpersonal relationships.

5. *Lack of motivation.* When the patient's discomfort regarding the disorder is greater than the patient's discomfort regarding treatment, there is greater motivation to change and comply with behavior therapy. However, lack of compliance does not always mean lack of motivation. Other reasons for noncompliance should be entertained, such as comorbid conditions, lack of support systems, or highly overvalued ideas (Foa et al. 1983b).

6. *Other immediate family members with OCD.* The presence of OCD in other family members may make treatment more difficult because the family's norms are similar to those of the patient. This limits the family's ability to help the patient change his or her cognition and behavior.

7. *Procrastination.* One of OCD's salient features is doubt and indecisiveness, and therefore, procrastination is common. It is often necessary that the therapist be directive in making appointments and pursuing patients.

Proposed Mechanism of Action

Although behavior therapy's efficacy has been demonstrated, the mechanism by which it works is not as well established. Psychophysiological studies have provided some clues to how the body responds during exposure and response prevention. Exposure without active avoidance behaviors (compulsions) produces habituation of anxiety. *Habituation* is when fatigue occurs as a result of constant neuronal stimulation. Groves and Lynch (1972) have stated that habituation of cellular activity occurs in the brain stem reticular formation, particularly in the mesencephalon.

Few researchers have investigated neurochemical changes as a function of behavior therapy, specifically exposure in vivo and exposure in imagination. Zohar et al. (1989) measured cerebral blood flow in 10 drug-free patients with washing compulsions. They used the xenon flow method in which small quantities of radioactive xenon gas are inhaled by patients so that blood flow and perfusion over the cerebral cortex's surface convexity can be estimated. After two placebo xenon test runs (done to diminish test situation anxiety), all subjects underwent xenon flow studies in a relaxation state, in an exposure in imagination state, and in an exposure in vivo state. To avoid a sequence presentation bias, the tests were reconducted 10 days later in a different order. No order effect was found. Symptom rating scores were highest during exposure in vivo and lowest during relaxation. In contrast, cerebral blood flow increased during relaxation and exposure in imagination but decreased during exposure in vivo. The findings were contrary to what the researchers expected. They speculated that during exposure in vivo, a high anxiety-provoking state, blood was directed away from the cortical areas of the brain to other areas, such as the caudate nucleus or orbital gyri, that cannot be visualized with the xenon flow method. They suggested positron-emission tomography (PET) blood flow, glucose, and oxygen extraction studies.

PET scan changes as a function of behavior therapy were investigated by Baxter et al. (1992). They found that changes in metabolic rates in the caudate nucleus decreased significantly compared with pretreatment values in responders to behavior therapy and fluoxetine. Behavior therapy consisted of exposure in vivo and response prevention. Nonresponders and control patients did not demonstrate caudate nucleus metabolic changes when compared with baseline. The percentage of change in OCD symptom ratings correlated significantly with the percentage of change in the caudate nucleus with drug therapy, and a trend was observed with behavior therapy. These findings are similar to Baxter et al.'s (1987) results, where patients who improved with pharmacotherapy had consistent decreases in caudate metabolic rates. Both studies suggest that after successful treatment, brain glucose consumption decreases to the normal range. Furthermore, these regions in the brain correlate with OCD symptoms (Baxter et al. 1987).

In our study on serotonin activity change in eight patients, platelet-poor plasma serotonin decreased and imipramine binding (B_{max}) and K_d (binding strength) affinity increased after 3 weeks of intensive behavior therapy (90-minute sessions, 5 days a week) (Neziroglu et al. 1990). At 4-week follow-up, platelet-poor plasma serotonin values returned to baseline, whereas B_{max} and K_d affinity remained the same as at posttreatment. These encouraging findings suggest that behavior therapy alone, without any medications, may modify biochemistry in OCD patients.

Course, Prognosis, and Follow-Up

The prognosis for OCD patients may be dictated by 1) the lapse between illness onset and first treatment; 2) severity and frequency of symptoms; 3) the presence, or lack thereof, of comorbidity; 4) type of treatment offered;

and 5) patient motivation and family participation in therapy. The frequency of sabotage practiced by patients or participant relatives may disappoint an optimistic therapist. If untreated, OCD follows a downhill course with acute exacerbation periods.

The prognosis for patients with obsessive premorbid personalities seems significantly less favorable than those without. These findings substantiated Straus's (1948) and Ingram's (1961) results, where they found that symptoms in childhood and obsessional acts were associated with a poor prognosis. Pollitt (1957) also believed that the obsessional premorbid personality influenced the prognosis unfavorably. Muller (1957), however, could not find any special effects. Both Muller (1957) and Kringlen (1965) indicated that aging may at times have a positive effect because patients no longer pay as much attention to their symptoms, and therefore they suffer less.

Nemiah (1975) stated that generally, with the exception of leukotomy cases, prognosis studies indicated that 15% of patients were well, 45% were improved, and 40% were unchanged or worse. Improved patients fall into two groups: 1) those whose symptoms lessened so that they were able to work and function socially, and 2) those who ran a fluctuating course, often with long periods of complete symptom remission. He did not indicate what type of therapy was administered.

Patients may not report OCD symptoms because they use different measures to evaluate what clinicians consider symptoms. Over time, patients' norms may change, and obsessing 25% of their waking hours may be considered normal. OCD may cause an extreme degree of dependency, primarily because of an inability to make decisions. In time, the patient may become dysfunctional intellectually, emotionally, and socially. After treatment this might be reversed, but learning how will take a long time, especially with a long-standing illness.

Nemiah (1975) stated that patient prognosis is better when 1) the symptoms' duration, before the patient is first seen, is shorter; 2) the element of environmental stress associated with the disorder's onset is greater; 3) the environment the patient returns to after treatment is better; and 4) general social adjustment and relationships are better.

Ingram (1961) indicated that there were four course types for symptom development: 1) constant with progressive worsening; 2) constant and static; 3) fluctuating but never symptom free; and 4) phasic, with one or more remissions. He also said that the majority of patients usually become progressively worse. Foa and Tillmanns (1979) suggested that progressive worsening involves two processes: 1) the number of contaminating stimuli increases with time and 2) the effort to counteract the multiplication of anxiety-provoking stimuli, the number of rituals, their duration, and intensity increases.

Some authors have reported a poor prognosis for obsessive-compulsive patients who become psychotic in the course of their OCD (Bleuler and Hess 1956; Gordon 1926; Kraepelin 1915; Kringlen 1965; Muller 1957; Stengel 1957). We briefly examined follow-up studies of six major OCD pathology researchers who preceded by many years the current work in OCD (Grimshaw 1965; Ingram 1961; Kringlen 1965; Lewis 1936; Muller 1957; Pollitt 1957; Rudin 1953). Their individual work encompassed a 29-year period (1936–1965). The patients received supportive therapy or drug therapy or underwent leukotomy. The average improvement was about 50%, which is similar to current results using anti–obsessive-compulsive agents. Two caveats to consider are the lack of consensus in diagnostic criteria and the absence of reliable assessment scales. However, these researchers consider their empirical findings reliable and valid because of their experience and knowledge (Table 2–1).

Psychopharmacological Directions

Because etiology is unknown, the most appropriate psychopharmacological approach is symptomatic, or target directed. Sometimes, after a drug trial, symptom suppression induces a new or dormant symptom. In fact, Petrilowitsch (1968b) observed that if therapeutic effects are not achieved within a certain time period, then intermediary syndromes, in part characterized as pathomorphoses, are brought to the surface by the drug. Some of these "silent syndromes" are either anancastic or phobic. Moreover, Petrilowitsch (1968a) asserted that the therapeutic procedure should be disease directed as long as these symptoms prevail over expression of individual structure.

Therapeutic Strategies

We use an integrationist or biopsychosocial model. The experience accumulated by OCD researchers and therapists indicates that one form of therapy may not be the answer. According to Sargant and Slater (1950), in obsessional neurosis, therapeutic confusion is at least as bad in any other field.

Table 2–1. Follow-up studies in OCD

Study	No. of patients	Follow-up (years)	% Much improved	% Improved	% Unchanged or worse
Grimshaw (1965)	100	6.08	40	24	29
Ingram (1961)	64	5.90	0	55[a]	45[a]
				38[b]	62
Kringlen (1965)	85	16.6	13	28	41
Lewis (1936)	50	5.0	46	20	
Muller (1957)	57	20–30	16	50	7
Pollitt (1957)	101	3.44	44	39[b]	15
			25	48[b]	26[b]
Rudin (1953)	130	2–20	33	34	33

Note. [a]Leukotomy. [b]Medication. The treatments used in other studies are unknown.

Fortunately, current anti–obsessive-compulsive agents enhance the therapeutic outlook.

It helps to explain to the patient the illness mechanism and the treatment program. This psychoeducational program should encompass pharmacotherapy, behavior therapy, family participation, and rehabilitation.

Clinicians should not practice replacement therapy but selection therapy and should try a different form of therapy only if one therapy fails. They also must remember that the wrong psychological approach can be as damaging as any biological therapy. Quality and quantity in treatment are both important. For example, if, during consultation, a patient declares that behavior therapy has failed, the clinician should consider whether the patient was treated with appropriate behavioral techniques. Furthermore, if a patient says that most psychopharmacological agents did not help, the clinician should ask, "Which medication was given, and what was the dosage and duration of treatment?" Furthermore, measuring drug plasma level concentrations may be useful in seeking the therapeutic range.

Conclusions

The prognosis for OCD patients may be dictated by the time from onset to treatment, by symptom severity and frequency, by the obsessive-compulsive condition, by the type of treatment offered, and by patient motivation and family participation in therapy. The amount of sabotage practiced by patients or participant relatives may disappoint therapists. If untreated, these disorders may worsen with periods of acute exacerbation. OCD is refractory to complete cure because it is a chronic illness. The goal is to target specific problems, such as emotionality, resocialization, and work adaptability.

Symptom severity, bizarreness, and symptom duration are three variables that might determine outcome (DeVeaugh-Geiss et al. 1990; Hoogduin et al. 1986; Lelliot et al. 1988). Poor outcome is found in those who drop out of treatment. Such patients list several reasons for discontinuing: environmental constraints, dissatisfaction with services, and the lack of a need for further assistance (Hansen et al. 1992). We also might add the need to sabotage treatment once the patient begins to improve. Poor treatment outcome is observed in OCD patients with schizotypal, borderline, and avoidant personality disorder (Baer et al. 1992).

Patients are eager to know whether they have to be on medication forever. In one study of clomipramine dosage reduction (i.e., a dosage of 165 mg/day), no significant changes in symptoms were observed (Pato et al. 1990), but completely discontinuing clomipramine caused the symptoms to return (Pato et al. 1988). This agrees with previous observations (Ananth 1986; Asberg et al. 1982; Capstick 1973; Flament et al. 1985; Thoren et al. 1980; Yaryura-Tobias et al. 1976).

One other important aspect should be managing psychopharmacological side effects, mainly those involving disturbed mentation and motor activity. Neuroleptics may cause obsessive symptoms or depression, whereas antidepressants may exacerbate the anxiety or produce agitation. Moreover, neurological side effects affecting the extrapyramidal system may distort the improvement of the disorders' motor components. Remembering these factors is imperative, as is sharing the implications of these factors with patients and their relatives, thereby avoiding unnecessary misunderstandings and aggravations.

Family Participation

Integral OCD treatment must include the family as one variable influencing therapeutic outcome. Many OCD patients' first-degree relatives may have psychopathology (Bellodi et al. 1992; S. W. Black et al. 1992; Insel and Pickar 1983; McKeon and Murray 1987; Neziroglu et al. 1994), and parents present a higher incidence of expressed emotions (Hibbs et al. 1991). In one study, parents showed a strong tendency toward anxiety, overprotectiveness, and compulsive behavior, and it was found that patient exposure to a strict, authoritarian upbringing contributed to the development of OCD, particularly when this was contradicted by overprotective parental behavior. In the same study, done in Germany, one-third of the families described themselves as deeply religious (Knolker 1983).

OCD patients display behavior that might interfere with family interaction. Patients may request or even demand family participation to answer repetitive questions in ritual performance—in general, to become an actor taking a role in the illness, rather than a witness. Leaving aside analytical considerations (i.e., symbiosis), it is common to observe the enmeshment between patient and family unfolding as the disease progresses. There are several components in the relationship between OCD adolescents and their families that are worth mentioning. In one study, family members of OCD adolescents held higher expectations of career achievements from their children (Clark and Bolton 1985). In another study, parents were more rejecting, overprotective, and less warm; the notion that compulsive checkers, as opposed to compulsive cleaners, emerge from two different child-rearing patterns was not sustained (Ehiobuche 1988). Some families come from cultures emphasizing cleanliness and perfection which may contribute to OCD development (Hoover and Insel 1984). OCD's invasive nature causes familial frustration and criticism. (Tynes et al. 1990).

In evident family pathology cases, family therapy might be indicated (Hafner 1992; Oppenheim and Rosenberger 1991). Moreover, a family member may operate as a co-therapist after appropriate training. This family approach results in greater improvement in anxiety, depression, obsessive symptoms, and social adjustment in occupational and household responsibilities (Mehta 1990). The severity of OCD seriously impaired functional ability, with disastrous economic consequences (Khanna et al. 1988). Therefore, social adjustment is an important variable and should be considered part of an integral therapeutic approach.

Marital problems are important OCD prognosis factor modifiers. Poor marital interaction may affect behavior therapy results. In this situation, use of the spouse as a co-therapist may improve the results (Hafner 1982). In contraposition, marital maladjustment does not influence behavior therapy outcome, even if the partner is an actively involved co-therapist (Emmelkamp et al. 1990).

Group Therapy

Cognitive-behavior therapy in the form of a group therapeutic program that introduced educational OCD material and instruction for self-treatment in a 36-patient sample resulted in significant improvement after 7 weeks (Krone et al. 1991). Contrarily, a 24-patient study suggested that the specific effects of such therapy in terms of reducing OCD symptoms were minimal (Enright 1991).

Self-Support Groups

In 1977 The Society for Obsessive-Compulsive Disorder in Long Island, New York, became the first organization to bring public attention to OCD. This society advocates the introduction of self-support groups and psychoeducational programs. The groups, which are conducted by patients, place special emphasis on symptoms and medication and its side effects, as well as on how to develop coping mechanisms. Each month professionals are invited to update the group in recent advancements. As a result, participating patients develop camaraderie, acquire coping mechanisms, and learn to socialize during the illness' acute period. Family members are encouraged to attend and to bring their input and concerns. In 1986 the Obsessive Compulsive Foundation was created in New Haven, Connecticut. This foundation has developed an impressive program to foster public awareness and research.

Psychoeducational and support groups offer a 10-week program consisting of OCD assessment and information on its learning and neurobiological basis and other pertinent issues. This format maintains clinical utility by offering support and information (Tynes et al. 1990). One group has done a survey of relevant OCD topics, such as symptoms and biographical data, as well as the family and social context of those in the group. Results indicated that members of the group had long-standing illness, received prolonged psychiatric treatment, and rated behavior therapy and individual psychotherapy the most effective forms of treatment (Hafner 1988).

Another group applied the Iowa model to their meetings. This model emphasizes patient education and emotional support (Black and Blum 1992). Psychoeducation may enhance treatment outcome by providing information.

The human occupation model was used as a frame of reference for one group of OCD patients. The following problem areas were identified: disruptions in habituation, available volition, and the ability to adapt and perform in their own environment (Bavaro 1991). In case of hospitalization, the nursing staff provides physical and emotional support, as well as education in drug therapy and side effects (Simoni 1991).

References

Akhtar S, Wig NN, Varma VK, et al: A phenomenological analysis of symptoms in obsessive-compulsive neurosis. Br J Psychiatry 127:342–348, 1975

Amabile G, Giacomini P, Giraldi R: Contributo alla terapia psico-farmacologica delle nevrosi ossessivo fobiche. Minerva Psichiatrica Psicologiea 14:238–245, 1973

Ananth J: Clomipramine: an antiobsessive drug. Can J Psychiatry 31:253–258, 1986

Ananth J, Van Den Steen N: Systematic studies in the treatment of obsessive compulsive neurosis with tricyclic antidepressants. Curr Ther Res Clin Exp 21: 495–501, 1977

Ananth J, Solyom L, Solyom C, et al: Doxepine in the treatment of obsessive-compulsive neurosis. Psychosomatics 16:185–187, 1975

Angst J, Theobald W: Tofranil. Bern, Switzerland, Stampfli & Cie, 1970, pp 31–32

Annesley PT: Nardil response in a chronic obsessive compulsive (letter). Br J Psychiatry 115:748, 1969

Ansseau M, Legros JJ, Mormont C, et al: Intranasal oxytocin in obsessive compulsive disorder. Psychoneuroendocrinology 12:231–236, 1987

Asberg M, Thoren P, Bertilsson L: Clomipramine treatment of obsessive disorder: biochemical and clinical aspects. Psychopharmacol Bull 18:13–21, 1982

Baer L, Jenike MA: Personality disorders in obsessive-compulsive disorder, in Obsessive-Compulsive Disorders: Theory and Management. Edited by Jenike MA, Baer L, Minichiello W. Chicago, IL, Year Book Medical, 1990, pp 76–88

Baer L, Minichiello WE: Behavior therapy for obsessive-compulsive disorder, in Obsessive-Compulsive Disorders: Theory and Management. Edited by Jenike MA, Baer L, Minichiello WE. Chicago, IL, Year Book Medical, 1990, pp 203–232

Baer L, Jenike MA, Black DW, et al: Effect of axis II diagnoses on treatment outcome with clomipramine in 55 patients with obsessive-compulsive disorder. Arch Gen Psychiatry 49:862–866, 1992

Baruk H, Launay J, Cournut J, et al: Le probleme des indications therapeutiques des doses, et des incidentes de traitment par l'imipramine apres une experience de 18 moins. Societé Moreau de Tours 1:14–28, 1959

Bauer G, Novack H: Doxepin ein nerves antidepressivum: Virkungsvergletch mit amitriptylin. Arzneimittelforschung 19:1642–1646, 1969

Baum M: Extinction of an avoidance response following a period of response prevention in the avoidance apparatus. Psychol Rep 18:55–64, 1966

Bavaro SM: Occupational therapy and obsessive-compulsive disorder. Am J Occup Ther 45:456–458, 1991

Baxter LR Jr: Two cases of obsessive compulsive disorder with depression responsive to trazodone. J Nerv Ment Dis 173:432–433, 1985

Baxter LR, Phelps ME, Mazziotta JC, et al: Local cerebral glucose metabolic rates in obsessive-compulsive disorder: a comparison with rates in unipolar depression and in normal control. Arch Gen Psychiatry 44:211–218, 1987

Baxter LR, Schwartz JM, Bergman KS, et al: Caudate glucose metabolic rate changes with both drug and behavior therapy for obsessive-compulsive disorder. Arch Gen Psychiatry 49:681–689, 1992

Bellodi L, Scuito G, Diaferia G, et al: Psychiatric disorders in the families of patients with obsessive-compulsive disorder. Psychiatry Res 42:111–120, 1992

Berlin I, Grimaldi A, Landault C, et al: Suspected postprandial hypoglycemia is associated with beta-adrenergic hypersensitivity and emotional distress. J Clin Endocrinol Metab 79:1428–1433, 1994

Bethune HC: A new compound in the treatment of severe anxiety states: report on the use of diazepam. N Z Med J 63:153–156, 1964

Black DW, Blum NS: Obsessive-compulsive disorder support groups: the Iowa model. Compr Psychiatry 33:65–71, 1992

Black SW, Noyes R, Goldstein RB: A family study of obsessive-compulsive disorder. Arch Gen Psychiatry 49:362–368, 1992

Bleuler M, Hess R: Psiquiatria Endocrinologica. Buenos Aires, Brazil, Intermedica, 1956, pp 390–393

Boersma K, Hengst S, Dekker J, et al: Exposure and response prevention in the natural environment: a comparison with obsessive compulsive patients. Behav Res Ther 14:19–24, 1976

Borenstein P, Dabbah M: Action du Tofranil sur l'electroencephalogramme. Ann Med Psychol 1:923–931, 1959

Boulougouris JC, Bassiakos L: Prolonged flooding in cases with obsessive-compulsive neurosis. Behav Res Ther 11:227–231, 1973

Breitner C: Drug therapy in obsessional states and other psychiatric problems. Dis Nerv Syst 21:31–35, 1960

Brown FW: Heredity in psychoneurosis. Proc R Soc Med 35:785–790, 1942

Burrell RH, Culpan RH, Newton KJ, et al: Use of clonazepam in obsessional phobic and related states. Curr Med Res Opin 2:430–436, 1974

Capstick N: Clomipramine in obsessional states: a pilot study. Psychosomatics 12:332–335, 1971

Capstick N: The Grayling well study. J Int Med Res 1:392–396, 1973

Carles Egea F: El empleo del tryptizol en el tratamiento ambulatorio de los sindromes depresivos timopaticos y astenicos. Farma Esp 62:292–294, 1963

Carr AT: Compulsive neurosis: a review of the literature. Psychol Bull 81:311–318, 1974

Catts S, McConaghy N: Ritual prevention in the treatment of obsessive-compulsive neurosis. Aust N Z J Psychiatry 9:37–41, 1975

Cheng JT, Gutman RA, Chen WY: Compulsive water drinking simulating diabetes insipidus. J Formos Med Assoc 67:182–189, 1968

Chouinard G: Sertraline in the treatment of obsessive-compulsive disorder: two double-blind placebo-controlled studies. Int Clin Psychopharmacol 7 (suppl 2):37–41, 1992

Chouinard G, Goodman W, Greist J, et al: Results of a double-blind placebo controlled trial of a new serotonin uptake inhibitor, sertraline, in the treatment of obsessive-compulsive disorder. Psychopharmacol Bull 26:279–284, 1990

Christensen H, Hadzi-Pavlovic D, Andrews G, et al: Behavior therapy and tricyclic medication in the treatment of obsessive-compulsive disorder: a quantitative review. J Consult Clin Psychol 55:701–711, 1987

Clark DA, Bolton D: Obsessive-compulsive adolescents and their parents: a psychometric study. J Child Psychol Psychiatry 26:267–276, 1985

Clomipramine Collaborative Study Group: Clomipramine in the treatment of patients with obsessive compulsive disorder. Arch Gen Psychiatry 48:730–738, 1991

Cottraux J, Mollard E, Bouvard M, et al: A controlled study of fluvoxamine and exposure in obsessive-compulsive disorder. Int Clin Psychopharmacol 5: 17–30, 1990

Coullaut Mendigutia R: El uso asociado de ipronizida y alcaloides de la rawolfia serpentina en enfermos mentales. Act Luso-Española de Neurología y Psiquiatría 19:130–133, 1960

Dally P: Chemistry of Psychiatric Disorders. London, Logos Press, 1967

DeVeaugh-Geiss J, Katz R, Landau P, et al: Clinical predictors of treatment response in obsessive compulsive disorder: exploratory analyses from multicenter trials of clomipramine. Psychopharmacol Bull 26:54–59, 1990

Dowson JH: The phenomenology of severe obsessive-compulsive neurosis. Br J Psychiatry 131:75–78, 1977

Dugas M, Velin J: Etude de l'activite therapeutique de la clomipramine chez l'enfant. Rev Neuropsychiatr Infant 20:785–790, 1972

Ehiobuche I: Obsessive-compulsive neurosis in relation to parental child-rearing patterns amongst the Greek, Italian, and Anglo-Australian subjects. Acta Psychiatr Scand Suppl 344:115–120, 1988

Eisenberg J, Asnis G: Lithium as an adjunct treatment in obsessive-compulsive disorder (letter). Am J Psychiatry 142:663, 1985

Emmelkamp PMG, Beens H: Cognitive therapy with obsesssive-compulsive disorder: a comparative evaluation. Behav Res Ther 29:293–300, 1991

Emmelkamp PMG, Giesselbach P: Treatment of obsessions: relevant versus irrelevant exposure. Behav Psychother 9:322–329, 1981

Emmelkamp PMG, Kraanen J: Therapist controlled exposure in-vivo versus self-controlled exposure in-vivo: a comparison with obsessive-compulsive patients. Behav Res Ther 21:341–346, 1977

Emmelkamp PMG, Kwee KG: Obsessional ruminations: a comparison between thought-stopping and prolonged exposure in imagination. Behav Res Ther 15:441–444, 1977

Emmelkamp PMG, Rabbie D: Psychological treatment of obsessive-compulsive disorder, in The Proceedings of the Third World Congress of Biological Psychiatry. Edited by Perris C, Striwe G, Jansson B. Amsterdam, The Netherlands, Elsevier, 1981, pp 1095–1102

Emmelkamp PMG, Van der Heyden H: Treatment of harming obsessions. Behavioural Analysis and Modification 4:28–35, 1980

Emmelkamp PMG, Van der Helm M, Van Zanten BL, et al: Contributions of self instructional training to the effectiveness of exposure in-vivo: a comparison with obsessive-compulsive patients. Behav Res Ther 18:61–66, 1980

Emmelkamp PMG, Visser S, Hoekstra RJ: Cognitive therapy versus exposure in-vivo in the treatment of obsessive-compulsives. Cognitive Therapy and Research 12:103–114, 1988

Emmelkamp PMG, de Haan E, Hoogduin CA: Marital adjustment and obsessive-compulsive disorder. Br J Psychiatry 156:55–60, 1990

Enright SJ: Group treatment for obsessive-compulsive disorder: an evaluation. Behavioral Psychotherapy 19:183–192, 1991

Enright SJ, Beech AR: Reduced cognitive inhibition in obsessive-compulsive disorder. Br J Clin Psychology 32 (pt 1): 67–74, 1993

Fallon BA, Campeas R, Schneier FR, et al: Open trial of intravenous clomipramine in five treatment refractory patients with obsessive compulsive disorder. J Neuropsychiatry Clin Neurosci 4:70–75, 1992

Fernández de Córdoba CE, López Ibor JJ: Monochlorimipramine in the treatment of psychiatric patients resistant to other therapies. Act Luso-Española de Neurología Psiquiatría 26:119–147, 1967

Flament MF, Rapoport JL, Berg CJ, et al: Clomipramine treatment of childhood obsessive-compulsive disorder: a double-blind controlled study. Arch Gen Psychiatry 42:977–983, 1985

Foa EB: Failures in treating obsessive-compulsives. Behav Res Ther 17:169–176, 1979

Foa EB, Goldstein A: Continuous exposure and complete response prevention in the treatment of obsessive-compulsive neurosis. Behav Ther 9:821–829, 1978

Foa EB, Steketee GS: Obsessive-compulsives: conceptual issues and treatment interventions. Prog Behav Modif 8:1–51, 1979

Foa EB, Steketee GS: Reply to letter to the editor: behavior therapy following drug administration. Arch Gen Psychiatry 41:107, 1984

Foa EB, Steketee G: Emergent fears during treatment of three obsessive-compulsives: symptom substitution or de-conditioning? J Behav Ther Exp Psychiatry 8: 353–358, 1987

Foa EB, Tillmanns A: The treatment of obsessive-compulsive neurosis, in Handbook of Behavioral Interventions: A Clinical Guide. Edited by Goldstein A, Foa EB. New York, Wiley, 1979, pp 241–262

Foa EB, Steketee G, Groves GA: The use of behavioral therapy and imipramine in a case of obsessive-compulsive neurosis with severe depression. Behav Modif 3:419–430, 1979

Foa EB, Steketee G, Milby JB: Differential effects of exposure and response prevention in obsessive-compulsive washers. J Consult Clin Psychol 48:71–79, 1980

Foa EB, Grayson JB, Steketee GS, et al: Success and failure in the behavioral treatment of obsessive-compulsives. J Consult Clin Psychol 51:287–297, 1983a

Foa EB, Steketee GS, Grayson JB, et al: Treatment of obsessive-compulsives: when do we fail? in Failures in Behavior Therapy. Edited by Foa EB, Emmelkamp PMG. New York, Wiley, 1983b, pp 10–34

Foa EB, Kozak MJ, Steketee GS, et al: Treatment of depressive and obsessive-compulsive symptoms in OCD by imipramine and behavior therapy. Br J Clin Psychol 31 (pt 3):279–292, 1992

Frenkel A, Rosenthal J, Nezu A, et al: Efficacy of long term fluoxetine treatment of obsessive compulsive disorder. Mt Sinai J Med 57:348–352, 1990

Geisler A, Schou M: Lithium treatment for obsessive compulsive neurosis. Nord Psykiatr Tidsskr 23:493–495, 1969

Giberti F, Gregoreti L: Studio farmacopsichiatrico di un caso di psiconevrosi ossessiva. Sist Nerv 9:275–288, 1957

Gittelson NL: Depressive psychosis in the obsessional neurotic. Br J Psychiatry 112:883–887, 1966a

Gittelson NL: The fate of obsessions in depressive psychosis. Br J Psychiatry 112: 705–709, 1966b

Gittelson NL: The phenomenology of obsessions in depressive psychosis. Br J Psychiatry 112:261–264, 1966c

Gittelson NL: The relationship between obsessions and suicidal attempts in depressive psychosis. Br J Psychiatry 112:889–890, 1966d

Goodman WK, Price LH, Delgado PL, et al: Specificity of serotonin reuptake inhibitors in the treatment of obsessive compulsive disorder. Comparison of fluvoxamine and desipramine. Arch Gen Psychiatry 47:577–585, 1990

Gordon A: Obsessions in their relations to psychosis. Am J Psychiatry 4:647–659, 1926

Gordon PK: Allocation of attention in obsessional disorder. Br J Clin Psychol 24: 101–107, 1985

Grady TA, Pigott TA, L'Heureux F, et al: Double-blind study of adjuvant buspirone for fluoxetine treated patients with obsessive compulsive disorder. Am J Psychiatry 150:819–821, 1993

Green RS, Rau JH: Treatment of compulsive eating disturbance with anticonvulsant medication. Am J Psychiatry 131:428–432, 1974

Grimshaw L: The outcome of obsessional disorder: a follow-up study of 100 cases. Br J Psychiatry 111:1051–1056, 1965

Groves PM, Lynch GS: Mechanisms of habituation in the brain stem. Psychol Rev 79:237–244, 1972

Guyotat J, Marin A, Dubor C, et al: L'imipramine en dehors des etats depressifs. Ann Med Psychol (Paris) 1:566–567, 1960

Hafner RJ: Marital interaction in persisting obsessive-compulsive disorder. Aust N Z J Psychiatry 16:171–178, 1982

Hafner RJ: Obsessive-compulsive disorder: a questionnaire survey of a self-help group. Int J Soc Psychiatry 34:310–315, 1988

Hafner RJ: Anxiety disorders and family therapy. Aus N Z J Family Ther 13:99–104, 1992

Hansen AM, Hoogduin CA, Schaap C, et al: Do drop-outs differ from successfully treated obsessive-compulsives? Behav Res Ther 30:547–550, 1992

Haward LRC: Effects of sodium diphenylhydantoinate and pemoline upon concentration: a comparative study, in Drugs and Cerebral Function. Edited by Smith W. Springfield, IL, Charles C Thomas, 1970, pp 103–120

Head D, Bolton D, Hymas N: Deficit in cognitive shifting ability in patients with obsessive-compulsive disorder. Biol Psychiatry 25:929–937, 1989

Headland K, MacDonald B: Rapid audio-tape treatment of obsessional ruminations: a case report. Behav Psychother 15:188–192, 1987

Hermesh H, Weizman A, Shahar A, et al: Vitamin B_{12} and folic acid serum levels in obsessive-compulsive disorder. Acta Psychiatr Scand 78:8–10, 1988

Hermesh H, Aizenberg D, Munitz H: Trazodone treatment in clomipramine-resistant obsessive compulsive disorder. Clin Neuropharmacol 13:322–328, 1990

Hesso R, Thorell LH: Lithium treatment for obsessive-compulsive neurosis. Nord Psykiatr Tidsskr 23:496–499, 1969

Hewlett WA, Vinogradov S, Agras WS: Clonazepam treatment of obsessions and compulsions. J Clin Psychiatry 51:158–161, 1990

Hewlett WA, Vinogradov S, Agras WS: Clomipramine, clonazepam, and clonidine treatment of obsessive-compulsive disorder. J Clin Psychopharmacol 12: 420–430, 1992

Hibbs ED, Hamburger SD, Lenane M, et al: Determinants of expressed emotion in families of disturbed and normal children. J Child Psychol Psychiatry 32: 757–770, 1991

Hoflich G, Kasper S, Moller HJ: Successful treatment of seasonal compulsive syndrome with phototherapy (German). Nervenarzt 63:701–704, 1992

Hollander E, DeCaria CM, Schneier FR, et al: Fenfluramine augmentation of serotonin reuptake blockade antiobsessional treatment. J Clin Psychiatry 51: 119–123, 1990

Hoogduin CAL, Hoogduin WA: The outpatient treatment of patients with an obsessive-compulsive disorder. Behav Res Ther 22:455–459, 1984

Hoogduin CA, deHaan E, Hoogduin WA: Severity and duration of obsessive-compulsive complaints. Results of treatment. Acta Psychiatr Belg 86:316–323, 1986

Hoogduin K, deHaan E, Schapp C: Exposure and response prevention in patients with obsessions. Acta Psychiatr Belg 87:640–653, 1987

Hoover CF, Insel TR: Families of origin in obsessive-compulsive disorder. J Nerv Ment Dis 172:207–215, 1984

Hussain MZ, Ahad A: Treatment of obsessive-compulsive neurosis. Can Med Assoc J (Toronto) 103:648–650, 1970

Ingram IM: Obsessional illness in mental hospital patients. Journal of Mental Science 107:382–396, 1961

Insel TR, Pickar D: Naloxone administration in obsessive-compulsive disorder: report of two cases. Am J Psychiatry 140:1219–1220, 1983

Isberg RS: A comparison of phenelzine and imipramine in an obsessive compulsive patient. Am J Psychiatry 138:1250–1251, 1981

Izikowitz S: Trial of catron therapy in compulsions and some other "nervous" states. Svensk Lakartidn 57:1993–2039, 1960

Jain VK, Swinson RP, Thomas JG: Phenelzine in obsessive neurosis. Br J Psychiatry 117:237–238, 1970

Janet P: Les Obsessions et la Psychasthenie. Paris, France, Alcan, 1903

Jenike MA: Drug treatment of obsessive-compulsive disorder, in Obsessive-Compulsive Disorders: Theory and Management. Edited by Jenike MA, Baer L, Minichiello WE. Chicago IL, Yearbook Medical, 1990, pp. 249–282

Jenike MA: Use of monoamine oxidase inhibitors in obsessive-compulsive disorder (letter). Br J Psychiatry 140:159, 1982

Jenike MA, Baer L, Minichiello WE: Concomitant obsessive-compulsive disorder and schizotypal personality disorder. Am J Psychiatry 143:530–532, 1986

Jenike MA, Baer L, Summergrad P, et al: Obsessive-compulsive disorder: a double-blind, placebo-controlled trial of clomipramine in 27 patients. Am J Psychiatry 146:1328–1330, 1989

Jenike MA, Baer L, Greist JH: Clomipramine versus fluoxetine in obsessive compulsive disorder: a retrospective comparison of side effects and efficacy. J Clin Psychopharmacol 10:122–124, 1990a

Jenike MA, Baer L, Summergrad P, et al: Sertraline in obsessive-compulsive disorder: a double-blind comparison with placebo. Am J Psychiatry 147:923–928, 1990b

Judd FK, Chua P, Lynch C, et al: Fenfluramine augmentation of clomipramine treatment of obsessive-compulsive disorder. Aust N Z J Psychiatry 25:412–414, 1991

Kahn RS, Westenberg HG, Jolles J: Zimeldine treatment of obsessive-compulsive disorder: biological and neuropsychological aspects. Acta Psychiatr Scand 69:259–261, 1984

Kasviskis Y, Marks IM: Clomipramine, self-exposure, and therapist-accompanied exposure in obsessive-compulsive ritualizers: two-year follow-up. Journal of Anxiety Disorders 2:291–298, 1988

Kendell RE, Discipio WJ: Obsessional symptoms and obsessional personality traits in patients with depressive illness. Psychol Med 1:65–72, 1970

Khanna S, Rajendra PN, Phannabasavanna SM: Social adjustment in obsessive-compulsive disorder. Int J Soc Psychiatry 34:118–122, 1988

Kirk JW: Behavioral treatment of obsessive-compulsive patients in clinical practice. Behav Res Ther 21:57–62, 1983

Knolker U: Zwangssyndrome bei Kindern und Jugendlichen: pathogentische Aspekte des familiaren Hintergrundes (Obsessive-compulsive disorders in children and adolescents: pathogenic aspects in the contact of family background). Z Kinder Jugenpsychiatr 11:317–327, 1983

Kraepelin E: Psychiatrie. Leipzig, Germany, Barth, 1915

Kringlen E: Obsessional neurotics. Br J Psychiatry 111:709–722, 1965

Krone KP, Himle JA, Nesse RM: A standardized behavioral group treatment program for obsessive-compulsive disorder: preliminary outcomes. Behav Res Ther 29:627–631, 1991

Lambertet P, Midenet P, Midenet J, et al: Traitement par la thioproperazine a haute dose de manifestations pseudo obsessives d'origine encephalitique. J Med Lyon 47:1219–1224, 1966

Lanfranchi R: Modificaciones de la evolucion de la neurosis obsesiva por la propericiazina. Paper presented at the Congress of the French Language. Paris, Clermont Ferrand, 1968

Lee MA, Cameron OG, Gurguis GN, et al: Alpha 2 adrenoreceptor status in obsessive–compulsive disorder. Biol Psychiatry 27:1083–1093, 1990

Lelliott PT, Noshirvani HF, Basoglu M, et al: Obsessive-compulsive beliefs and treatment outcome. Psychol Med 18:697–702, 1988

Leonard HL, Rapoport JL: Relief of obsessive-compulsive symptoms by LSD and psilocin. Am J Psychiatry 144:1239–1240, 1987

Lewis A: Problems of obsessional illness. Proc R Soc Med 29:325–336, 1936

Lewis AJ: Obsessional illness. Acta Neuropsiquíatrica Argentina 3:323–335, 1957

Likiermein H, Rachman S: Obsessions: an experimental investigation of thought stopping and habituation training. Behavioral Psychotherapy 10:324–338, 1982

López Ibor JJ: Anxiety states and their treatment by intravenous acetylcholine. Proc R Soc Med 45:511–516, 1952

López Ibor Alino JJ, López Ibor Alino JM: Tratamiento psico-farmacologico de las neurosis obsessivas. Act Luso Esp Neurol Psiq Cien Afines 1:767–774, 1973

López Ibor Alino JJ, López Ibor Alino JM: Die Psychopharma-kologische Behandlung von Zwangsneurosen. Arzneimittelforschung 24:1119–1122, 1974

Maier NRF: Frustration: The Study of Behavior Without a Goal. New York, McGraw-Hill, 1949

Malik SC, Chainia S: Clinical trials with protriptyline in depressive reactions. Current Medical Practice (Bombay) 12:525–526, 1968

Mallya GK, White K, Waternaux C, et al: Short and long-term treatment of obsessive compulsive disorder with fluvoxamine. Ann Clin Psychiatry 4:77–80, 1992

Markovitz PJ, Stagno SJ, Calabrese JR: Buspirone augmentation of fluoxetine in obsessive compulsive disorder. Am J Psychiatry 147:798–800, 1990

Marks IM: Behavior psychotherapy in obsessive-compulsive disorders. Encephale 16 (spec no):341–346, 1990

Marks IM, Hodgson R, Rachman S: Treatment of obsessive-compulsive neurosis by in-vivo exposure: a two-year follow-up and issues in treatment. Br J Psychiatry 127:349–364, 1975

Marks IM, Stern RS, Mawson D, et al: Clomipramine and exposure for obsessive-compulsive rituals: I. Br J Psychiatry 136:1–25, 1980

Marshall WK, Micev V: Clomipramine in the treatment of obsessional illness and phobic anxiety states. J Int Med Res 1:403–412, 1973

Mattes JA: A pilot study of combined trazodone and tryptophan in obsessive-compulsive disorder. Int Clin Psychopharmacol 1:170–173, 1986

Mavissakalian M, Turner SM, Michelson L: Future directions in the assessment and treatment of obsessive-compulsive disorder, in Obsessive-Compulsive Disorder: Psychological and Pharmacological Treatment. Edited by Mavissakalian M, Turnes SM, Michelson L. New York, Plenum, 1985, pp 213–228

Mavissakalian MR, Jones B, Olson S, et al: Clomipramine on obsessive-compulsive disorder: clinical response and plasma levels. J Clin Psychopharmacol 10: 261–268, 1990

Mawson D, Marks IM, Romm L: Clomipramine and exposure for chronic obsessive-compulsive disorder: two-year follow-up and further findings. Br J Psychiatry 140:11–18, 1982

McDougle CJ, Price LH, Goodman WK, et al: A controlled trial of lithium augmentation in fluvoxamine refractory obsessive-compulsive disorder: lack of efficacy. J Clin Psychopharmacol 11:175–184, 1991

McDougle CJ, Goodman WK, Leckman JF: Limited therapeutic effect of addition of buspirone in fluvoxamine refractory obsessive-compulsive disorder. Am J Psychiatry 150:647–649, 1993

McFall ME, Wollershein JP: Obsessive-compulsive neurosis: a cognitive-behavioral formulation and approach to treatment. Cognitive Therapy and Research 3: 333–348, 1979

McKay D, Danyko S, Neziroglu F, et al: Factor structure of the Yale-Brown Obsessive-Compulsive Scale: a two dimensional measure. Behav Res Ther 33:865–869, 1995

McKay D, Neziroglu F, Todaro J, et al: Changes in personality disorders following behavior therapy for obsessive compulsive disorder. Journal of Anxiety Disorders 10:47–57, 1996

McKeon P, Murray R: Familial aspects of obsessive-compulsive neurosis. Br J Psychiatry 151:528–534, 1987

Mehta M: A comparative study of family-based and patient-based behavioral management in obsessive-compulsive disorders. Br J Psychiatry 157:133–135, 1990

Mellman LA, Gorman JM: Successful treatment of obsessive-compulsive disorder with ECT. Am J Psychiatry 141:596–597, 1984

Meyer V: Modification of expectations in cases with obsessional rituals. Behav Res Ther 4:273–280, 1966

Meyer V, Levy R, Schnurer A: The behavioral treatment of obsessive-compulsive disorders, in Obsessional States. Edited by Beech HR. London, Methuen, 1974, pp 238–258

Minichiello WE, Baer L, Jenike MA: Schizotypal personality disorder: a poor prognostic indicator for behavior therapy in the treatment of obsessive-compulsive disorder. Journal of Anxiety Disorders 1:273–276, 1987

Minkowski E, Citrome P: Resultats d'une cure de sommeil dans un cas d'obsession. Ann Med Psychol 111:400–401, 1953

Modell JG, Himle J, Nesse RM, et al: Sequential trials of fluoxetine, phenelzine, and tranylcypromine in the treatment of obsessive compulsive disorder. Journal of Anxiety Disorders 3:287–293, 1989

Monteiro WO, Noshirvani HF, Marks IM, et al: Anorgasmia from clomipramine on obsessive-compulsive disorder: a controlled trial. Br J Psychiatry 151:107–112, 1987

Moreau de Tours JJ: 1845. Cited in Caldwell AE: History of psychopharmacology, in: Principles of Psychopharmacology. Edited by Clark WG, del Giudice J. New York, Academic Press, 1970, pp 9–30.

Muller C: Weitere Beobachtungen zum Verlauf der Zwangskrankheit. Psychiatr Neurol (Basel) 133:80–94, 1957

Navarro F: Trattamento delle nevrosi ossisive con un iminodibenzil-derivato. Rass Int Clin Ter 40:616–619, 1960

Needleman HL, Waber D: The use of amitriptyline in anorexia nervosa, in Anorexia Nervosa. Edited by Vigersky RA. New York, Raven, 1977, pp 357–368

Nemiah JC: Obsessive-compulsive neurosis, in Comprehensive Textbook of Psychiatry, 2nd Edition, Vol 1. Edited by Freedman A, Kaplan H, Ladock B. Baltimore, MD, Williams & Wilkins, 1975, pp 1241–1255

Neziroglu F: A combined behavioral-pharmocotherapy approach to obsessive-compulsive disorders, in Biological Psychiatry Today. Edited by Obiols J, Ballus C, Gonzales-Monclus E, et al. Amsterdam, the Netherlands, Elsevier North-Holland, 1979, pp 591–596

Neziroglu F: Complexities and lesser know aspects of obsessive compulsive and related disorder. Cognitive and Behavioral Practice 1:133–156, 1994

Neziroglu F, Neuman J: Three approaches to the treatment of obsessions. International Journal of Cognitive Therapy 4:371–392, 1990

Neziroglu FA, Yaryura-Tobias JA: Follow-up study on obsessive-compulsive patients on chlorimipramine and behavior therapy. Pharmaceutical Medicine 1:170–173, 1980

Neziroglu F, Yaryura-Tobias JA: Obsessive compulsive disorder, in The Counseling Sourcebook: A Practical Reference on Contemporary Issues. Edited by Judah JL, Ornum WV, Stillwell N. New York, Crossroad Publishing, 1994, pp 425–436

Neziroglu F, Yaryura-Tobias JA: Over and Over Again: Understanding Obsessive Compulsive Disorder (updated and revised). New York, Lexington Books, 1995

Neziroglu FA, Steele J, Yaryura-Tobias JA, et al: Effect of behavior therapy on serotonin level in obsessive-compulsive disorder, in Psychiatry: A World Perspective, Vol 3. Edited by Stefanis CN. New York, Elsevier, 1990, pp 707–710

Neziroglu FA, Yaryura-Tobias JA, Lemli JM, et al: Estudio demografico del trastorno obseso compulsivo. Acta Psiquiatr Psicol Am Lat 40:217–223, 1994

Okuma T, Nakao T, Ogura C, et al: Effect of 7-bromo-5-(2-pyridyl-3H-1,4-benzo-diazepin-2(1H)-one, bromazepam (Ro 5-3350), a new minor tranquilizer, on psychoneurosis with special reference to the obsessive-compulsive symptoms. Folia Psychiatr Neurol Jpn (Tokyo) 25:181–193, 1971

Oppenheim S, Rosenberger J: Treatment of a case of obsessional disorder: family systems and object relations approaches. American Journal of Family Therapy 19:327–333, 1991

Orvin GH: Treatment of the phobic obsessive compulsive patient with oxazepam, an unproved benzodiazepine compound. Psychosomatics 8:278–280, 1967

O'Sullivan G, Noshirvani H, Marks I, et al: Six-year follow-up after exposure and clomipramine therapy for obsessive-compulsive disorder. J Clin Psychiatry 52:150–155, 1991

Papart P, Ansseau M: Milnacipran in obsessive-compulsive disorder: study in one case (in French). Psychiatrie and Psychobiologie 5:325–327, 1990

Pato MT, Zohar-Kadouch R, Zohar J, et al: Return of symptoms after discontinuation of clomipramine in patients with obsessive-compulsive disorder. Am J Psychiatry 145:1521–1525, 1988

Pato MT, Hill JL, Murphy DL: A clomipramine dosage reduction study in the course of long-term treatment of obsessive-compulsive disorder patients. Psychopharmacol Bull 26:211–214, 1990

Pato MT, Pigott TA, Hill JL, et al: Controlled comparison of buspirone and clomipramine in obsessive compulsive disorder. Am J Psychiatry 148:127–129, 1991

Pearson J, Foa EB: Processing of fearful and neutral information by obsessive-compulsives. Behav Res Ther 22:259–265, 1984

Petrilowitsch N: Der Zeitfaktor in der Pharmakopsychiatrie, in Psychiatrische Krankheitslehre und Psychiatrische Pharmakotherapie. Basel, S Karger, 1968a, pp 64–90

Petrilowitsch N: Die Ganzheitliche und die "Atomistische" Betrachtungsweise in der Pharmakotherapie. Zielsyndrome oder Zielsymptoms? in Psychiatrische Krankheitslehre und Psychiatrische Pharmakotherapie. Basel, S Karger, 1968b, pp 42–63

Pigott TA, Pato MT, Bernstein SE, et al: Controlled comparisons of clomipramine and fluoxetine in the treatment of obsessive compulsive disorder. Arch Gen Psychiatry 47:926–932, 1990

Pigott TA, Pato MT, L'Heureux F, et al: A controlled comparison of adjuvant lithium carbonate or thyroid hormone in clomipramine treated patients with obsessive compulsive disorder. J Clin Psychopharmacology 11:242–248, 1991

Pigott TA, L'Heureux F, Hill JL, et al: A double blind study of adjuvant buspirone hydrochloride in clomipramine treated patients with obsessive compulsive disorder. J Clin Psychopharmacol 12:11–18, 1992a

Pigott TA, L'Heureux F, Rubenstein CS, et al: A double-blind, placebo controlled study of trazodone in patients with obsessive compulsive disorder. J Clin Psychopharmacol 12:156–162, 1992b

Pollitt J: Natural history of obsessional states: a study of 150 cases. BMJ 1:194–198, 1957

Porta Biosca A, Vallejo Ruiloba J: Aportacion a la terapeutica de los cuadros obsesivos por la monoclorimipramina. Revista de Psiquiatría y Psicología Medica 3: 157–176, 1971

Price J, Grunhaus LJ: Treatment of clomipramine induced anorgasmia with yohimbine: a case report. J Clin Psychiatry 51:32–33, 1990

Rabavilas AD, Boulougouris JC, Stefanis D: Duration of flooding session in the treatment of obsessive-compulsive patients. Behav Res Ther 14:349–355, 1976

Rachman SJ: Obstacles to the successful treatment of obsessions, in Failures in Behavior Therapy. Edited by Foa EB, Emmelkamp PMG. New York, Wiley, 1983, pp 35–57

Rasmussen SA: Lithium and tryptophan augmentation in clomipramine resistant obsessive-compulsive disorder. Am J Psychiatry 141:1283–1285, 1984

Rego A, Guimon J, Sanchez Vega J, et al: Tratamiento de las psicosis cronicas y neurosis obsesivas graves con monoclorimipramina. Revista de Psiqiatría y Psicología Medica de Europa y América Latina 9:340–357, 1970

Rippere V: Can hypoglycemia cause obsessions and ruminations? Medical Hypothesis 15:3–13, 1984

Rojo Sierra M: Tratamiento de la neurosis obsesiva por los derivados del tropano. Consecuencias psicologicas. Revista de Psiquiatría y Psicología Médica de Europa y América Latina 1:354–373, 1954

Rojo Sierra M: Terapeutica lisergica en ciertos sindromes obsesivos y neurosis sexuales. IV Congreso Internacional de Psicoterapia. Actas Luso-Esp de Neurol y Psiq 18:108–113, 1959

Roper G, Rachman SJ, Marks IM: Passive and participant modelling in exposure treatment of obsessive-compulsive neurotics. Behav Res Ther 13:271–279, 1975

Rousal J, Brichoin S: Pripad Myzofilie. Cesk Psychiatr 67:176–180, 1971

Rubin RD: Clinical use of retrograde amnesia produced by electroconvulsive shock. Can Psychiatr Assoc J 21:87–90, 1976

Rudin E: Ein Beitrag zur Frage der Zwang Krankheit, Insbesondere ihrer Hereditaren Bezielungen. Arch Psychiatr Nervenkr 191:14–54, 1953

Ruegg RG, Evans DL, Comer WS, et al: Lithium augments fluoxetine treatment of obsessive-compulsive disorder. Lithium 3:69–71, 1992

Sakai T: Clinico-genetic study on obsessive-compulsive neurosis. Bull Osaka Med Sch Suppl 12:323–331, 1967

Salkovskis PM: Treatment of an obsession. Br J Clin Psychol 22:311–313, 1985

Salkovskis PM, Warwick HMC: Cognitive therapy of obsessive-compulsive disorder: treating treatment failures. Behav Psychother 13:243–255, 1985

Salkovskis PM, Westbrook D: Behaviour therapy and obsessional ruminations: can failure be turned into success? Behav Res Ther 27:149–160, 1989

Salzman C: Electroconvulsive therapy, in The Harvard Guide to Modern Psychiatry. Edited by Nicholi AM. Cambridge, MA, Harvard University Press/Belknap Press, 1978, pp 475–476

Sargant W, Slater E: Discussion on the treatment of obsessional neuroses. Proc R Soc Med 43:1007–1010, 1950

Simoni PS: Obsessive-compulsive disorder. The effect of research on nursing care. Psychosocial Nursing and Mental Health Services 29:19–23, 1991

Smeraldi E, Erzegovesi S, Bianchi I, et al: Fluvoxamine vs clomipramine treatment in obsessive compulsive disorder: a preliminary study. New Trends in Experimental and Clinical Psychiatry 8:63–65, 1992

Solyom L, Sookman D: A comparison of clomipramine hydrochloride (Anafranil) and behavior therapy in the treatment of obsessive neurosis. J Int Med Res 5:49–61, 1977

Steketee GS: Personality traits and diagnosis in obsessive compulsive disorder. Paper presented at the meeting of the Association for Advancement of Behavior Therapy, New York, November 1988

Steketee GS, Foa EB, Grayson JB: Recent advances in the treatment of obsessive-compulsives. Arch Gen Psychiatry 39:1365–1371, 1982

Stengel E: The significance of obsessional symptoms in schizophrenia. International Congress of Psychiatry (Zurich) 1:318–321, 1957

Stern RS, Marks IM, Mawson D, et al: Clomipramine and exposure for compulsive rituals: II. plasma levels, side effects and outcome. Br J Psychiatry 136: 161–166, 1980

Straus EW: On obsession: a clinical and methodological study. Nervous Mental Diseases Monography New York, 73:1–92, 1948

Symonds RL: An obsessional patient treated with clomipramine. Br J Psychiatry 123:255–258, 1973

Tamini RR, Mavissakalian MR, Jones B, et al: Clomipramine versus fluvoxamine in obsessive-compulsive disorder. Ann Clin Psychiatry 3:275–279, 1991

Tapia F: Haldol in the treatment of children with tics and stutters, and an incidental finding. Psychiatr Q 43:647–649, 1969

Tellenbach H: Uber die Behandlung Phobischer und Anankasticher Zustande mit Imipramin. Nervenarzt 34:133–138, 1963

Tesar GE, Jenike MA: Alprazolam as treatment for a case of obsessive-compulsive disorder. Am J Psychiatry 141:689–690, 1984

Thakur AK, Remillard AJ, Meldrum LH, et al: Intravenous clomipramine and obsessive-compulsive disorder. Can J Psychiatry 36:521–524, 1991

Thoren P, Asberg M, Cronholm B, et al: Clomipramine treatment of obsessive-compulsive disorder. I: a controlled clinical trial. Arch Gen Psychiatry 37: 1281–1285, 1980

Thyer B: Audiotaped exposure therapy in a case of obsessional neurosis. J Behav Ther Exp Psychiatry 16:271–273, 1985

Tollefson G: Alprazolam in the treatment of obsessive symptoms. J Clin Psychopharmacol 5:39–42, 1985

Trabucci C, Zuanazzi GF, Caceffo G: Nostre experienze sulla cura con Tofranil. Riv Sper Freniatr 83:328–335, 1959

Tynes LL, Salins C, Winstead DK: Obsessive-compulsive patients: familial frustration/criticism. J La State Med Soc 142:24–26, 1990

Vallejo J, Olivares J, Marcos T, et al: Clomipramine versus phenelzine in obsessive-compulsive disorder: a controlled clinical trial. Br J Psychiatry 161:665–670, 1992

Van Reynynghe De Voxurie G: Anafranil (G.34586) in obsessive neurosis. Acta Neurol Belg 68:787–792, 1968

Venkoba Roa A: A controlled trial with "Valium" in obsessive-compulsive state. J Indian Med Assoc 42:564–567, 1964

Vidal G, Vidal B: Imipramine et obsessions. Encephale 52:167–180, 1965

Visser S, Hoekstra RJ, Emmelkamp PMG: Follow-up study on behavioral treatment of obsessive-compulsive disorders, in Perspectives and Promises of Clinical Psychology. Edited by Ehlers A, Fiegenbaum W, Florin I, et al. New York, Plenum, 1991, pp 152–170

Volavka J, Neziroglu F, Yaryura-Tobias JA: Clomipramine and imipramine in obsessive-compulsive disorder. Psychiatry Res 14:85–93, 1985

Warneke LB: The use of intravenous chlorimipramine in the treatment of obsessive-compulsive disorder. Can J Psychiatry 29:135–141, 1984

Wolpe J: Psychotherapy by Reciprocal Inhibition. Stanford, CA, Stanford University Press, 1958

Yaryura-Tobias JA: Clinical observations on L-tryptophan in the treatment of obsessive compulsive disorders, in Abstracts of the Third World Congress of Biological Psychiatry. Edited by Struve G. Stockholm, Sweden, 1981, pp 5–410

Yaryura-Tobias JA: Desorden obseso-compulsivo primario. Aspectos bioquimicos, in Psiquiatria Biologica. Edited by Ciprian-Ollivier J. Buenos Aires, Brazil, Cierntifica Interamericana, 1988, pp 121–127

Yaryura-Tobias JA, Bhagavan HN: L-Tryptophan in obsessive-compulsive disorders. Am J Psychiatry 134:1298–1299, 1977

Yaryura-Tobias JA, Neziroglu F: The action of chlorimipramine in obsessive-compulsive neurosis: a pilot study. Curr Ther Res Clin Exp 17:111–116, 1975

Yaryura-Tobias JA, Neziroglu F: Compulsions, aggressions, and self-mutilation: a hypothalamic disorder? Journal of Orthomolecular Psychiatry 7:114–117, 1978

Yaryura-Tobias JA, Neziroglu F: Follow-up study on obsessive-compulsive patients on chlorimipramine and behavior therapy. Pharmaceutical Medicine 1:170–173, 1979

Yaryura-Tobias JA, Neziroglu FA: Biological therapy, in Obsessive-Compulsive Disorders: Pathogenesis, Diagnosis, and Treatment. Edited by Yaryura-Tobias JA, Neziroglu FA. New York, Marcel Dekker, 1983, pp 173–194

Yaryura-Tobias JA, Neziroglu FA: Over and Over Again: Understanding Obsessive Compulsive Disorder (paperback edition). New York, Simon & Shuster, 1995

Yaryura-Tobias JA, Neziroglu F, Bergman L: Chlorimipramine for obsessive-compulsive neurosis: an organic approach. Curr Ther Res Clin Exp 20: 541–548, 1976

Yoney TH, Pigott TA, L'Heureux F, et al: Seasonal variation in obsessive-compulsive disorder: preliminary experience with light treatment. Am J Psychiatry 148: 1727–1729, 1991

Zhao JP: A control study of clomipramine and amitriptyline for treating obsessive-compulsive disorder (in Chinese). Chung Hua Shen Ching Ching Shen Ko Tsa Chih 24:68–70, 123, 1991

Zohar J, Insel TR, Berman KF, et al: Anxiety and cerebral blood flow during behavioral challenge: dissociation of central from peripheral and subjective measures. Arch Gen Psychiatry 46:505–510, 1989

Chapter 3
Obsessive-Compulsive Disorders of Childhood

Although obsessive-compulsive disorders (OCDs) usually start in childhood or adolescence, much of the literature has discussed phenomenological aspects and treatment in adults. As with any disorder, the recognition of its symptoms and early intervention may prevent its proliferation. The ability of clinicians, teachers, and parents to note the early signs of OCD will assist in helping children achieve their full potential. When OCD is not prevented from unfolding, generalization of symptoms occurs, and the individual's functioning is impaired. In this chapter we acquaint the readers with the early signs of OCD in children and adolescents so that treatment strategies can be implemented early.

Epidemiology

The prevalence rate of OCD in children is 1%, and about 200,000 American children and adolescents are affected (Piacentini et al. 1992). Worldwide studies indicate a wide range of prevalence rates that may be attributed to different populations studied. For example, in a study in Japan, 5% of 1,293 patients younger than 18 years old had OCD (Honjo et al. 1989). In The Netherlands, 1.33% of 4,594 Danish children and adolescents had OCD (Thomsen and Mikkelson 1991). In Israel, 3.6% of 562 Army inductees had OCD (Zohar et al. 1992). In a United States study of two self-contained classrooms of emotionally handicapped children, 3% had OCD (Silver 1984).

When a specific population is studied, the distribution will be skewed. Epidemiological data should be based on childhood disorder prevalence rates in the normal population. An OCD prevalence rate of 1% (± 0.5%) has been found in the general adolescent population, with a 1.9% (± 0.7%) lifetime prevalence rate. These rates are slightly lower than the 2.5% lifetime prevalence rate in adults (Flament 1990).

The consensus is that onset of this disorder is rare before puberty (Judd 1965; Neziroglu et al. 1994). The disorder's course is chronic and unremitting for both children and adults (Swedo et al. 1992).

Phenomenology

Childhood OCD differs from normal developmental rituals and superstitions in its severity, content, and associated distress. When 38 children with severe primary OCD were compared with 22 matched control subjects, the number and type of superstitions did not differ. However, parents of children with OCD reported more "marked" early ritualistic behavior patterns than parents of normal control subjects (Leonard et al. 1990). Other researchers found that anxiety, affective disorder and compulsive personality disorders were associated features for many children with OCD (King and Tonge 1991). It is hard to determine whether the children develop the compulsive personality to control their disorder or whether it precedes the disorder. We believe the associated depressive affective state is secondary to the disorder. Depression is a consequence of the resulting disorder problems (i.e., poor peer relations, academic problems, and inability to actualize one's potential).

Many children engage in rituals or superstitious games (e.g., not stepping on cracks, counting cars of a certain color, or touching every third fence post). However, these are games rather than compulsions and can be stopped without anxiety. Children and adolescents with OCD generally do not share their symptoms with family members until the distress is beyond what they can handle. They are usually embarrassed and try to conceal the compulsions. Sometimes they cannot hide them, and teachers or parents notice "strange" behaviors. Unfortunately, these behaviors are often attributed to normal childhood and adolescent habits; if investigated, many of them would be considered persistent, pervasive, and distressing symptoms for the child. The children are silently crying for help.

Simons (1974) reported that some compulsive behaviors appear around age 2 in normal children and continue for 4 to 5 years. He further noted that changes in physical surroundings or daily routines normally upset 2-year-old children who want order. Such rigidity may be attributed to the child's attempt to control his or her demanding environment. The child may ritualize daily activities, such as eating, dressing, and washing, and then make them distorted reflections of parental demands. Our clinical observations are that normal childhood compulsive behaviors usually revolve around bedtime rituals. The rituals commence between ages 3 and 6. These iterative rituals may focus on checking or touching various objects; saying goodnight to parents; or following a sequence of events, such as touching drawers several times, going to the bathroom, getting a glass of water and putting it by the bed, saying prayers in a particular manner, placing slippers at a chosen side of the bed, fixing the pillow, and so on, before finally getting in bed. In most children these rituals disappear rapidly.

Normally children's play is full of ritualistic and compulsive behavior. Many people observe children meticulously stepping or attempting not to step on sidewalk cracks, tapping every other mailbox or fence post, touching certain street signs, and counting objects or particular license plates.

Between ages 2 and 3, complicated ritualistic symptoms develop (Gesell 1925, 1930, 1940). These rituals help children define their environment and help them develop new abilities. Abnormal obsessions and compulsions differ from normal ones in that they create distress and interfere in the child's life. With normal obsessions and compulsions, children perceive the rituals as part of their lives and are not disturbed. The percentage of children falling into the normal obsessive-compulsive category is unknown.

A common question is whether OCD in children and adolescents is different from OCD in adults. There seem to be no symptom differences in the phenomenology literature. Rettew et al. (1992) reported no significant age-related trends with any type of symptom, although patients with early illness onset (before age 6) were more likely to have compulsions. In their sample of patients studied over an 8-year span, approximately 47% displayed both washing and checking compulsions. No patient maintained the same symptom constellation. No intercultural differences were found in obsessional thought content and compulsive behavior among children and adolescents from Denmark, India, and Japan (Thomsen 1991).

Early Signs of OCD

There are certain behaviors that may indicate to teachers and parents that a child either has or is developing OCD. Some of the overt signs that should be further investigated are the following: daydreaming; red hands; declining grades; increased reactions and concerns regarding minor issues; slowness on tests, simple tasks, projects, or reading; walking back and forth in hallways; excessive/poorly explained absences; excessive time in the bathroom; repetitive questions; excessive need for reassurance; avoidance of art/playground; and complaints of fatigue or of life being too stressful. If these warning signs are noticed, it is important to question the child to elicit the obsessions or compulsions that may be provoking these behaviors. Once the problem is identified, treatment should be sought before the symptoms generalize and the child becomes more engrossed in them.

Psychiatric Interfaces

OCD and Psychosis

As early as 1954, Piaget identified normal obsessive-compulsive behavior and OCD in infants. He stated that the latter may develop into psychosis. The relationship between OCD and schizophrenia is controversial. The main difference between obsessive-compulsive neurosis and childhood schizophrenia is intact reality testing in the former (Despert 1955). Moreover, the concomitant presence of childhood schizophrenia with compulsive symptoms may indicate two illnesses in one, rather than one illness leading to the other (Despert 1955). Although it may sometimes be difficult to determine the extent of an overvalued idea and to know whether the thoughts are delusional, on average, we do not find that OCD develops into psychosis.

OCD and Depression

According to Regner (1959), during childhood depression, obsessive-compulsive symptoms may appear as a phobia extension. He believed an OCD diagnosis in childhood could prevent the illness continuing in adult life. However, Vikar (1977) believed that a childhood obsessional disorder in childhood did not necessarily result in an adult form. In our experience, OCD treated during childhood may or may not continue into adulthood. Some children and adolescents that we treated more than 15 years before follow-up did not have any symptoms during their adulthood, although they had occasional thoughts or urges that quickly faded away. However, others were successfully treated and went into remission, but their symptoms reappeared later on during adulthood. Regardless of the long-term outcome, the symptoms should be treated as soon as they appear.

OCD, Autism, and Fire Setting

Two other obsessive-compulsive behaviors noted in children are fire setting and autism. Childhood fire setting was not described in the psychiatric literature until 1940 (Gessell 1940). Although most childhood fire setting interpretations are linked to enuresis and sexual disturbances, the symptomatology includes obsessive-compulsive behavior. Unlike other obsessive-compulsive individuals, these children usually have low IQs. In our opinion those children with OCD who also are hyperactive have a greater propensity toward acting out behavior, as seen in fire setting. On average, most OCD children are not fire setters nor do they engage in impulsive behaviors. On the contrary, they are extremely intelligent, verbal, and assertive rather than aggressive. They usually show a need to please rather than rebel.

Compulsive, iterative behaviors are common in autism. Reference to compulsive behavior in autism is found in most childhood psychosis studies. Kanner (1951) has stated:

> The autistic child desires to live in a static world, a world in which no change is tolerated. The status quo must be maintained at all costs. Only the child himself may sometimes take it upon himself to modify existing combination. But no one else may do so without arousing unhappiness and anger. It is remarkable to what extent the children will go to assure the preservation of sameness. The totality of an experience that comes to the child from the outside must be reiterated, often with all its constituent details, in complete photographic and phonographic identity. No one part of this totality may be altered in terms of shape, sequence, or space. The slightest change of arrangement, sometimes so minute that it is hardly perceived by others, may evoke a violent outburst of rage. This behavior differs from ordinary obsessive ritualism in one significant respect: The autistic child forces the people in his world to be even more obsessive than he is himself. While he may make occasional concessions, he does not grant this privilege to others. He is a stern and unrelenting judge and critic. When one watches such a child for any length of time, it becomes evident that, unless he is completely alone, most of his activities go into

the job as serious, solemn, sacerdotal enforcement of the maintenance of sameness, of absolute identity. (p. 24)

In summary, it can be said that autistic children show a peculiar type of obsessiveness that forces them to imperiously postulate a static, unchanged environment. Any modification is met with perplexity and major discomfort. The patients find security in sameness, but this security is tenuous, because changes occur constantly. Therefore, the children are perpetually threatened and try intensely to ward off this threat to their security.

The autistic child seems excessively preoccupied with names, watches, maps, calendar dates, and so forth. Despert (1965) attributed autistic children's compulsive behavior (i.e., rocking, twirling, compulsive handling of objects) to anxiety defenses. Rutter and Lockyer (1967) also discussed compulsive locomotion along with decreased pain sensitivity in autism. Simons (1974) indicated that compulsive behavior and anxiety may be related at different points in the autistic child's development. Anxiety may have been present initially when the child faced a frightening world. He or she thus coped with this anxiety by becoming self-involved. Once the child withdraws, there is no evidence of anxiety. Only when the child becomes aware of others does the anxiety reappear. To cope with these new feelings, Simons asserted, the child resorts to compulsive behavior. Furthermore, Simon noted that the desire to maintain sameness is different from OCD compulsions. In the former, when "sameness" is achieved (i.e., furniture, toys, and so forth, in their right places), the child moves to new activities. In the latter, the child clings to compulsions and cannot engage in other activities.

Certainly some autism symptoms present characteristics similar to those in OCD. However, this similitude may not be sufficient to classify autism as an OCD variant. It seems that in autism, essential subjective data (relating to unwantedness, distress, resistance, senselessness, and egodystonia) are not available (Baron-Cohen 1989). Autistic children are unable to contemplate and become aware of their own mental status. This inability limits the phenomenological interpretation of collected information, and thus the examiner must use the findings cautiously. Although patients with various illnesses may display symptoms of OCD, it is important not to categorize these patients as having OCD. The dissimilarities between autism and OCD at this point seem to be greater than the similarities. Until further research indicates otherwise, it seems more prudent to indicate that autism demonstrates some symptoms found in OCD.

Attention-Deficit/Hyperactivity Disorder

The relationship among attention-deficit disorder (ADD), attention-deficit/ hyperactivity disorder (ADHD), and OCD has not been widely studied. Most of the literature discusses Tourette's syndrome and its relationship to ADD and ADHD. It has been reported that OCD and ADD are part of the continuum of Tourette's syndrome (Drake et al. 1992).

In our practice, about 25% of the adult OCD patients report having been diagnosed as having ADD or ADHD. Thus, the percentage of patients with OCD may be an overestimation owing to misdiagnosis. Often children with OCD may behave similarly to children with ADD and therefore be diagnosed incorrectly. Children with OCD are easily distracted, appear to be daydreaming, seem "spacey," do not do well on tests, and function below their intelligence. These characteristics are similar to those of children with ADD. However, children with ADD may engage in compulsions to compensate for their distractibility and feelings of being out of control. Of course, a child may have both OCD and ADD or OCD and ADHD. The fact that a child can focus and engage in compulsions endlessly does not rule out the diagnosis of ADD. A child may be compulsive in certain areas and yet have difficulty concentrating, learning, and focusing on other things.

Cognitive-behavior treatment for patients with OCD and ADD may be more difficult. Behavior therapy is based on learning, and individuals with ADD or ADHD have difficulty focusing long enough to learn the principles necessary to generalize from one situation to another. Therefore, treatment may take longer. Also, individuals with ADD concentrate on short-term consequences, whereas long-term gains with behavior therapy are made by concentrating on long-term consequences. Clinicians may often give up if their patients do not comply quickly, interpreting their patients' inability to focus as resistance, stubbornness, or lack of effort. Perhaps the ADD must be addressed before the OCD. As indicated before, currently there is little information about the phenomenology and treatment of patients with both OCD and ADD or ADHD. Another question that needs to be addressed is whether those patients with comorbid ADD or ADHD are more prone to alcohol and substance abuse.

Mental Retardation

Mental retardation is a neuropsychiatric disorder that can manifest as a result of any of a vast number of cerebral abnormalities. Its connection with

OCD mostly relates to the presence of compulsive behavior, including self-mutilation (see Chapter 11). When examining a child or adult with mental retardation, it is common to find double-checking, rituals, and hair pulling (Hurley and Sovner 1984).

In one report, a mildly retarded woman had had trichotillomania and trichophagia since childhood and, as a consequence, had multiple complications, including malnutrition and trichobezoar, which caused intestinal obstruction (Wadlington et al. 1992). Treatment consisted of psychotherapy behavior modification and various medications, without success.

Differential diagnosis may be required to differentiate OCD from Asperger's syndrome. This syndrome, a rare form of pervasive developmental disorder, is characterized by eccentricities, emotional lability, anxiety, repetitive behavior, fixed habits, and poor social functioning. Ryan (1992) emphasized the need for differential diagnosis in treatment-resistant patients.

In two Down's syndrome patients with obsessive-compulsive symptoms, one experienced abrupt OCD onset on starting a new school, and the other had sudden onset after a sexual assault (O'Dwyer et al. 1992). Note that in both cases the onset was sudden, which is unusual in primary OCD.

Course of Illness

The question is often raised as to whether adult disorders are extensions of childhood disorders. Although some investigators consider childhood disorders a separate entity with different symptoms and etiology, others view them as precursors of adulthood disorders. We believe childhood and adult OCDs are similar; both adults and children have the subjective urge to perform a particular ritual and then experience anxiety if they do not. Furthermore, annoyance results from performing the rituals, and both children and adults often try to resist the compulsion.

If OCDs are viewed as a conditioning process and a biochemical predisposition, then it seems logical to assume that age is only one factor in their development. For instance, childhood symptoms may reappear in adults, perhaps as a result of the neurological, biochemical, and hormonal changes later on. Later, stress may precipitate alterations in an individual's biological makeup. From a psychological perspective, children may succeed in struggling to resist the urges and may be able to extinguish the compulsions. The reappearance of symptoms may be a function of a learned avoidance response (ritual performance) in the presence of stress. Elkins et al. (1980) proposed a neurobiological hypothesis based on a review of the literature.

Although symptoms may vary from childhood to adulthood, this variance may be attributed to the different stimuli an individual encounters at various ages. However, not every childhood disorder continues into adulthood, although follow-up studies suggest that most children and adolescents with OCD continue to experience the disorder as adults (Allsopp and Verduyn 1989; Berg et al. 1989; Flament et al. 1990).

Treatments

Behavior Therapy

There is little literature on the psychological treatment of childhood OCD. The few reports that exist are uncontrolled case studies and usually discuss a combination of treatments. Although the efficacy of behavior therapy—specifically, exposure and response prevention—has been demonstrated in the treatment of adult OCD, it has been overlooked in the treatment of childhood and adolescent OCD. It is probably more accurate to state that there are few published studies using exposure and response prevention than to claim that this form of therapy is not used with children. Case studies indicate that it is effective (Bolton et al. 1983; Harris and Wiebe 1992; Phillips and Wolpe 1981; Thyer 1991). However, other adolescent problems often interfere with the application of behavior therapy; such problems include acting out behavior, rebelliousness, and overall lack of compliance with treatment.

In conjunction with behavior and drug therapy, several researchers consider family and milieu therapy important (Adams 1985; Apter and Tyano 1988; Bolton et al. 1983; de-Haan and Hoogduin 1992; King and Tonge 1991). Even studies reporting a positive outcome with behavior therapy are not pure behavior therapy treatment outcome studies, because myriad therapies have been used.

In our experience, behavior therapy is necessary for any OCD treatment program, although its application in children may vary somewhat from that in adults. We find that adolescents, like adults, are compliant with treatment, even when a conduct disorder is present. However, children younger than 15 years often need positive reinforcement when they comply. We often use behavior modification programs, devise games to make behavior therapy more enjoyable, and include the family in every phase.

A review of the literature indicates that many more studies have been conducted with medications than with psychological treatments. Controlled studies investigating different treatment approaches to childhood OCD are needed.

Pharmacological Treatment

Before starting a drug program to treat children and adolescents with OCD, the issues that should be considered include 1) treatment rationale, 2) degree of illness severity, 3) drug of choice, 4) dosage, 5) side effects, 6) toxicity, 7) alternative therapy (e.g., behavior therapy), and 8) clinical management.

Therapists must explain to the parents the pros and cons of the treatment suggested; if necessary, written authorization to prescribe medication should be requested. It should be remembered that psychopharmacotherapy in children is a controversial issue (Gadow 1991).

Two medications, clomipramine and fluoxetine, appear to be the treatment choices. It has been suggested that fluoxetine is better for long-term improvement, because it has a lower rate of relapse (Piacentini et al. 1992).

Clomipramine had a good success rate and efficacy when compared with placebo (DeVaugh-Geiss et al. 1992; Flament et al. 1985; Leonard and Rapoport 1989) or to desipramine (Gordon et al. 1993; Leonard et al. 1989, 1991). An adolescent with a severe case of OCD was successfully treated with intravenous clomipramine (Warneke 1985).

When clomipramine and fluoxetine are combined, required dosages of both medications are reduced, thus reducing the incidence of untoward effects (Simeon et al. 1990). Satisfactory results were obtained with fluoxetine in an OCD patient group (Riddle et al. 1992) and in a group of patients with OCD and Tourette's syndrome (Riddle et al. 1990). In the latter group, agitation was reported in 40% of the sample. In a sample of Tourette's syndrome patients with comorbidity (e.g., primary anorexia nervosa) and OCD, administration of clomipramine seemed beneficial (Yaryura-Tobias 1975, 1979; Yaryura-Tobias and Neziroglu 1977).

Overall, the ideal treatment is using partial (clomipramine) or selective serotonin reuptake inhibitors. However, one group of side effects that concerns us consists of agitation, hyperactivity, and acting out behavior. These may be caused by an increase in and increased availability of serotonin. The effectiveness of antidepressants may be hindered by the presence of anxiety (Ambrosini et al. 1993).

Our therapeutic approach is to avoid medication if possible and start treatment with behavior therapy. A combined approach renders good response and fewer side effects, because less medication is required. Medication should be titrated, beginning with small doses, followed by gradual increments. This may avoid side effects and allow the patient's fear of medication to diminish or dissipate all together. Finally, we corroborate suggestions emphasizing the need for a dosing strategy (Schatzberg 1991).

References

Adams PL: The obsessive child: a therapy update. Am J Psychother 39:301–313, 1985

Allsopp M, Verduyn C: A follow-up of adolescents with obsessive-compulsive disorder. Br J Psychiatry 154:829–834, 1989

Ambrosini PJ, Pianchi MD, Rabinovich H, et al: Antidepressant treatments in children and adolescents: II. anxiety, physical, and behavioral disorders. J Am Acad Child Adolesc Psychiatry 32:483–493, 1993

Apter A, Tyano S: Obsessive-compulsive disorders in adolescence. J Adolesc 11: 183–194, 1988

Baron-Cohen S: Do autistic children have obsessions and compulsions? Br J Clin Psychol 28:193–200, 1989

Berg CZ, Rapoport JL, Whitaker A, et al: Childhood obsessive-compulsive disorders: a two-year prospective follow-up of a community sample. J Am Acad Child Adolesc Psychiatry 28:528–533, 1989

Bolton D, Collins S, Steinberg D: The treatment of obsessive-compulsive disorder in adolescence: a report of fifteen cases. Br J Psychiatry 142:456–464, 1983

de-Haan E, Hoogduin CA: The treatment of children with obsessive-compulsive disorder. Acta Paedopsychiatr 55:93–97, 1992

Despert JL: Differential diagnosis between obsessive-compulsive neurosis and schizophrenia in children, in Psychopathology of Childhood. Edited by Hoch PH, Zubin J. New York, Grune & Stratton, 1955, pp 240–253

Despert JL: The Emotionally Disturbed Child—Then and Now. New York, Robert Brunner, 1965

DeVaugh-Geiss J, Moroz G, Biederman J, et al: Clomipramine hydrochloride in childhood and adolescent obsessive-compulsive disorder—a multicenter trial. J Am Acad Child Adolesc Psychiatry 31:45–49, 1992

Drake ME Jr, Hietter SA, Padamadan H, et al: Auditory evoked potentials in Gilles de la Tourette syndrome. Clin Electroencephalogr 23:19–23, 1992

Elkins R, Rapoport J, Lipsky A: Childhood obsessive-compulsive disorder: a neurobiological viewpoint. J Am Acad Child Psychiatry 19:551–554, 1980

Flament M: Epidemiology of obsessive compulsive disorders in children and adolescents (in French). Encephale 16:311–316, 1990

Flament MF, Rapoport JL, Berg CJ, et al: Clomipramine treatment of childhood obsessive-compulsive disorder. Arch Gen Psychiatry 42:977–983, 1985

Flament MF, Koby E, Rapoport JL, et al: Childhood obsessive-compulsive disorder: a prospective follow-up study. J Child Psychol Psychiatry 31:363–380, 1990

Gadow KD: Clinical issues in child and adolescent psychopharmacology. J Consult Clin Psychol 59:842–852, 1991

Gesell AL: Mental Growth of the Pre-School Child. New York, Macmillan, 1925

Gesell AL: First Five Years of Life. New York, Harper Brothers, 1930

Gesell AL: Guidance of Mental Growth in the Infant and Child. New York, Macmillan, 1940

Gordon CT, State RC, Nelson JE, et al: A double-blind comparison of clomipramine, desipramine, and placebo in the treatment of autistic disorder. Arch Gen Psychiatry 50:441–457, 1993

Harris CV, Wiebe DJ: An analysis of response prevention and flooding procedures in the treatment of adolescent obsessive-compulsive disorder. J Behav Ther Exp Psychiatry 23:107–115, 1992

Honjo S, Hirane C, Murase S, et al: Obsessive-compulsive symptoms in childhood and adolescence. Acta Psychiatr Scand 80:83–91, 1989

Hurley AD, Sovner R: Diagnosis and treatment of compulsive behaviors in mentally retarded persons. Psychiatric Aspects of Mental Retardation Reviews 3:37–40, 1984

Judd LL: Obsessive-compulsive states in childhood. Arch Gen Psychiatry 12:136–143, 1965

Kanner L: The concepts of wholes and parts in early infantile autism. Am J Psychiatry 108:23–26, 1951

King NJ, Tonge BJ: Obsessive-compulsive disorder in children and adolescents: clinical syndrome and treatment. Scand J Behav Ther 20:91–99, 1991

Leonard HL, Rapoport JL: Pharmacotherapy of childhood obsessive-compulsive disorder. Psychiatr Clin North Am 12:963–970, 1989

Leonard HL, Swedo SE, Rapoport JL, et al: Treatment of obsessive-compulsive disorder with clomipramine and desipramine in children and adolescents: a double-blind crossover comparison. Arch Gen Psychiatry 46:1088–1092, 1989

Leonard HL, Goldberger EL, Rapoport JL, et al: Childhood rituals: normal development or obsessive-compulsive symptoms? J Am Acad Child Adolesc Psychiatry 29:17–23, 1990

Leonard HL, Swedo SE, Lenane MC, et al: A double-blind desipramine substitution during long-term clomipramine treatment in children and adolescents with obsessive-compulsive disorder. Arch Gen Psychiatry 48:922–927, 1991

Neziroglu FA, Yaryura-Tobias JA, Lemli J, et al: Estudio demografico del trastorno obseso compulsivo. Acta Psiquiatr Psicol Am Lat 40:217–223, 1994

O'Dwyer J, Holmes J, Collacott RA: Two cases of obsessive-compulsive disorder in individuals with Down's syndrome. J Nerv Ment Dis 180:603–604, 1992

Phillips B, Wolpe S: Multiple behavioral techniques in severe separation anxiety of a twelve year-old. J Behav Ther Exp Psychiatry 12:329–332, 1981

Piacentini J, Jeffer M, Gitow A, et al: Psychopharmacologic treatment of child and adolescent obsessive-compulsive disorders. Psychiatr Clin North Am 15: 87–107, 1992

Piaget J: Construction of Reality in Children. New York, Basic Books, 1954

Regner IG: Obsessive-compulsive neurosis in children. Acta Psychiatr Neurol 34:110–125, 1959

Rettew DC, Swedo SE, Leonard HL, et al: Obsession and compulsions across time in 79 children and adolescents with obsessive compulsive disorders. J Am Acad Child Adolesc Psychiatry 1:1050–1056, 1992

Riddle MA, Hardin MT, Ling R, et al: Fluoxetine treatment of children and adolescents with Tourette's and obsessive-compulsive disorder: preliminary clinical experience. J Am Acad Child Adolesc Psychiatry 29:45–48, 1990

Riddle MA, Scahill L, King RA, et al: Double-blind, cross-over trial of fluoxetine and placebo in children and adolescents with obsessive-compulsive disorder. J Am Acad Child Adolesc Psychiatry 31:1062–1069, 1992

Rutter M, Lockyer L: A five-to-fifteen year follow-up study of infantile psychosis: description of sample. Br J Psychiatry 113:1169–1182, 1967

Ryan RM: Treatment-resistant chronic mental illness: is it Asperger's syndrome? Hosp Community Psychiatry 43:807–811, 1992

Schatzberg AF: Dosing strategies for antidepressant agents. J Clin Psychiatry 52: 14–20, 1991

Silver AA: Children in classes for the severely emotionally handicapped. J Dev Behav Pediatr 5:49–54, 1984

Simeon JG, Thatte S, Wiggins D: Treatment of adolescent obsessive-compulsive disorder with a clomipramine-fluoxetine combination. Psychopharmacol Bull 26:285–290, 1990

Simons JM: Observations on compulsive behavior in autism. J Autism Child Schizophr 4:1–10, 1974

Swedo SE, Leonard HL, Rapoport JL: Childhood-onset obsessive-compulsive disorder. Psychiatr Clin North Am 15:767–775, 1992

Thomsen PH: Obsessive-compulsive symptoms in children and adolescents: a phenomenological analysis of 61 Danish cases. Psychopathology 24:12–18, 1991

Thomsen PH, Mikkelson HU: Children and adolescents with obsessive-compulsive disorders: the demographic and diagnostic characteristics of 61 Danish patients. Acta Pediatr Scand 83:262–266, 1991

Thyer BA: Diagnosis and treatment of child and adolescent anxiety disorders. Behav Modif 15:310–325, 1991

Vikar G: Zwangsneurose und Kinheit. Psyche 31:1133–1143, 1977

Wadlington WB, Rose M, Holcomb GW: Complications of trichobezoars: a 30-year experience. South Med J 85:1020–1022, 1992

Warneke LB: Intravenous chlorimipramine in the treatment of obsessional disorder in an adolescence case report. J Clin Psychiatry 46:100–103, 1985

Yaryura-Tobias JA: Chlorimipramine in Gilles de la Tourette's syndrome (letter). Am J Psychiatry 132:1221, 1975

Yaryura-Tobias JA: Gilles de la Tourette's syndrome: interactions with other neuropsychiatric disorders. Acta Psychiatr Scand 59:9–16, 1979

Yaryura-Tobias JA, Neziroglu FA: Gilles de la Tourette's syndrome: a new clinico-therapeutic approach. Prog Neuropsychopharmacol 1:335–338, 1977

Zohar AH, Ratzoni G, Pauls DL: An epidemiological study of obsessive-compulsive disorders and related disorders in Israeli adolescents. J Am Acad Child Adolesc Psychiatry 31:1057–1061, 1992

Chapter 4
Assessment Tools

Blood Chemistry Tests and Urinalyses

Routine blood chemistry tests and urinalyses of patients with obsessive-compulsive disorder (OCD) are done to obtain a baseline for future reference or to rule out any biological malfunction (e.g., liver abnormality) that may interfere with treatment. Results of these tests, including red and white blood cell count; liver profile; lipid profile; and determinations of electrolyte, urea, glucose, and iron levels, are usually within normal ranges. In most OCD patients, the thyroid profile, including thyroid-stimulating hormone levels, also appears to be normal. A 5-hour oral glucose tolerance test, which is a measure of the ability to metabolize carbohydrates, often yields a functional hypoglycemic response.

Vitamins, as a coenzyme function, have been measured in several studies, and deficiencies or dependency on them have been reported. In a 30-patient sample with OCD, vitamin B_{12} serum levels were found to be abnormally low (20% below normal) (Hermesh et al. 1988). In another study, vitamin B_6 status and levels of its coenzyme pyridoxal phosphate were altered in a small sample of four patients with OCD (Russ et al. 1983).

Biological Markers

Amine Profile

The serotonin OCD hypothesis initiated many studies searching for biological markers that could cast light on OCD pathology. Neurotransmitter levels were the leading factors assessed; blood levels of serotonin, norepinephrine, L-tryptophan, 5-hydroxytryptophan, and phenylethylamine were measured. Neurotransmitters and their metabolites also have been measured in the urine and spinal fluid (see Chapter 13).

Biological Challenges

Biological challenges aim to study OCD pathophysiology by measuring responses to substances known to modify biological parameters that are theoretically associated with OCD. These challenges are used to study depression and other neuropsychiatric conditions. The dexamethasone suppression test, which is widely used in major affective disorders, also was tested in OCD patients, with equivocal results. So far, no pathognomonic assay has been shown to be valid (see Chapter 13).

Electroencephalography

Most of the seminal work done by applying electroencephalography (EEG) in OCD has detected an association between OCD and seizure disorders (see Chapter 12). Topographic brain mapping indicates a left hemispherical dysfunction, mostly localized in the temporal region (Okasha and Raafat 1990), the left posterior frontal to mid-temporal region (Perros et al. 1992), and the bitemporal region (Aslanov 1970). Of a 12–OCD patient sample, one-third had temporal abnormalities (Jenike and Brotman 1984). In elderly individuals with OCD, quantitative electroencephalogram revealed lower log absolute power in the δ, β_1, and β_2 bandwidths at frontal and right hemisphere locations in OCD patients. OCD patients displayed greater hemispheric asymmetries indicative of severe right hemispheric EEG hypoactivity (Kuskowski et al. 1993). A controlled clinical study using EEG power spectra results in OCD children and adolescents indicated a frontotemporal dysfunction in both females and males (Knolker 1988). Further temporal lobe abnormality evidence was found in a family with three children suffering from OCD (Silverman and Loychik 1990). One report on EEG and sleeping patterns showed that REM latency is reduced in OCD patients (Souetre 1990).

In general, the clinical EEG is nonspecific for OCD. However, a baseline EEG helps rule out a seizure disorder, the presence of cortical hyperexcitability, or an anatomical brain lesion and is beneficial when prescribing an anti–obsessive-compulsive medication that may trigger a seizure (e.g., clomipramine).

Neuroradiology

The development of equipment that makes a brain image accessible to the naked eye was a milestone in neuropsychiatry. OCD research has benefited from it, and gradually clinical applications are being drawn.

Magnetic resonance imaging (MRI) is helpful in observing structural changes in the brain of OCD patients. MRI scans in patients with OCD show prolongation of the spin-lattice relaxation time (T1) and greater right-minus-left differences for frontal white matter. Furthermore, right-minus-left T1 differences in the orbital frontal cortex strongly correlate with symptom severity (Garber et al. 1989).

Computed tomography was used to analyze the brain volume of severe OCD patients with OCD and showed that the caudate nucleus volume was significantly less in OCD patients than in control subjects (Luxenburg et al. 1988). Another study shows that the bicaudate ratio, the bifrontal ratio, and the bifrontal distance divided by the bicaudate distance are fairly good measures of caudate atrophy but poor measures of caudate size when no atrophy is present (Aylward et al. 1991). Patients studied include those with autism, Huntington's disease, and OCD. Huntington's disease patients have the largest bicaudate ratio, bifrontal ratio, and frontal horn area. Some clinical comments pertaining to Huntington's disease and OCD are made in Chapter 12.

In one study, no significant differences were reported between patients with major psychiatric disorders, including OCD, and a control group, except for patients with major depression (Brown et al. 1992). Another report on 12 OCD patients showed no differences in brain structures (head of the caudate nucleus, cingulate gyrus thickness, intracaudate-to-frontal horn ratio, and area of the corpus callosum) when compared with a control group (Kellner et al. 1991).

Indications for MRI or computed tomography include 1) to rule a brain lesion in patients with late-onset OCD (after age 50 years), 2) in cases refractory to treatment, 3) in patients with concrete thinking or illness indifference, and 4) in OCD patients with concomitant neurological disorders or mental retardation.

Assessment Tools

To date, there are few reliable and valid OCD tests. The earliest psychological instruments used were the Minnesota Multiphasic Personality Inventory (Hathaway and McKinley 1951), the Cornell Health Questionnaire (Brodman et al. 1956), and the Maudsley Personality Inventory (Eysenck 1959). These tests contain several items pertaining to obsessional or perfectionistic traits, but none adequately covers the wide range of OCD symptoms. In addition, none were developed to diagnose or assess the severity of OCD.

In 1960 Sandler and Hazari developed the Tavistock Self-Assessment Inventory. However, the items' content was nonspecific; hence, Cooper (1970) developed the Leyton Obsessional Inventory, in which he included some of Sandler and Hazari's items.

Before proceeding with the most commonly used scales in assessing OCD and related disorders, it is important to state that any test used must demonstrate reliability and validity. Scales may be divided into two types; self-rated and clinician administered. The major problem with self-rated scales is they rely on the patient's self-perception. Self-rating scales are often unreliable, because patients do not accurately report their symptoms and the responses often are biased. The problem most frequently found in OCD patients is their indecisiveness, which interferes with the ability to report symptoms. They doubt their responses and keep changing them or explain them at great length.

Self-Rated Scales

Leyton Obsessional Inventory. The Leyton Obsessional Inventory is a card-sorting procedure requiring a simple yes/no reply to 69 questions (Cooper 1970). It diagnoses obsessional symptoms and personality traits. However, Cooper has suggested that it also may assess change in obsessional symptoms during treatment. Thus, although unintended, it has clinical usage. Compared with previously published questionnaires, it gives more detailed and extensive coverage to obsessional complaints. It places particular emphasis on domestic topics, such as household cleanliness and tidiness, and less on more unusual symptoms, such as aggressive, sexual, and religious obsessions.

The questions can be categorized as 1) symptom questions (thoughts, checking, dirt and contamination, dangerous objects, personal cleanliness and tidiness, order and routine, repetition, overconscientiousness and lack of satisfaction, and indecision) or 2) trait questions (hoarding, cleanliness, meanness, irritability and moroseness, rigidity, health, regularity, and punctuality).

The original card-sorting procedure was modified into a written test to facilitate administration (Snowdon 1980), but many clinicians still use the old procedure. The Leyton Obsessional Inventory obtains three different scores: 1) a "yes" score for symptoms and traits, 2) a resistance score, and 3) an interference score. The obsessional symptom score differentiates among various diagnostic groups, whereas resistance and interference scores are additional aids in discriminating between high-scoring nonobsessive patients and the few low-scoring obsessional patients.

Table 4–1 reviews this scale's positive and negative aspects. The disadvantages seem to outweigh the advantages.

Maudsley Obsessive-Compulsive Inventory. The Maudsley Obsessive-Compulsive Inventory (MOCI) is a 30-item true/false self-rated questionnaire devised by Hodgson and Rachman (1977). The items were selected from a larger pool of 65 items that differentiate obsessional patients from control patients and obsessional symptoms from obsessional personality traits. A possible acquiescent response set was avoided by having half the items keyed true and half keyed false. A principal components analysis performed on the MOCI, using 100 severe obsessional patients, identified checking, cleaning, slowness, and doubting. A fifth component was ignored because it comprised two items concerning ruminations and unwanted thoughts.

The MOCI yields a total obsessionality score and four subtotal scores reflecting checking, cleaning, slowness, and doubting. The total score's test-retest reliability was determined by giving the test to 50 night school attenders. The questionnaire was given on two occasions 1 month apart. The test-retest reliability may be questioned because it was determined in night school attenders rather than in an obsessive-compulsive group, whose reliability

Table 4–1.   Critical evaluation of the Leyton Obsessional Inventory

Positive aspects	Negative aspects
1. Comprehensive.	1. Requires 2 hours to administer.

2. Gives three scores:
  a. Symptom, trait
  b. Resistance
  c. Interference.
	2. Lacks reliability.

3. Extensive usage and more comprehensive than preceding questionnaires.	3. Lacks validity.
	4. Omits morbid thought questions.
	5. Omits direct hand washing.
	6. Total score may be misleading.
	7. Not developed for obsessive-compulsive patients.
	8. Does not give accurate reflection of change with treatment.
	9. Lacks questions on bizarre symptoms.

might be different. For example, considering that obsessive-compulsive individuals are indecisive, their answers may differ on two testing occasions.

The total score's validity was determined by correlating it with the Leyton Obsessional Inventory symptoms score ($r = .60$). Hodgson and Rachman further validated the questionnaire by assessing how sensitive it was to obsessive-compulsive behavior changes after treatment. The difference between 40 patients' pretreatment and posttreatment scores was correlated with improvement ratings by both patients and two therapists. With pretreatment scores covaried out, correlations ranged from .53 to .74. Hodgson and Rachman attempted to validate subtest scores; although they discussed four components, they considered only checking and cleaning subtest scores to be accurate. Both slowness and doubting have only two strongly loaded items and two to three other items that pertain to these subtests. For slowness, the two strongest loading items concern ruminations, both loaded negatively; three questions pertain directly to slowness. Thus, it is questionable whether the component should be labeled "slowness," based on these three questions. The doubting component has only two high-loading items related directly to doubting and two concerned with honesty. Because item selection is biased toward checking and cleaning compulsions, patients with these problems may score higher than those with other obsessions and/or compulsions, even though the latter group may be just as severely ill. The MOCI does not seem sensitive to treatment change. In two fluvoxamine drug trial studies, there was a small but significant decrease in MOCI scores (Goodman et al. 1989a; Perse et al. 1987). The lack of sensitivity may be attributed to the test's true/false structure. The questionnaire's negative and positive aspects are shown in Table 4–2.

Neziroglu–Yaryura-Tobias Obsessive-Compulsive Questionnaire. After carefully evaluating several OCD rating scales, we observed that many did not assess several aspects of the broad OCD spectrum. These aspects include abnormal cognitive processes, speech pattern changes, compulsive eating habits, abnormal movements, dysperceptions, and morbid thoughts, among others. Consequently, in 1979 we began to construct the Neziroglu–Yaryura-Tobias (NYT) Obsessive-Compulsive Questionnaire. A Likert-type scale was designed consisting of 70 items, with questions directed at assessing compulsivity, obsessionality, perceptual deficits, and personality factors consistent with OCD. To establish test-retest reliability, the questionnaire was administered 2 weeks apart to 50 OCD patients, and a .98 correlation

Table 4–2. Critical evaluation of the Maudsley Obsessive-Compulsive
Questionnaire

Positive aspects	Negative aspects
1. Easy and quick to administer.	1. Paucity of time sampling.
2. Reliability and validity established.	2. Ruminations and unwanted thoughts not represented.
	3. Two of the four components are not accurately assessed.
	4. Reliability not determined in an obsessive-compulsive population.
	5. Too many items pertain to checking and cleaning.
	6. Not sensitive enough to change with treatment.

was found. In addition, 143 patients with OCD rated themselves on the NYT Obsessive-Compulsive Questionnaire and the MOCI. Exploratory factor analysis suggested that a four-factor solution exists for the constructed scale, encompassing the four proposed scales. Cronbach's α suggests that the perceptual subscale is most reliable ($r = .92$), with compulsions ($r = .86$) and obsessions ($r = .79$) also demonstrating adequate reliability. The personality subscale was not adequate ($r = .58$). A path analysis was conducted to better establish the scales' relationship. The model suggested that obsessions relate significantly to perceptual deficits ($r = .77$). None of the scales significantly relates to the MOCI (Neziroglu F, Yaryura-Tobias JA, McKay D, unpublished manuscript, September 1994) Based on these analyses, the constructed scale seems reliable but assesses aspects of OCD that are unrelated to traditional conceptions of the condition. This finding is consistent with current literature identifying OCD as a disorder sharing more of its pathology with perceptual and cognitive aberrations and less with anxiety disorders (Yaryura-Tobias et al. 1994). Because this questionnaire was not used and tested extensively, evaluation of its advantages and disadvantages is premature.

Compulsive Activity Checklist. The Compulsive Activity Checklist was developed by Hallam and then published by Philpott (1975). It consists of 62 items of daily activities that OCD patients may have difficulty performing. Patients rate, on a 1- to 4-point scale, the degree to which their obsessive-compulsive behavior interferes with their functioning. The scale has been used effectively in many studies to assess treatment effect (Foa and Steketee

1984). A shorter version consisting of 38 items was devised by Freund et al. (1987). For this version, the test-retest reliability (*r*) was .68, and internal consistency was high ($\alpha = 0.91$). Their factor analysis revealed two components: washing/cleanliness and checking/repetitive acts. To establish normative data that may be important in evaluating clinical significance, the Compulsive Activity Checklist was administered to 579 American college students (Sternberger and Burns 1990). Internal consistency was good ($\alpha = 0.86$), and three factors were found: washing, checking, and personal hygiene. The checklist helps assess performance difficulties and changes with treatment, and it is easy to administer. However, it does not evaluate many important symptoms that are unrelated to daily activities.

Behavior Measurement Chart (fear thermometer). The Behavior Measurement Chart, or Self Monitoring Rituals Scale, was devised by Foa and Steketee at Temple University (E. B. Foa and G. Steketee, personal communication, June 1978). Patients record their activities for each day, from the time they awaken to when they go to sleep; any obsession or compulsion they engage in, the amount of time spent, and the degree of discomfort are rated on a scale of 1 to 10 (Wolpe 1958). The behavior measurement chart is kept for 1 week to attain a fair estimate of the patient's discomfort level and symptom severity. We often find that patients do not record their passive avoidance activities and consequently underestimate their dysfunctionality. For example, patients who avoid touching contaminated objects, therefore avoiding washing and appear to function better than they actually do function. For this reason, we advise patients to record not only their obsessions and compulsions, but also any normal activity they avoid. Reliability and validity measures are not available for this instrument. However, it is informative for spectrum disorders.

Clinician-Administered Tests

Yale-Brown Obsessive Compulsive Scale. The Yale-Brown Obsessive Compulsive Scale (Y-BOCS), currently the most popular scale, measures symptom severity and assesses change with treatment without being influenced by the number and type of obsessions and compulsions (Goodman et al. 1989a, 1989b, 1989c). It is a 16-item scale, 10 of which make up the scale's core. Five of these 10 items pertain to obsessions and five to compulsions. The sum of the 10 items is reported as the total score. The other six items include insight (overvalued ideation), avoidance, indecisiveness, sense of responsibility, slowness, and pathological doubt. The first five questions of each subscale assess time spent on obsessions or compulsions, interference, distress, resistance, and control. Each item is rated on a 0 to 4 scale, where 0 corresponds to no symptoms and 4 to extreme symptoms. An asset of this scale is that it relies not on symptom quantity, but quality. Because it does not describe OCD symptoms, the clinician administering the Y-BOCS must be well versed with the disorder to properly evaluate patients and score items. A symptom checklist allows the clinician to review symptoms with patients, but unless he or she is acquainted with OCD symptoms, it is hard to make an assessment. In formulating this scale, Goodman et al. (1989b, 1989c) reported high interrater reliability ($r = .98$) and internal consistency ($\alpha = 0.89$). To establish discriminant and convergent validity, the Y-BOCS was compared with the MOCI; the National Institute of Mental Health Global Obsessive-Compulsive Scale (Insel et al. 1983a; Murphy et al. 1982); the Clinical Global Impression Scale, adapted for OCD (Guy 1976); and the Hamilton Scales for Anxiety (Hamilton 1959) and Depression (Hamilton 1960). The validity data have moderate correlations (range, $r = .67–.74$). These data are limited to the extent the factor structure is delineated, and the sample was small for several correlations. This limitation has not prevented widespread application of this scale and modified versions of it to OCD-related disorders.

Stanley et al. (1992) reported the reliability of the Y-BOCS in assessing trichotillomania. McKay and Neziroglu (1993) and Neziroglu et al. (1993) discussed the utility of the Y-BOCS for assessing hypochondriasis and body dysmorphic disorder, respectively, and suggested modifying particular items, because the scale does not adequately address the particulars of these disorders' symptom complex.

These studies also call for more basic psychometric research into the nature of the Y-BOCS and its relation to other scales commonly used to assess OCD. A factor analysis study of the Y-BOCS with patients indicated that its structure is robust for a two-factor model (McKay et al. 1993). This finding contradicts the current Y-BOCS structure and suggests that the total scale score is a poor index. Instead, the obsessions and compulsions subscales should be viewed as distinct constructs possessing overlapping features. This finding is important, because clinical significance with the Y-BOCS is generally assessed by the total score and must be established against the separate constructs. This finding lends greater credence to OCD's multidimensionality (Yaryura-Tobias and Neziroglu 1983) and substantiates Neziroglu–Yaryura-Tobias Obsessive-Compulsive Questionnaire findings that OCD is more than the composite of obsessions and compulsions.

The Y-BOCS has been converted to an interactive computer-administered format (Rosenfeld et al. 1992), and it correlates highly with the clinician-administered version and may be preferred by some patients. It is a good instrument for assessing OCD severity. Its positive and negative aspects are shown in Table 4–3.

Overvalued Ideas Scale.   To assess the degree to which OCD patients with body dysmorphic disorder and hypochondriasis hold on to their fears and/or beliefs, a scale was devised by F. Neziroglu, J. A. Yaryura-Tobias, and D. McKay (personal communication, January 1994). Patients report their three main obsessional beliefs (e.g., "my nose is too big"; "I am contaminated by germs or AIDS"; "if I don't check the stove, I will start a fire"). They then rate themselves, on a scale of 1 to 10, on the following questions:

- How strong is your belief?
- How reasonable is your belief?
- In the past week, what was the lowest rating for these beliefs?
- In the past week, what was the highest rating for these beliefs?
- How inaccurate is your belief?
- How likely is it that others have the same beliefs about your situation?
- If other people do not have these beliefs, to what do you attribute this?

Table 4–3.   Critical evaluation of the Yale-Brown Obsessive Compulsive Scale (Y-BOCS)

Positive aspects	Negative aspects
1. Reliability established.	1. Clinician must be well versed in symptoms of obsessive-compulsive disorder.
2. Validity partly established.	2. Validity data correlations are moderate, and sample sizes are small.
3. Not dependent on number	3. Total score is a poor index. or type of symptoms to derive severity.
4. Allows assessment of change with treatment.	

- What is the likelihood or probability of your compulsions/ritualistic behaviors being effective?
- Compared with others, how unusual is your belief?

This rating is done for each of the nine beliefs. A score for each and a total score for all beliefs are obtained. Test-retest reliability, internal consistency, and validity constructs are currently being established.

Other Relevant Tests

Exposure test.   The exposure test is similar to the avoidance test. The patient is exposed to his or her most feared item, situation, or person. Discomfort levels may be obtained by varying exposure according to 1) the distance in feet from the feared item, 2) the amount of hand insulation before touching the item (e.g., the number of paper towels used), or 3) the amount of time in direct contact with the feared item.

Social Adjustment Scale.   Gelder and Marks (1966) evaluated the social adjustment of phobic patients in several spheres. The patient's symptom interference was assessed in the following areas: sexual activities, family relationships, social and private leisure activities, home management, and work interference. Each item on the scale is rated from 0 to 8, with five headings: not at all, slightly, definitely, markedly, and severely.

Rachman et al. (1971) used the same scale with an obsessive-compulsive population. The reliability coefficient was not determined for the OCD group. However, Gelder and Marks (1966) found that the correlation coefficient for phobic patients in the various functional areas ranged from .73 to .58. Although these are fairly low correlation coefficients, they may not be the same for obsessional patients.

Certainly instruments for assessing functioning level need to be developed and used in all studies investigating treatment change. This is an important but grossly neglected area.

Neuropsychological testing.   Neuropsychological test data have made significant contributions to the development of hypotheses about abnormal brain structure and function in patients with psychiatric disorders. Although neuroimaging better diagnoses abnormal brain structure, neuropsychological tests are useful in providing treatment strategies tailored for an individual's specific cognitive strengths and deficits (Keefe 1995).

Neuropsychological OCD studies may help identify the cognitive impairments most associated with the development of OCD or the specific brain areas impaired by OCD. Two impaired areas in OCD patients are the frontal lobe and memory. The link between frontal lobe dysfunction and OCD was presented by Flor Henry (1983) and Malloy (1987). Flor Henry suggested a loss of inhibitory processes in the dominant frontal lobe in OCD. Malloy stated that OCD is a consequence of orbital medial dysfunction or an interruption in the dorsolateral limbic pathways. His hypothesis was substantiated by evoked potential differences in OCD patients compared with control patients (Malloy 1987) and by increased glucose metabolism in the left orbitofrontal gyrus and the caudate nucleus (Baxter et al. 1987).

Neuropsychological test findings indicate bilateral left frontal dysfunction (Behar et al. 1984; Flor Henry et al. 1979; Malloy 1987). None of these authors found memory deficits. However, Sher et al. (1983, 1984, 1989) found that incidental memory for actions assessed by the Cognitive Failures Questionnaire (Broadbent et al. 1982) was poorer in students and patients with high-frequency checking behavior. This test is a self-report measure of deficits in memory, perception, and motor functioning in natural settings. However, these findings did not hold for general memory deficit. The difference between researchers who found memory impairment in OCD patients and those who did not may be attributed to the assessment method used, rather than to actual differences in memory dysfunction in the patients studied. Individuals are more likely to report memory problems on self-report measures than on tests that rely on performance.

Frontal lobe dysfunction may interrupt communication of action completion to the subcortical systems. In addition to frontal lobe dysfunction and memory, the basal ganglia's role was investigated (Baxter et al. 1987, 1988; Luxenburg et al. 1988; Modell et al. 1989; Pitman 1989; Weilburg et al. 1989). The basal ganglia is crucial in regulating sensory input to motor output; thus, disrupting it results in an inability to discard irrelevant information and to process incoming stimuli properly. Consequently, individuals may exhibit inappropriate cognitive and emotional responses, resulting in obsessive-compulsive behaviors. In the basal ganglia, the caudate nucleus, along with the frontal lobe, is the primary location of OCD pathogenesis.

Few studies report on the neuropsychological test findings of OCD patients. Insel et al. (1983a) found impairment on the tactual performance of the Halstead-Reitan Neuropsychological Test Battery (Reitan 1979), suggesting a possible spatial perception deficit. Consistent with neuropsychological deficits, they also noted a large verbal-minus-performance IQ difference on the Wechsler Adult Intelligence Scale and a high

Halstead-Reitan Battery average impairment rating in a four-patient subgroup. In another study using the Halstead-Reitan Neuropsychological Test Battery, 53% of OCD patients were in the borderline range for brain damage (Neziroglu et al. 1988). There was impairment in the tests of tactual performance, finger oscillation, and category. The tactual performance test's time component also was impaired. Unlike Insel et al.'s (1983a) study using the Wechsler Adult Intelligence Scale—Revised (Wechsler 1987), no difference was noted between the verbal (mean score = 102) and performance (mean score = 95) subtests. Historically, it was believed that OCD patients had superior intelligence, primarily in verbal function. Left hemisphere functions were considered more dominant than right hemisphere functions. Given the limited evidence for left hemispheric overactivation and superior performance on verbal tasks, the role of hemispheric laterality in mediating visuospatial deficits also is less convincing (Otto 1992). Neuropsychological data are far from consistent regarding hemispheric malfunctioning. Flor Henry et al. (1979) reported a left frontal malfunction, but this result has not been replicated. Later, a right hemisphere malfunction (Behar et al. 1984) was reported, yet others found no lateralized dysfunctions (Insel et al. 1983a).

Neuropsychological performances on the Luria Nebraska Neuropsychological Battery in 10 OCD patients, 10 schizophrenic patients, and 10 control patients indicated no differences between OCD patients and control patients (Bellini et al. 1989). The schizophrenic group showed the poorest performance on the localization and right temporal scales compared with the OCD and control groups. It seems that despite the current research investigating the similarities in cognitive functions of patients with OCD and schizophrenia, the two groups do not demonstrate similar performance on neuropsychological tests.

Neuropsychological functioning was examined in 18 nondepressed 18-year-old OCD patients along with education- and gender-matched control patients (Christensen et al. 1992). From performance on timed and untimed construct measures, it appears that OCD patients score more poorly than control patients when testing speed. Although performance on a timed tactual spatial motor test also is impaired in OCD patients, it is unclear whether this deficit is attributable to nonverbal memory, speed deficits, or both. We observed that timed tasks are difficult for patients, and when given extra time, they successfully complete them. Thus, impairment most often relates to speed. In another neuropsychological study, impairment was observed on visual-spatial recall tests, recognition, and sequencing (Zielinski et al. 1991). Patients performed as well as control subjects on verbal tasks and measures of frontal lobe functioning.

One study investigated neuropsychological test performance in patients with trichotillomania, one of the obsessive-compulsive spectrum disorders (Rettew et al. 1991). Two tests—the Road Map Test (Money et al. 1965) and the Stylus Maze—were administered to patients with trichotillomania, to sex-matched groups with OCD or other anxiety disorders, and to control subjects. The trichotillomania group had significantly more errors than control patients on the Stylus Maze but not on the Road Map test. In the trichotillomania group, errors on the two tasks correlated with symptom severity and clomipramine improvement. The OCD group also broke more Stylus Maze rules compared with the control group. Similarities were noted between response style of the OCD and trichotillomania groups, suggesting a link between the two.

References

Aslanov AS: Correlation between cortical potentials in patients with obsessive neuroses, in Electrophysiology of the Central Nervous System. Edited by VS Rusinov. Translated by Haigh B. New York, Plenum, 1970, pp 39–47

Aylward EH, Schwartz J, Machlin S, et al: Bicaudate ratio as a measure of caudate volume on MR images. Am J Neuroradiol 12:1217–1222, 1991

Baxter LR, Phelps ME, Mazziotta TC: Local cerebral glucose metabolic rates in obsessive-compulsive disorder. Arch Gen Psychiatry 44:211–218, 1987

Baxter LR, Schwartz JM, Mazziotta JC, et al: Cerebral glucose metabolic rates in nondepressed patients with obsessive-compulsive disorder. Am J Psychiatry 145:1560–1563, 1988

Behar D, Rapoport JL, Berg CJ, et al: Computerized tomography and neuropsychological test measures in adolescents with obsessive-compulsive disorder. Am J Psychiatry 141:363–369, 1984

Bellini L, Massironi R, Palladino F, et al: Obsessive-compulsive disorders. Neurofunctional Assessment Research Communications in Psychology, Psychiatry and Behavior 14:73–83, 1989

Broadbent D, Cooper P, Fitzgerald P, et al: The Cognitive Failures Questionnaire (CFQ) and its correlates. Br J Clin Psychol 21:1–16, 1982

Brodman K, Deutschenberger J, Wolff HG: Manual for the Cornell Medical Index Health Questionnaire. New York, Cornell University Medical College, 1956

Brown FW, Lewine RJ, Hudgins PA, et al: White matter hyperintensity signals in psychiatric and nonpsychiatric subjects. Am J Psychiatry 149:620–625, 1992

Christensen KJ, Kim SW, Dysken MW, et al: Neuropsychological performance in obsessive-compulsive disorder. Biol Psychiatry 31:4–18, 1992

Cooper JE: The Leyton Obsessional Inventory. Psychol Med 1:48–64, 1970

Eysenck HJ: Manual of the Maudsley Personality Inventory. London, Methuen, 1959

Flor Henry P: Cerebral Basis of Psychopathology. Boston, MA, John Wright, 1983

Flor Henry P, Yeudall LT, Koles ZJ, et al: Neuropsychological and power spectral EEG investigations of the obsessive-compulsive syndrome. Biol Psychiatry 14:119–130, 1979

Foa EB, Steketee G: Behavioral treatment of obsessive-compulsive ritualizers, in New Findings in Obsessive-Compulsive Disorder. Edited by Insel TR. Washington, DC, American Psychiatric Press, 1984, pp 46–69

Freund B, Steketee GS, Foa EB: Compulsive Activity Checklist (CAC): psychometric analysis with obsessive-compulsive disorder. Behavioral Assessment 9: 67–79, 1987

Garber HJ, Ananth JV, Chiu LC, et al: Nuclear magnetic resonance study of obsessive-compulsive disorder. Am J Psychiatry 146:1001–1005, 1989

Gelder MG, Marks IM: Severe agoraphobia: a controlled prospective trial of behavior therapy. Br J Psychiatry 112:309–319, 1966

Goodman WK, Price LH, Rasmussen SA, et al: Efficacy of fluvoxamine in obsessive-compulsive disorder: a double blind comparison with placebo. Arch Gen Psychiatry 46:36–44, 1989a

Goodman WK, Price LH, Rasmussen SA, et al: The Yale-Brown Obsessive-Compulsive Scale (Y-BOCS). Part 1: development, use, and reliability. Arch Gen Psychiatry 46:1006–1011, 1989b

Goodman WK, Price LH, Rasmussen SA, et al: The Yale-Brown Obsessive-Compulsive Scale (Y-BOCS). Part 2: validity. Arch Gen Psychiatry 46:1012–1016, 1989c

Guy W: ECDEU Assessment Manual for Psychopharmacology (Publ no 76-338). Washington, DC, U.S. Department of Health, Education and Welfare, 1976

Hamilton M: The assessment of anxiety states by ratings. Br J Med Psychiatry 32: 50–55, 1959

Hamilton M: A rating scale for depression. J Neurol Neurosurg Psychiatry 23: 56–62, 1960

Hathaway SR, McKinley JC: The MMPI Manual. New York, Psychological Corporation, 1951

Hermesh H, Weizman A, Shahar A, et al: Vitamin B-12 and folic acid serum levels in obsessive-compulsive disorder. Acta Psychiatr Scand 78:8–10, 1988

Hodgson RJ, Rachman S: Obsessional-compulsive complaints. Behav Res Ther 15:389–395, 1977

Insel TR, Donnelly EF, Lalakea ML, et al: Neurological and neuropsychological studies of patients with obsessive-compulsive disorder. Biol Psychiatry 18: 741–751, 1983a

Insel TR, Murphy DL, Cohen RM, et al: Obsessive-compulsive disorder: a double trial of clomipramine and clorgyline. Arch Gen Psychiatry 40:605–612, 1983b

Jenike MA, Brotman AW: The EEG in obsessive-compulsive disorder. J Clin Psychiatry 45:122–124, 1984

Keefe RSE: The contribution of neuropsychology to psychiatry. Am J Psychiatry 152:6–15, 1995

Kellner CH, Jolley RR, Holgate RC, et al: Brain MRI in obsessive-compulsive disorder. Psychiatry Res 36:45–49, 1991

Knolker U: EEG frequency analyses in children and adolescents with obsessive-compulsive neuroses. Z Kinder Jugenpsychiatr 16:180–185, 1988

Kuskowski MA, Malone SM, Kim SW, et al: Quantitative EEG in obsessive-compulsive disorder. Biol Psychiatry 33:423–430, 1993

Luxenburg JS, Swedo SE, Flament MF, et al: Neuroanatomical abnormalities in obsessive-compulsive disorder detected with quantitative x-ray computed tomography. Am J Psychiatry 145:1089–1093, 1988

Malloy P: Frontal lobe dysfunction in obsessive-compulsive disorder, in The Frontal Lobes Revisited. Edited by Perecman E.

McKay D, Neziroglu FA: Hypochondriases: common pathways to obsessive-compulsive disorder. Paper presented at the convention of the Association for Advancement of Behavior Therapy, Atlanta, GA, November 1993

McKay D, Danyko S, Neziroglu F, et al: Factor structure of the Yale-Brown Obsessive Compulsive Scale: a two dimensional measure. Behav Res Ther 33: 865–869, 1993

Modell JG, Mountz JM, Curtis G, et al: Neuropsychologic dysfunction in basal ganglia/limbic striatal and thalamocortical circuits as a pathogenic mechanism of obsessive-compulsive disorder. J Neuropsychiatry 1:27–36, 1989

Money J, Walker HT, Duane A: Development of direction sense and three syndromes of impairment. Slow Learning Child 11:145–155, 1965

Murphy D, Pickar D, Alterman J: Methods for the qualitative assessment of depression and manic behavior, in The Behavior of Psychiatric Patients: Quantitative Techniques for Evaluation. Edited by Burdock E, Sudilovsky A, Gershon S. New York, Marcel Dekker, 1982, pp 355–392

Neziroglu F, Penzel F, Vasquez J, et al: Neuropsychological studies in obsessive-compulsive disorder. Paper presented at the meeting of the Association for Advancement of Behavior Therapy, New York, November 1988

Neziroglu F, McKay D, Yaryura-Tobias JA: Body dysmorphic disorder: is it obsessive-compulsive disorder and should it be treated the same? Paper presented at the convention of the Association for Advancement of Behavior Therapy, Atlanta, GA, November 1993

Okasha A, Raafat M: Neurophysiological substrate of obsessive-compulsive disorder: an evidence from topographic EEG. Egypt J Psychiatry 13:97–106, 1990

Otto MH: Normal and abnormal information proceeding. A neuropsychological perspective on obsessive-compulsive disorder. Psychiatr Clin North Am 15: 825–848, 1992

Perros P, Young ES, Ritson JJ, et al: Power spectral EEG analysis and EEG variability in obsessive-compulsive disorder. Brain Topogr 4:187–192, 1992

Perse TL, Griest JH, Jefferson JW, et al: Fluvoxamine treatment of obsessive-compulsive disorder. Am J Psychiatry 144:1543–1548, 1987

Philpott R: Recent advances in the behavioral measurement of obsessional illness difficulties common to these and other measures. Scott Med J 20:33–40, 1975

Pitman RK: Animal models of compulsive behavior. Biol Psychiatry 26:189–198, 1989

Rachman S, Hodgson R, Marks IM: The treatment of chronic obsessive-compulsive neurosis. Behav Res Ther 9:237–247, 1971

Reitan RM: Halstead-Reitan Neuropsychological Test Battery. Tucson, AZ, Neuro-psychology Laboratory, University of Arizona, 1979

Rettew DC, Cheslow DL, Rapoport JL, et al: Neuropsychological test performance in trichotillomania: a further link with obsessive-compulsive disorder. Journal of Anxiety Disorders 5:225–235, 1991

Rosenfeld R, Dar R, Anderson D, et al: A computer administered version of the Yale-Brown Obsessive-Compulsive Scale. Psychological Assessment 4:329–332, 1992

Russ CS, Thelma A, Hendricks BM, et al: Vitamin B-6 status of depressed and obsessive-compulsive patients. Nutrition Reports International 27:867–873, 1983

Sandler J, Hazari A: The obsessional: on the psychological classification of obsessional character traits and symptoms. Br J Med Psychol 23:113–122, 1960

Sher KJ, Frost RO, Otto R: Cognitive deficits in compulsive checkers: an exploratory study. Behav Res Ther 21:357–363, 1983

Sher KJ, Mann B, Frost RO: Cognitive dysfunction in compulsive checkers: further exploration. Behav Res Ther 22:493–502, 1984

Sher KJ, Frost RO, Kushner M, et al: Memory deficits in compulsive checkers: replication and extension in a clinical sample. Behav Res Ther 27:65–69, 1989

Silverman JS, Loychik SG: Brain-mapping abnormalities in a family with three obsessive-compulsive children. J Neuropsychiatry Clin Neurosci 2:319–322, 1990

Snowdon J: A comparison of written and postbox forms of the Leyton Obsessional Inventory. Psychol Med 10:165–170, 1980

Souetre E: Sleep disorders related to anxiety. Presse Med 19:1839–1841, 1990

Stanley MA, Swann AC, Bowers TC, et al: A comparison of clinical features in trichotillomania and obsessive-compulsive disorder. Behav Res Ther 30:39–44, 1992

Sternberger LG, Burns GL: Compulsive Activity Checklist and Maudsley Obsessional-Compulsive Inventory: psychometric properties of two measures of obsessive-compulsive disorder. Behavior Therapy 21:117–127, 1990

Wechsler D: Wechsler Memory Scale—Revised. San Antonio, TX, Psychological Corporation, 1987

Weilburg JB, Mesulam M, Weintraub S, et al: Focal striatal abnormalities in a patient with obsessive-compulsive disorder. Arch Neurol 46:233–235, 1989

Wolpe J: Psychotherapy by Reciprocal Inhibition. Stanford, CA, Stanford University Press, 1958

Yaryura-Tobias JA, Neziroglu F: Psychological diagnostic assessment, in Obsessive
    Compulsive Disorders: Pathogenesis Diagnosis Treatment. Edited by Yaryura-
    Tobias JA, Neziroglu FA. New York, Marcel Dekker, 1983, pp 51–64

Yaryura-Tobias JA, Campisi TH, McKay D: Unified aspects of obsessive-compulsive
    disorder and schizophrenia. Paper presented at American Psychiatric Associa-
    tion meeting, Philadelphia, PA, May 1994

Zielinski C, Carole M, Taylor M, et al: Neuropsychological deficits in obsessive-
    compulsive disorder. Neuropsychiatry, Neuropsychology and Behavioral Neu-
    rology 4:110–126, 1991

Section II

Neuropsychiatric Disorders Associated With OCD

Section II consists of neuropsychiatric disorders that manifest obsessions and compulsions in their phenomenology. A major characteristic of these disorders is the constant presence of abnormal thought, perception, and motor activity. Their epidemiological history connotes clinical forms compatible as comorbid conditions. However, comorbidity may not be the most important point of their pathology. We believe the association of phenomenological, anatomical, hormonal, and neurohistochemical factors constitutes the main OCD spectrum core. This core may emerge not as comorbidity, but as the representation of one single disease. Another aspect is the integration of the highly developed cortical brain and the primitive brain, as seen in observable behaviors (e.g., compulsions, self-harm).

Chapter 5
Obsessive-Compulsive Disorder and Schizophrenia

Obsessive-compulsive disorder (OCD) and schizophrenia may present clinical or pathophysiological similarities that require attention. These similarities may be found in thought process mechanisms, perceptual changes, motor impairment, confluence of anatomical pathways, and neurotransmitter utilization. Moreover, both conditions may have, in the course of their evolution, a severe psychosocial and economic impact on the patient's wellness.

As we will see in this chapter, a growing interest in the interfaces of these two disorders is taking place. This is a remarkable event, because current investigation may answer questions posted long ago.

Sufficient evidence is available to state that OCD and schizophrenia share some clinical aspects. These aspects include thought, perceptual, and motor pathology. Confirmation of OCD and schizophrenia interfaces or comorbidity is provided by a cohort of clinical studies and epidemiological data. Finally, the concomitant presence of both OCD and schizophrenia calls for therapeutic consideration.

Symptom Manifestation and Alternative Course

Historically, OCD and schizophrenia sometimes coexist or alternate in patients with clinical symptoms attributed to either one of these two entities (Bumke 1906; Claude et al. 1941; Eggers 1969; Jahrreiss 1926; Mignard 1913; Sadoun 1957; Schneider 1939; Stengel 1931; Stern 1930; Sullivan 1956). The main differences between schizophrenia and an OCD are that, in the latter, reality remains intact, insight and awareness of illness are present, symptoms perceived as unreasonable cannot be resisted, and there is an absence of delusions and hallucinations. However, these differences may not be clearly elicited when obsessions, compulsions, and schizophrenic symptoms are detected in both entities. For example, Bleuler (1955), Diathelm

(1955), Wooley (1937), and others have indicated an intimate relationship between both conditions and have implied that obsessive-compulsive neuroses are a function of latent schizophrenia. According to Achkova (1976), an obsessional syndrome may become schizophrenia; therefore, he recommended observing the patient continuously.

The relationship between schizophrenia and OCD also interested Sullivan (1956), who asserted that either condition could shift to the other and then back again. For Rosen (1957) obsessive-compulsive symptoms could appear at the onset or during the course of schizophrenia, and schizophrenic symptoms could appear in an advanced obsessional neurosis. Although Bleuler (1911) and Mayer-Gross (1932) suggested that some patients having chronic obsessional symptoms are schizophrenic, others have stated that compulsive neurosis can be followed by schizophrenia (Gordon 1926; Kringlen 1965; Muller 1953; Rudin 1953; Stengel 1945). The coexistence of both entities also was observed by Birnie and Littmann (1978). Sometimes OCD includes neurotic and psychotic symptoms (Eisen and Rasmussen 1993; Lewis 1936; Pujol and Savy 1968) or appears as an atypical psychosis (Solyom et al. 1985). However, Bratfos et al. (1969), after examining the history of 6,983 patients, concluded that a neurosis rarely generates a psychosis.

We agree with Blanc (1956) that the presence of an obsession as an isolated symptom and without other obsessive-compulsive symptomatology cannot conform a syndrome, which requires the presence of a cluster of symptoms. For example, in the obsessional form of a schizophrenic syndrome, the schizophrenia develops from an obsessional thought, excessive preoccupation, and parasitic ideas. This thought appears alone and the patient's attitude lacks the emotional content seen in obsessive patients. Gradually the patient presents additional symptoms characteristic of schizophrenia. For Sadoun (1957), this onset is common and basically consists of obsessions and moderate amounts of compulsions.

Perhaps an understanding of the basic symptoms of schizophrenia and its reversibility or irreversibility may cast a light on the comorbidity issue. This issue is indirectly addressed in the long-term project of the Bonn Schizophrenia Study (Gross et al. 1986a), which was started by Huber in an inpatient population admitted between 1945 and 1959 with a clear-cut diagnosis of schizophrenia. Part of this study has shown that during the schizophrenia prodromal phase, patients may manifest obsessional perseveration of thoughts and obsessive-compulsive phenomena (Huber and Gross 1989). These findings corroborated previous observations of Westphal (1878). Furthermore,

OCD may appear at different clinical phases of schizophrenia (Huber and Gross 1989).

It has been stated that when compulsive ideation occurs in conjunction with schizophrenia, the symptoms of the latter have an early onset and become prominent among other symptoms (Bleuler 1955). In these cases, once schizophrenia is ruled out, obsessive-compulsive ideas are rarely formed in combination with a true psychosis. Although some authors reject the admixture of OCD and schizophrenia, others accept coexistence as a clinical form (Birnie and Littman 1978; Hwang and Hollander 1993; Insel and Akiskal 1986).

In a current long-term study assessing thought and perceptual pathology in patients with primary OCD or primary schizophrenia without comorbidity, statistically significant similarities have been found in both thought and perceptual pathology. The thought process was characterized by obsessionality, overvalued ideas, and delusions. Dysperceptions were reported as changes in smell and sight, tactile hyperarousal, and bodily changes in shape and size (Yaryura-Tobias et al. 1994, 1995). Of note, symptoms of obsessional melodies or sounds or dysperceptions could be classified as eidetic hallucinations (Ey 1973). This pathology may precede or eventually evolve into an hallucinatory process, as seen in the typical patient with psychosis or schizophrenia. Perception and thought factors also can be associated with the motor disturbances observed in both OCD and schizophrenia. We believe that thought, perception, and motor symptoms may fluctuate from one condition to the next. Body dysmorphic disorder also is a condition that might relate to perceptual and thought changes as manifested in OCD and schizophrenia (Figure 5–1).

Lewis et al. (1991) discussed the dual diagnosis of OCD and schizophrenia in three consecutive twin pairs and concluded that despite the large degree of overlap between these disorders, it may be accurate to consider OCD and schizophrenia separate disorders when symptoms of each exist in the same patient. Rosen (1957) observed more than 800 patients with schizophrenia and reported that 3.5% had obsessive-compulsive symptoms, but only 7 of 30 patients had obsessions that became delusions.

Thought Pathology

In 1951 Rapaport edited a collection on thought pathology. We agree with his preface: "The knowledge that thinking has conquered for humanity is vast, yet our knowledge of thinking is scant" (p. vii).

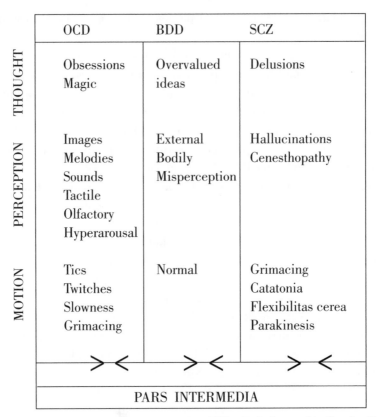

	OCD	BDD	SCZ
THOUGHT	Obsessions Magic	Overvalued ideas	Delusions
PERCEPTION	Images Melodies Sounds Tactile Olfactory Hyperarousal	External Bodily Misperception	Hallucinations Cenesthopathy
MOTION	Tics Twitches Slowness Grimacing	Normal	Grimacing Catatonia Flexibilitas cerea Parakinesis

PARS INTERMEDIA

Figure 5–1.   Putative symptom progression. BDD = Body dysmorphic disorder; SCZ = schizophrenia.

The obsessive thought may be impregnated by a doubtful belief that is clearly independent or interchangeable, whereas the schizophrenic thought is characterized by a belief that is irreplaceable. Nonetheless, the patient with OCD may display pathological beliefs similar to those seen in schizophrenia patients.

There are several types of pathological beliefs or ideas: delusional ideas, delirious ideas, overvalued ideas, and fixed ideas. A *delusional idea* stems from primary pathological experiences or drastic personality changes. A *delirious idea* stems from a psychic process without the personality changes seen in emotions, wishes, fears, and instincts; such ideas include transient misinterpretations, melancholic or manic beliefs (e.g., delusions of sinful nihilism, impoverishment, etc.), and overvalued ideas (Jaspers 1913/1955). An *overvalued idea* (Wernicke 1900) is a transient, strong belief built on an affective foundation, thereby forming a strong bond between the personality and the idea. Overvalued ideas may be seen in healthy or diseased individuals; for example a jealous person, a social reformer, an inventor, and an OCD patient may all have overvalued ideas. A delusional idea is unchangeable, but an overvalued idea is isolated, representing a binding of personality and situation. Finally, a *fixed idea* is an unchangeable thought that usually does not affect the person's everyday life.

As early as 1913, Mignard stated delusions of influence could be present in emotional obsessions; later, Lewis (1936) and Gordon (1960) described a transformation of an obsession into a delusion, an observation that could not be shown by the investigations of Mayer-Gross (1932) and Stengel (1945).

Of note, the OCD and paranoia diagnosis is not adequately addressed conceptually or phenomenologically, as, for example, when dealing with a monosymptomatic hypochondriacal psychosis (Ross et al. 1987) or, as observed, in the fixed ideation of paranoia or paranoic syndromes. We believe that some obsessive patients appear to show an impairment of comprehension that may lead to a misinterpretation of events, which in turn may lead to a pseudoparanoid behavior of distrust and isolation. It also should be remembered that a monosymptomatic obsession is comparable in quality with the paranoid fixed idea. However, the doubtful nature of the obsession, as opposed to the conviction of the paranoid fixed idea, will allow differentiation between them.

The term *paranoid* often is used ambiguously and applied to a variety of processes that should be better differentiated. There are three paranoid processes that have genetic and dynamic sources: 1) paranoid processes resulting from guilt, 2) paranoid processes resulting from low self-esteem, and 3) paranoid processes resulting from a sense of persecution. This topology helps to distinguish a monothematic obsession from a paranoid idea. The persecutory type pertains mostly to the schizophrenic world. Patients with mental automatism remain passive in a situation that they blame on external forces.

Sometimes, in paranoid schizophrenic patients, intrusive and repetitive thinking is similar to the obsessive thinking of obsessive-compulsive patients. In addition, it has been observed that obsessive patients may have a low self-esteem comparable with that described in a paranoid subgroup (Roskin et al. 1977). Moreover, an intense sense of self-consciousness in public may be mistaken for ideas of reference, commonly seen in paranoid disorders.

These beliefs relate to the concept of reality in time and space and become interspersed with reality-unreality cycles that prevent the patient from performing. As a consequence, the schizophrenic patient's world is an accepted chronic, ruined catastrophe, whereas the obsessional patient's world is a chronic interrogation of an apparently harmful society. The schizophrenic patient has a paucity of reality; the obsessive patient preserves his or her reality. The schizophrenic patient withdraws from society for protection; the obsessive patient elaborates defenses by attempting to control it.

One other aspect pertaining to both conditions is "magic thinking." This type of thought has a strong, grandiose quality that puts the patient closer to a divine state and behavior. Paraphrasing Descartes, an OCD patient may say, "I think, ergo I control." The patient then expects that by thinking, he or she may prevent harm. Ritualization can further manifest this omnipotent thought. Furthermore, patients having grandiose delusions may believe they are God.

Finally, one definite schizophrenia characteristic is losing "my-ness" (i.e., thought insertion, broadcasting, commanding voices), whereas in OCD, the thought, although intrusive and against the will, is the patient's.

Case 1

Hank, a 17-year-old male student, comes for consultation because of intense obsessionality and compulsive checking. His symptoms have gradually worsened, making it difficult for him to function well. However, his school work is unaffected, and he is able to socialize with his peer group. Interestingly, his symptoms flare up at home. In his house, he remains in his bedroom; he locks the door when he walks into the bedroom, and he locks the door with a padlock when he walks out. No member of his family is allowed in his bedroom. Inside he keeps the room in almost complete darkness and places towels and papers in the door threshold to prevent light or "others" from entering in his bedroom. When asked who those "others" are, he is elusive. Eventually he admits that it is unrealistic to believe that someone will come in. He does have an impending fear of threat.

Hank wants help and wishes to be healthy like other teenagers. Diagnosed with OCD with delusional features, he is placed on fluoxetine, 80 mg/day, for more than 6 months, along with cognitive therapy. Hank recovers from the delusional experience, and his obsessive-compulsive symptoms decrease significantly.

Case 2

Rose Marie is a 16-year-old student who needs to remain in the dark of her bedroom but does not lock the door. When she goes to the bathroom, she covers the windows with blankets so that no one will look inside. The bathroom is on the second floor, and there is no way to access or look into it from the outside. She complains of horrific obsessions related to diseases and death. She has mental compulsions (arithmomania), need for symmetry, touching compulsions, and iterative questioning. She feels ugly (although she is pretty), inadequate, and sad. She experiences outbursts of anger, and she cannot socialize. The intensity of her symptoms forced her to quit school. There is a psychiatric family history of bipolar disorder and perhaps schizophrenia. When Rose Marie is asked about the need for darkness, she cannot offer a logical answer. She only says, "I have to do it."

A diagnosis of primary OCD with depressive symptomatology is made. The patient failed to adhere to treatment and never came back for follow-up.

Case 3

This is a brief history of a family of four. The parents brought one son, age 24, and a daughter, age 27, for diagnosis and treatment. Both were intelligent, successful people who had OCD. While assessing the family mental status, we found that both parents experienced OCD as well. One winter day, the daughter complained to us that the mother always kept the house in complete darkness, and both children had to go out while she was cooking. The mother developed a ritual of darkness and of cooking without the children in the house. A very cold winter triggered the consultation. Once again, we were faced with the need of some patients to live in darkness. Their father was an uninvolved person, quite passive, who tended to remain silent and without any ostensible power to modify these behaviors. Overall, the family was pervaded by intense anger, which was manifested through verbal fights among themselves and passively with their therapists. The course of treatment was partially satisfactory, but we were unable to control all of the variables in play, and finally the family gave up.

What is the meaning of darkness in these cases? What is or are the beliefs behind these behaviors? What is the relationship between darkness and OCD? If there is a paranoid component, how strong is it? Is darkness a manifestation of an attempt to conceal aspects of one's life? We have not reached any acceptable conclusion with regard to such cases.

Perception

Another topic in schizophrenia is a change in a perception's meaning, also known as *dysperception.* However, dysperception is not seen in schizophrenia exclusively; it also is seen in OCD, eating disorders, and body dysmorphic disorders.

Motoric Aspects: Catatonia and Slowness

Schizophrenia patients present with an association disorder (incoherence) and blocking of thought, motility, action, memory, and perception. In OCD, rather than blocking, certain patients have partial inhibition, or slowness. Schizophrenic patients handle words and objects; obsessive patients tend to use words and abstractions as objects. These phenomenological aspects might help dissipate hesitations when elaborating on a differential diagnosis in complex OCD-schizophrenia cases.

These two entities also seem to share motoric symptoms, among them stereotypy, grimacing, twitches, tics, and even (although rare) catatonia. Abnormal motor activity might be an expression of cerebral anatomical involvement affecting the basal region and the motoric areas of the brain. The clinical representation of this anatomical complex may be found in schizophrenia, OCD, Tourette's syndrome, and the choreas, among others. This psychomotor participation does not necessarily mean comorbidity but a condition that originates in or affects the same cerebral region.

Two cases of schizophrenia, catatonia type, were described by Arieti (1955). Another study described two OCD patients with severe catatonic symptoms (Hermesh et al. 1989). These two patients responded well to anti–obsessive-compulsive agents, but not to neuroleptics.

Of 59 patients diagnosed with OCD, 17 experienced significant slowness. In this population, a neurological examination yielded loss of motor fluency, hesitancy of initiation of limb movements, speech and gait abnormalities, cogwheel rigidity, complex repetitive movements, and tics. The authors suggest a dysfunction in the frontal-basal ganglia loop system (Hymas et al. 1991). These findings substantiate somewhat the OCD-schizophrenia-Parkinson's connection (see Chapter 12).

In the following text, three cases resembling a catatonic state with a presumptive OCD diagnosis are presented.

Case 1

A 35-year-old single woman with a high school diploma had incapacitating OCD symptoms, including "motor freezing behavior," in which the patient could stay motionless for hours in a standing position. These episodes took place in coffee shops, stores, and theaters, with obvious embarrassing consequences.

Case 2

A 23-year-old single man had quit college when his obsessions became overwhelming as well as emotionally and physically debilitating. To control his obsessions, he first designed a program in which his thought content consisted of the same short sentence, and he sat in the same chair all day in a room devoid of furniture to prevent any compulsive behavior. On examination, it was decided that he had severe OCD with catatonic features, placing him in an OCD subset of patients with motoric psychotic features. After several sessions where we discussed the dynamics of the condition and therapeutic strategies, he accepted the use of clomipramine, combined with a behavioral-cognitive approach to challenge his effective, yet unreasonable, program for controlling his severe symptomatology.

Case 3

A 17-year-old male student had developed OCD at age 6 years. Precipitating factors consisted of a subclinical encephalitis at age 5 years, followed by attention-deficit/hyperactive disorder. This patient could not move without writing a full description of the movement. He became more immobile and eventually completely catatonic. We lost contact with this patient, who came to us only for a second opinion. His symptoms seem to exemplify the OCD continuum, having a subclinical encephalitis, followed by a hyperactive disorder with subsequent OCD symptoms, and finally manifesting what could be a rare form of catatonia-like syndrome. Was this case the prodromal phase of a schizophrenic process?

The diagnosis of these cases requires differentiation of obsessional slowness from schizophrenic catatonia. Slowness might be associated with meticulosity, double-checking, and ruminations. Probably severe slowness is mistaken for catatonia. OCD slowness alone has been considered a primary dysfunction (Rachman 1974), although this was later disputed (Hodgson and Rachman 1976; Kendell and Zealley 1983; Marks 1981). In general, obsessive slowness is an infrequent yet disabling symptom (Ratnasuriya et al. 1991; Veale 1993).

Schizoaffective Psychoses

Schizoaffective psychoses have been described as rapid-onset disorders that are followed by complete remission (Kasanin 1933). The research diagnostic criteria (Spitzer et al. 1978) differ in definition only in that a psychoreactive start is not included. The presence of altered affect, one of Schneider's (1980) first-rank symptoms, is required to arrive at a diagnosis of schizoaffective disorder.

Sometimes a differential diagnosis among OCD, schizoaffective psychoses, and schizotypal personality disorder must be established. In OCD, the depression affect is a well-known reactive response. Also, some OCD forms are clearly preceded by depression. Our question is whether obsessive-compulsive symptoms participate in this group of psychoses (Gross et al. 1986b).

Personality Disorders

Diagnosis of schizotypal personality disorder in the presence of obsessive-compulsive symptoms may pose a problem. In a sample of refractory OCD patients, a substantial number manifested schizotypal symptoms. These symptoms included magic thinking, ideas of reference, paranoia or distrust, odd speech, derealization, depersonalization, illusions, social isolation, undue social anxiety, and hypersensitivity to criticism (Jenike et al. 1986). Another study concluded that the incidence of schizotypal personality disorder coexisting with OCD is small (8%), whereas the incidence of schizotypal features in OCD is large (28%) (Stanley et al. 1990). Both studies indicated the need to isolate this subset of patients for treatment purposes.

In Russia, two studies investigated the relationship between OCD and schizophrenia. Shakhlamov (1988) reported some variants in OCD-schizophrenic boundaries and observed a schizophrenic progression into anancastic and hysterical forms of schizophrenia. The second report showed six types of OCD typology starting during childhood and adolescence, the first being primary OCD, then slowly progressing into various forms, including one schizophrenic, one hypochondriac, and three depressive forms (Kalinina 1991).

Differential Diagnosis Issues

A well-defined cluster of symptoms is necessary to arrive at a correct diagnosis. The question is how to go about such diagnosis. We can start by reading the available classifications, which are wide in scope and therefore imbricate with other neuropsychiatric disorders. For OCD classifications, we can use those in Chapter 1. The most complete classifications of schizophrenias are those described by Leonhard (1968). A command of both OCD and schizophrenia classifications will be helpful to establish a solid diagnosis.

Argenta and Pichini (1968) reported that after reexamining 2,500 case histories bearing the diagnosis of schizophrenia, anancastia was found among the preschizophrenic symptomatology. The psychopharmacological response to treatment becomes a useful tool in establishing a differential diagnosis. In schizophrenic patients, the response to neuroleptic treatment is good, whereas in OCD patients, it is negative.

A differential diagnosis might require evolution of the disorder to permit emergent symptoms. Differential diagnosis in both OCD and schizophrenia calls for proper, universally accepted, diagnostic systems so that comparative notes can be exchanged. Doran et al. (1986) have conducted a comprehensive review indicating the necessity of establishing a universally accepted nomenclature.

Can clinicians validate the available information and reach an acceptable diagnosis? In a cross-validation study, patients having "obsessive psychosis" were evaluated with the same tests given to patients having compulsive neurosis. These tests were the Wechsler-Bellevue Intelligence Test Form II (Wechsler 1946), The Weigl-Goldstein-Scheerer Color-Form Sorting Test (Goldstein and Scheerer 1942), the Bender Visual-Motor Gestalt Test (Bender 1938), Benton's Visual Retention Test Form C (Benton 1963), and the Rorschach Test (Rorschach 1921). These test batteries helped discern both conditions (Weiss et al. 1975). Investigation of putative, inhibitory mechanisms in selective attention was able to distinguish between OCD and other anxiety disorders, whereas OCD patients scored close to the group of schizophrenia patients (Enright and Beech 1990). Finally, there are three major disorders—OCD, schizophrenia, and body dysmorphic disorder—that seem to share some thought and perceptual aspects that might call for consideration when investigating or treating these conditions.

Somnography

It has been reported that the sleep alterations in schizophrenia and OCD have features in common, but there are obvious differences in the magnitude of the changes. Schizophrenic patients have marked insomnia, whereas patients with OCD have only a small increase in wakefulness (Gaillard et al. 1984).

Epidemiology

Demographic studies of OCD and schizophrenic patients seem to reinforce the boundaries of the two conditions, without much evidence of crossover. However, OCD has a higher celibacy rate and lower fertility rate than other neuroses and in these respects resembles schizophrenia (Greenberg 1980; Hare et al. 1972). A follow-up of three monozygotic twin pairs who were concordant for OCD and discordant for schizophrenia or schizoaffective disorder showed that all had a schizotypal personality disorder (Lewis et al. 1991).

Some epidemiological studies have reported a 1.1% incidence of OCD in patients with schizophrenia (N = 1,000) (Jahrreiss 1926), whereas Rosen (1957) reported a 3.5% incidence of OCD in a population of 848 patients with schizophrenia. More recent studies have indicated an incidence of OCD in schizophrenia ranging from 10% (Boyd et al. 1984; Rasmussen and Tsuang 1986) to 12.2% (Karno et al. 1988).

Treatment

The concomitant treatment of both disorders undoubtedly presents a conflict of interest. Will an antipsychotic agent aggravate OCD? Will an anti–obsessive-compulsive agent aggravate the schizophrenia?

An old psychoanalytical axiom indicates that obsessive-compulsive symptoms present in schizophrenia constitute a mechanism of defense and therefore should not be treated. This empirical observation is partially substantiated by anecdotal reports. Interestingly, we have reported aggravation of schizophrenia without OCD in patients treated with clomipramine (Yaryura-Tobias et al. 1976).

Treatment must be tailored to the needs of each individual patient. The therapist must first isolate the major symptoms pertaining to the thought disorder (i.e., obsession, overvalue ideation, or delusion). A pharmacotherapeutic approach is the best choice. The questions are: Can we challenge these beliefs? Which therapy is more effective? The aim is to reduce the belief's intensity and frequency to permit the introduction of other therapeutic forms. In addition, the medication dose must be balanced to neutralize the possibility of worsening either condition.

Two case reports are worth reviewing. In the first case, an OCD patient progressed into schizophrenia and was subsequently treated with thioridazine and electroconvulsive therapy (ECT). The schizophrenic symptoms were replaced by OCD symptomatology. In a second case, a patient was diagnosed with schizophrenia, paranoid type. The treatment consisted of thioridazine and ECT. After initial improvement, obsessions, doubting, and double-checking were observed. The patient was then treated with neuroleptics and iproniazid, with complete remission of OCD symptoms, resulting in a psychotic relapse (Prat et al. 1971).

The onset of paranoid and aggressive behavior has been reported in two OCD adolescents treated with clomipramine, indicating the possibility of a serotonin dysfunction (Alarcon et al. 1991).

In one OCD case, successful treatment of psychotic symptoms with haloperidol, diazepam, buspirone, and fluoxetine was reported (Deckert and Malone 1990). The addition of neuroleptic medication in fluvoxamine-refractory OCD comorbid with tic spectrum disorder or schizotypal personality was associated with a better response (McDougle et al. 1990). In 43 treatment-resistant OCD patients, those with schizotypal personality disorder had an extremely high treatment failure rate (Jenike et al. 1986).

Pimozide, a potent antipsychotic agent used to treat Tourette's syndrome, body dysmorphic disorder, and hypochondriasis, has been administered to patients with OCD (Opler and Feinberg 1991). An unusual report described two cases of schizophrenia in which OCD developed after treatment with clozapine, a potent antagonist of serotonin receptors (Patil 1992).

To validate these reports, better diagnostic criteria and larger samples are required. This bring us back to the need to maintain the neurotransmitter equilibrium. Maintaining equilibrium permits us to manage the variety of symptoms present in both conditions to prevent predominance of either.

Behavioral techniques are best for obsessionality with severe compulsive symptoms. Cognitive therapy seems efficacious when delusions are prominent symptoms, because it is used in schizophrenia in general (Brenner et al. 1989). Improved cognition allows patients to process information more reasonably as they challenge the obsession or false belief. Meanwhile, new anti–obsessive-compulsive agents, the introduction of novel antipsychotic agents, and the combination of these compounds with coadjuvant medications (e.g., lithium, fenfluramine, carbamazepine, phenytoin, buspirone, L-tryptophan, 5-hydroxytryptophan) have assisted in developing a better therapeutic model.

Prognosis

What is the outcome of OCD-schizophrenia comorbidity, of OCD with schizophrenic symptoms, and of schizophrenia with OCD symptoms? Prognosis is guarded, considering the complex pathology involved.

No conclusive research allows certainty about the prognosis. In one study, the presence of obsessive-compulsive symptoms indicated poor prognosis for patients with schizophrenia (Fenton and McGlashan 1986).

References

Achkova M: Neurotic-like and psychopathic-like forms of schizophrenia in children and teenagers (in Bulgarian). Neurol Psikhiatr Neurokhir (Sofia) 15:326–332, 1976

Alarcon RD, Johnson BR, Lucas JP: Paranoid and aggressive behavior in two obsessive compulsive adolescents treated with clomipramine. J Am Acad Child Adolesc Psychiatry 30:999–1002, 1991

Argenta G, Pichini F: Gli inizi della schizofrenia. Rivista di Psichiatria (Roma) 3: 27–45, 1968

Arieti S: Study of catatonic patients, in Interpretation of Schizophrenia. New York, Robert Brunner, 1955, pp 108–129

Bender L: A Visual-Motor Gestalt Test and its Clinical Use, No 3. New York, American Orthopsychiatric Association of New York, Research monographs, 1938

Benton, AL: The Revised Visual Retention Test, 3rd Edition. New York, Psychological Corporation, 1963

Birnie WA, Littmann SK: Obsessionality and schizophrenia. Can Psychiatr Assoc J 23:77–81, 1978

Blanc M: Ner obsess et syndromes obsession. Rev Prat 6:935–947, 1956

Bleuler E: Textbook of Psychiatry. Translated by Brill AA. New York, Macmillan, 1911

Bleuler E: The theory of symptoms, in Dementia Praecox or Group of Schizophrenia. Translated by Zinkin J. New York, International Universities Press, 1955, pp 348–461

Boyd JH, Burke JD, Groenberg E, et al: Exclusion criteria of DSM-III: a study of co-occurence of hierarchy-free syndromes. Arch Gen Psychiatry 41:983–989, 1984

Bratfos O: Transition of neuroses and other Minor mental disorders into psychoses. Acta Psychiatr, Scand 46:35–49, 1969

Bratfos O: Transition of neuroses and other minor mental disorders into psychoses. Acta Psychiatr Scand 46:35–49, 1970

Brenner HD, Boker W, Hodel B, et al: Cognitive treatment of basic pervasive dysfunctions in schizophrenia, in Schizophrenia: Scientific Progress. Edited by Schulz SC, Tamminga CA. New York, Oxford University Press, 1989, pp 358–367

Bumke O: Die psychischen Zwangerscheinungen. Allgemeine Zeitschrift Fur Psychiatrie und Psychisch-Gerichtliche Medicine 63:138–148, 1906

Claude H, Vidart L, Longeut Y: Le journal d'un schizoide. Reflexions sur les rapport de la psychasthenie, la schizoidie et la schizophrenie. Encephale 2:323–338, 1941

Deckert DW, Malone DA: Treatment of psychotic symptoms in OCD patients (letter). J Clin Psychiatry 51:259, 1990

Diathelm O: Treatment in Psychiatry, 3rd Edition. Springfield, IL, Charles C Thomas, 1955

Doran AR, Breier A, Roy A: Differential diagnosis and diagnostic systems in schizophrenia. Psychiatr Clin North Am 9:17–33, 1986

Eggers C: Zwang und jugendliche Psychosen. Prax Kinderpsychologie 118:202–208, 1969

Eisen JL, Rasmussen SA: Obsessive compulsive disorder with psychotic features. J Clin Psychiatry 54:373–379, 1993

Enright SJ, Beech AR: Obsessional states: anxiety disorders or schizotypes? An information processing and personality assessment. Psychol Med 20:621–627, 1990

Ey H: Les eidolies hallucinosiques, in Traite des Hallucinations, Vol. 1. Paris, France, Masson et Cie, 1973, pp 329–377

Fenton WS, McGlashan TH: The prognostic significance of obsessive-compulsive symptoms in schizophrenia. Am J Psychiatry 143:437–441, 1986

Gaillard JM, Iorio G, Campajola P, et al: Temporal organization of sleep in schizophrenics and patients with obsessive-compulsive disorder. Advances in Biological Psychiatry 15:76–83, 1984

Goldstein K, Scheerer M: Abstract and Concrete Behavior. Evanston, IL, American Psychological Association, 1942

Gordon A: Obsessions in their relation to psychoses. Am J Psychiatry 5:647–659, 1926

Gordon A: Transitions of obsessions into delusions. Am J Psychiatry 107:455–458, 1960

Greenberg ED: Obsessive-compulsive neurosis and season of birth. Biol Psychiatry 16:513–516, 1980

Gross G, Huber G, Armbruster B: Schizoaffective psychoses—long term prognosis and symptomatology, in Schizoaffective Psychoses. Edited by Marneros A, Tsuang MT. Berlin, Germany, Springer-Verlag, 1986a, pp 188–203

Gross G, Huber G, Schuttler R: Long term course of Schneiderian Schizophrenia, in Schizoaffective Psychoses. Edited by Marneros A, Tsuang MT. Berlin, Germany, Springer-Verlag, 1986b, pp 164–178

Hare EH, Price JS, Slater ET: Fertility in obsessional neurosis. Br J Psychiatry 121:197–205, 1972

Hermesh H, Hoffnung RA, Aizenberg D, et al: Catatonic signs in severe obsessive compulsive disorder. J Clin Psychiatry 50:303–305, 1989

Hodgson RJ, Rachman S: Obsessive-compulsive complaints. Behav Res Ther 15: 389–395, 1976

Huber G, Gross G: The concept of basic symptoms in schizophrenic and schizoaffective psychoses. Recenti Prog Med 80:646–652, 1989

Hwang MY, Hollander E: Schizo-obsessive disorders. Psychiatric Annals 23: 396–401, 1993

Hymas N, Lees A, Bolton D, et al: The neurology of obsessional slowness. Brain 114:2203–2233, 1991

Insel TR, Akiskal HS: Obsessive-compulsive disorder with psychotic features: a phenomenologic analysis. Am J Psychiatry 143:1527–1533, 1986

Jahrreiss W: Chronic systematized compulsive disease. Arch Psychiatr Nervenkr 77:596–612, 1926

Jaspers K: Psicopatologia General (Allgemeine Psychopatologie) (1913). Translated by Saubidet RO. Buenos Aires, Argentina, Beta, 1955, pp 116–132

Jenike MA, Baer L, Minichiello W, et al: Concomitant obsessive-compulsive disorder and schizotypal personality disorder. Am J Psychiatry 143:530–532, 1986

Kalinina MA: Clinical characteristics and typology of the obsessive-compulsive disorder in slowly-progressing recurrent schizophrenia with the onset in childhood and adolescence. Zh Nevropatol Psikhiatr Im S S Korsakova 91:104–107, 1991

Karno M, Golding JM, Sorenson SB, Burnam MA: The epidemiology of obsessive compulsive disorder in five U.S. communities. Arch Gen Psychiatry 45:1094–1099, 1988

Kasanin J: The acute schizo-affective psychoses. Am J Psychiatry 13:97–126, 1933

Kendell RE, Zealley AK: Companion to Psychiatric Studies. Edinburgh, Scotland, Churchill Livingstone, 1983

Kringlen E: Obsessional neurotics. Br J Psychiatry 111:709–722, 1965

Leonhard K: Le Psicosi Endogene. Milan, Italy, Feltrinelli, 1968

Lewis A: Problems of obsessional illness. Proc R Soc Med 29:325–336, 1936

Lewis SW, Chitkara B, Reveley AM: Obsessive-compulsive disorder and schizophrenia in three identical twin pairs. Psychol Med 21:135–141, 1991

Marks I: Cure and Care of Neurosis: Theory and Practice of Behavior Psychotherapy. New York, Wiley, 1981

Mayer-Gross W: Handbuch der Greistes-Krankenheiten, Vol 9. Edited by Bumke O. Berlin, Springer, 1932, p 459

McDougle CJ, Goodman WK, Price LH, et al: Neuroleptic addition in fluvoxamine-refractory obsessive-compulsive disorder. Am J Psychiatry 147:652–654, 1990

Mignard M: De l'obsess: emotive au delire d'influence. Ann Med Psychol (Paris) 71:333–343, 1913

Muller CH: Vorlaufige mitteilung zur langen katamneseder zwangsskranken. Nervenarzt 24:112–115, 1953

Opler LA, Feinberg SS: The role of pimozide in clinical psychiatry: a review. J Clin Psychiatry 52:221–233, 1991

Patil VJ: Development of transient obsessive-compulsive symptoms during treatment with clozapine (letter). Am J Psychiatry 149:272, 1992

Prat J, Porta A, Vallejo J: Sindromes obsesivoides en psiquiatria, in Patologia Obsesiva. Edited by Montserrat S, Esteve JM, Costa M, et al. Malaga, Spain, Malaga Graficasa Publishers, 1971, pp 313–337

Pujol R, Savy A: Le devenir de l'obsede. Marseille, France, Masson & Cie, 1968

Rachman S: Primary obsessive slowness. Behav Res Ther 11:463–471, 1974

Rapaport D: Organization and Pathology of Thought. Selected Sources. New York, Columbia University Press, 1951

Rasmussen SA, Tsuang MT: Clinical characteristics and family history in DSM-III obsessive compulsive disorder. Am J Psychiatry 143:317–322, 1986

Ratnasuriya RH, Marks IM, Forshaw DM, et al: Obsessive slowness revisited. Br J Psychiatry 159:273–274, 1991

Rorschach H: Psychodiaghostik, 6. Bern, Aufl. H. Heuber, 1921

Rosen I: The clinical significance of obsessions in schizophrenia. Journal of Mental Science 103:773–785, 1957

Roskin G, Rabiner CJ, Blum MH, et al: Three types of paranoid processes. Dis Nerv Syst 38:269–271, 1977

Ross CA, Siddiqui AR, Matas M: DSM-III: problems in diagnosis of paranoia and obsessive-compulsive disorder. Can J Psychiatry 32:146–148, 1987

Rudin G: Ein Beitrag zur Frage der Zwang Krankheit, Insbesondere ihrer Hereditären Bezielungen. Arch Psychiatr Nervenkr 191:14–54, 1953

Sadoun R: Formes cliniques et diagnostic des modes de debut de la schizophrenie. Encephale 46:1–7, 9–14, 1957

Schneider K: Begriffliche Untersuchung uber den Zwang. Allgemeine Zeitschrift der Psychiatrie und Ihre Grenze. 112:17–24, 1939

Schneider K: Klinische Psychopathologie, 12th edition. Stuttgart, Germany, Thieme, 1980

Shakhlamov AV: One of the variants of schizophrenia with obsession. Zh Nevropatol Psikhiatr Im S S Korsakova 88:87–92, 1988

Solyom L, DeNicola VF, Phil M, Sookman D, Luchins D: Is there an obsessive psychosis? Aetiological and prognostic factors of an atypical form of obsessive-compulsive disorder. Can J Psychiatry 30:372–380, 1985

Spitzer RL, Endicott J, Robins E: Research diagnostic criteria. Arch Gen Psychiatry 35:773–782, 1978

Stanley MA, Turner SM, Borden JW: Schizotypal features in obsessive-compulsive disorder. Compr Psychiatry 31:511–518, 1990

Stengel E: Zur Kenntnis der Beziehungen zwischen Zwangsneurose und Paranoia. Arch Psychiatr Nervenkr 95:8–23, 1931

Stengel E: A study on some clinical aspects of the relationship between obsessional neurosis and psychotic types. Journal of Mental Science 91:166–187, 1945

Stern E: Zwang und Schizophrenie. Monatsschrift fur Psychiatrie und Neurologie 77:283–297, 1930

Sullivan HS: Clinical Studies in Psychiatry. Edited by Gawel HS, Gibbon M. New York, WW Norton, 1956

Veale D: Classification and treatment of obsessional slowness. Br J Psychiatry 162:198–203, 1993

Wechsler D: The Wechsler-Bellevue Intelligence Scale Form II. New York, Psychological Corporation, 1946

Weiss AA, Robinson Sh, Winnik HZ: Obsessive psychosis—a cross validation study. Isr Ann Psychiatry Relat Discip 13:137–141, 1975

Wernicke C: Grundrisse der Psychiatrie. Leipzig, Germany, Thieme, 1900

Westphal K: Uber Zwangsvorstellungen. Archiv fur Psychiatr und Nervenkr 8:734–750, 1878

Wooley LR: Studies on obsessive ruminative tension states. Etiology, dynamics and genesis. Psychoanal Q 11:654–676, 1937

Yaryura-Tobias JA, Neziroglu F, Bergman L: Chlorimipramine for obsessive-compulsive neurosis: an organic approach. Curr Ther Res Clin Exp 20: 541–548, 1976

Yaryura-Tobias JA, Campisi TH, McKay D: Unified aspects of obsessive-compulsive disorder and schizophrenia. Paper presented at the American Psychiatric Association meeting, Philadelphia, PA, May 1994

Yaryura-Tobias JA, Campisi T, McKay D, et al: Schizophrenia and obsessive-compulsive disorder: shared aspects of pathology. Neurology, Psychiatry and Brain Research 3:143–148, 1995

Chapter 6

Major Depression, Manic-Depressive Illness, and OCD

The association between major depression or manic-depressive illness and obsessive-compulsive disorder (OCD) has drawn the attention of many researchers. One of the problems encountered is the difficulty in establishing a clear clinical relationship. This difficulty is a result of the inability to identify a depression as a sign, as an endogenous syndrome, or as a reactive disorder. Gradually, the different criteria adopted by various groups in North America and Europe to classify the different types of depression are reaching an agreement. This agreement will benefit the understanding of the nosology of depression. Consequently, a better interpretation of the OCD-depression correlation may occur.

There are several areas that should be addressed to study the interaction of both OCD and major affective disorders. First, clinical variants have been reported for more than 150 years (Morel 1860). Second, similar structural anatomical changes have been observed in both conditions. Third, modifications in cerebral metabolism affect both disorders. Finally, the closeness of neurotransmitters shared by both disorders and the therapeutic response to the same family of drugs should be investigated.

Major Depression

Traditional North American and European concepts of depression have been subjected to periodic revisions. DSM-IV (American Psychiatric Association 1994) divides mood disorders into three parts. The first part consists of mood episodes (major depressive episode, manic episode, mixed episode, and hypomanic episode). These episodes constitute the building blocks for the disorder diagnosis. The second part comprises the criteria to diagnose mood disorders (i.e., depressive disorders, bipolar disorders, mood disorder caused by a general medical condition, substance-induced mood disorder). The third part includes the specifiers that describe either the most recent mood episode or the course of recurrent episodes. The European school follows basically a nosological order that includes 1) somatogenic depressions, 2) endogenous depressions, and 3) psychogenic depressions (Huber 1994). Two other conditions include cyclothymic depression and mania.

Major depression and OCD have been associated for many years. At times, the presence of comorbidity has been an important observation for those interested in the pathogenesis and treatment of both conditions. In one study, a major depressive episode was diagnosed in 56.9% of patents with OCD occurring first (Karno et al. 1988). Depression also has been reported as the most common form of comorbidity (Rasmussen and Tsuang 1986).

Although long-term follow-up studies suggest that OCD is commonly associated with depression, a review of the literature shows weakness in the current methodology. The instruments used to measure severity lack reliability and sensitivity to change (Zitterl et al. 1990). Overall we agree with the viewpoint of Zitterl et al. (1990). We believe that secondary depression is the most important form of depression present in OCD and that depression is not a comorbid entity. Secondary depression is a common symptom in OCD and is a result of the devastation and incapacity affecting patients in their work, in their emotionality, and in their social interactions. We have estimated in a previous study that 90% of patients with OCD experience secondary depression (Yaryura-Tobias and Neziroglu 1983). We accept the presence of major depression as a comorbid condition but with a minor prevalence, as shown in epidemiological studies.

For almost a century, depression and OCD have shared a combined form of nosology, although no good descriptions have been made to distinguish endogenous depression from reactive depression (Ballet 1902; Seva Diaz 1964; Soukanoff 1904). Obsessionality, a more unusual clinical form of OCD, combined with depression was reported in one study (Kendell and Discipio 1970), and symptoms of endogenous depression were elicited as background symptoms of OCD (Payk 1976). Others have indicated the presence of ruminations, obsessions, or obsessive-compulsive symptoms accompanied by depression (Peselow et al. 1990; Rasmussen and Eisen 1990; Vaughan 1976).

Eight patients have been reported who shared the combination of bilateral basal ganglia lesions and a frontal lobe–like syndrome. The main features were inertia and loss of motivation, with perseveration of intellectual functions. Some patients presented stereotyped activities with obsessive-compulsive behavior. These symptom similarities to major depression and OCD suggest a structural link between these two conditions (Laplane et al. 1989), a theory further supported in a review done by Cummings (1993). Positron-emission tomographic imaging in OCD with and without depression has indicated functional anatomical changes affecting the association of both conditions (Baxter et al. 1990).

Two other points should be made. One is that major depression and OCD share the indolaminergic and catecholaminergic pathways that seem involved in the pathogenesis of these conditions. The second point is that certain pharmacological agents are efficacious in both disorders.

Manic-Depressive Illness

The association between OCD and depression, or manic-depressive illness, has been described as an interface, as a response to the primary illness' severity (OCD), and as a continuum. Attempts were made to classify OCD as a form of depression. In fact, the efficacy of antidepressants in OCD reinforced the concept that OCD is indeed a form of depression. Nonetheless, OCD patients without depression show good therapeutic results with the use of antidepressants (e.g., tricyclic agents and selective serotonin reuptake inhibitors), raising the question of whether OCD's efficacious response to antidepressants is the result of OCD being an affective disorder.

Interfacing manic-depressive illness and OCD provides clinicians and researchers excellent clinical cues for better diagnosis and subsequent treatment. This variant has two phases: a manic phase that replaces the obsessive phase and an obsessive phase that replaces the manic phase (Bonhoeffer 1913; Marchand 1912; McKay et al. 1994; Michaux and Gallot 1965; Yaryura-Tobias and Neziroglu 1983).

We treated OCD patients who, after the administration of clomipramine, went into a subacute manic state or a hypomanic state. We thought these were hypomanic side effects induced by the use of tricyclic antidepressants, but in subsequent interviews we found an underlying manic-depressive illness, manic type (Yaryura-Tobias and Neziroglu 1983; Yaryura-Tobias et al. 1979). Some patients complain of bouts of mind racing, decreased sleep, feeling extremely energetic, and feeling in a rather good mood. These reports are not mediated by depressive symptoms. Depression is found only when obsessions and compulsions are intense and interfere with daily activities. This condition responds well to lithium alone (900 mg/day) or in combination with partial serotonin blockers.

References

American Psychiatric Association: Diagnostic and Statistical Manual of Mental Disorders, 4th Edition. Washington, DC, American Psychiatric Association, 1994

Ballet G: La melancolie intermittente. Presse Med 4:460, 1902

Baxter LR, Schwartz JM, Guze BH, et al: PET imaging in obsessive compulsive disorder with and without depression. J Clin Psychiatry 51 (suppl):61–69, 1990

Bonhoeffer K: Uber die Beziehung der Zwangvorst, zum Manisch-Depressiven. Monatsschr F Psych U Neurol 33:354–357, 1913

Cummings JL: Frontal-subcortical circuits and human behavior. Arch Neurol 50: 873–880, 1993

Huber G: Psychiatrie. Lehrbuch flir Studenten und Arzte, 5th Edition. Stuttgart, Germany, Schattauer, 1994

Karno M, Goldin JM, Sorenson SB, et al: The epidemiology of obsessive compulsive disorder in five U. S. communities. Arch Gen Psychiatry 45:1094–1099, 1988

Kendell RE, Discipio WJ: Obsessional symptoms and obsessional personality traits in patients with depressive illness. Psychol Med 1:65–72, 1970

Laplane D, Levasseur M, Pillon B, et al: Obsessive-compulsive disorder and other behavioural changes with bilateral basal ganglia lesions. Brain 112:699–725, 1989

Marchand L: Les access melancoliques des obsedes douteurs. Ann Med Psychol (Paris) 70:488–503, 1912

McKay DR, Yaryura-Tobias JA, Neziroglu FA: Obsessive-compulsive disorder and bipolar disorder: preliminary outcome data. Biol Psychiatry 35:615–747, 1994

Michaux L, Gallot HM: Les confins de la nevrose obsessionnelle. Rev Prat 15: 823–829, 1965

Morel: Du delire emotif. Neurose du systeme nerveux ganglionaire visceral. Arch Gen Med 1:385, 530, 700, 1236, 1860

Payk TR: Zwangssymptome in verlauf endogener depressionen. Nervenarzt 47: 343–346, 1976

Peselow ED, Figlia C, Fieve RR: Obsessive-compulsive symptoms in patients with major depression: frequency and response to the antidepressant treatment. Paper presented at the annual meeting of the American College of Neuropsychopharmacology, San Juan, Puerto Rico, December 1990

Rasmussen SA, Eisen JL: Epidemiological and clinical features of obsessive-compulsive disorder, in Obsessive-Compulsive Disorders: Theory and Management, 2nd Edition. Edited by Jenike MA, Baer LB, Minichiello WE. Chicago, IL, Year Book Medical, 1990, pp 10–27

Rasmussen SA, Tsuang MT: Clinical characteristics and family history in DSM III obsessive-compulsive disorder. Am J Psychiatry 143:317–322, 1986

Seva Diaz A: Investigaciones en torno al fenomeno obsesivo. Actas Luso Esp Neurol Pisquiatr 23:260–271, 1964

Soukanoff S: Sur les associatons psychiques obsedantes de contraste dans les estates melancoliques. Arch Neurol 18:305–312, 1904

Vaughan M: The relationships between obsessional personality, obsessions in depression, and symptoms of depression. Br J Psychiatry 129:36–39, 1976

Yaryura-Tobias JA, Neziroglu FA: Classification, in Obsessive-Compulsive Disorder: Pathogenesis, Diagnosis, Treatment. Edited by Yaryura-Tobias JA, Neziroglu FA. New York, Marcel Dekker, 1983, pp 37–50

Yaryura-Tobias JA, Neziroglu FA, Bhagavan HN: Biochemical correlates in obsessive-compulsive disorder, in Biological Psychiatry Today. Edited by Obiols J, Ballus C, Gonzalez-Monclus E, et al. Amsterdam, The Netherlands, Elsevier North-Holland, 1979, pp 574–580

Zitterl W, Lenz G, Mairhofer A, et al: Obsessive-compulsive disorder: course and interaction with depression. Psychopathology 23:73–80, 1990

Chapter 7
Alcohol and Substance Abuse

OCD, Alcohol, and Substance Abuse

The combination of the consumption of drugs and alcohol in general and the presence of comorbidity in particular has recently become an area of concern. Alcohol and drug consumption is on the increase, thereby creating a serious social problem. In addition, its presence in OCD complicates the clinical picture and poses treatment management difficulties (Hoffman 1994).

There are two major aspects of managing obsessive-compulsive disorder (OCD) and substance abuse that require attention. One is operational, and the other one is pharmacological. For operational purposes, a conceptualization of a compulsion and an addiction is deemed necessary. The therapeutic problem is pharmacological—that is, how to combine anti-obsessive agents in the presence of alcohol and/or illegal drugs. What drug interactions must one manage?

Addiction and Compulsion

Better clinical awareness of the presence of these three entities—OCD, alcoholism, and drug abuse—indicates the need to address the following issues pertinent to diagnosis and treatment:

- What is the difference between a compulsion and an addiction?
- What are the overlapping symptoms?
- Do these entities share a neurobiological pattern or a biopsychosocial profile?
- What treatment program is appropriate?

A *compulsion* is a state in which a person is compelled to perform mental or motor tasks against his or her will; it is unpleasant and anxiogenic. By comparison, an *addiction* is an uncontrollable inclination to seek pleasure. Addictions are pleasant behaviors that, unless satisfied, will produce untoward effects. There is some evidence that enzymatic and opiate factors predispose certain individuals to become addicts.

A person who simultaneously has a psychiatric illness and an addiction has a dual disorder. This classification suggests that an addiction has not only biological, but also psychosocial components. Current research indicates that genetic factors and biological parameters are altered in alcoholism and cocainism (Anton 1995; Wyatt et al. 1988). Therefore, it is sensible to think of neurobiological pathways and psychosocial determinants. The neurobiological pathways seem to be associated with pleasure centers and are mediated via opiate, noradrenergic, and serotoninergic circuits.

One issue is whether an addict is psychologically or physically dependent. There is no clear evidence for either side. We consider addictions as serious conditions, usually refractory to treatment. A sudden discontinuation of drugs or alcohol results in emotional, behavioral, and physical symptoms.

Chronic rewarding of the pleasure centers makes it difficult to interrupt the use or abuse of drugs and alcohol. In a sample of 2,471 patients with a lifetime diagnosis of agoraphobia, panic disorder, agoraphobia with panic, social phobia, simple phobia, and OCD, about 12% had a lifetime history of alcohol abuse, alcohol dependence, or both. The highest risk was among patients with agoraphobia and panic (Himle and Hill 1991).

An assessment of 50 alcoholic patients revealed that 12% had OCD, a prevalence rate that is five to six times greater than that in the general population. Although OCD is considered rare among blacks, four of six alcoholic patients with OCD were black (Rieman et al. 1992). A previous report indicated that 6% of the patients with alcoholism met the criteria for OCD; this prevalence is three times the lifetime prevalence for OCD found in the general population (Eisen and Rasmussen 1989).

In an epidemiological study involving 157 patients with OCD, there were statistically significantly fewer alcoholic and drug abusing patients when compared with the general population of the state of New York (Neziroglu et al. 1994).

Psychotic episode risk in alcohol and drug abuse was studied in a population of 4,994 adult household residents. The risk of alcohol addiction was eight times greater in men and three times greater in women than in the general population. The psychotic episode risk also increased in cocaine and marijuana users. Baseline depressive episodes, manic episodes, agoraphobia, and OCD also were associated with increased risk of onset of psychotic experiences (Tien and Anthony 1990).

Obsessive-compulsive symptoms in drug addicts and alcoholics were found in alcohol dependence (Edwards and Gross 1976), heroin dependence (Goldstein 1972), and compulsive self-injection by drug users (Levine 1974). Motor compulsions and choreiform movements were reported in those addicted to psychostimulants (Rylander 1972), and repetitive compulsive behavior has been observed in drug-dependent personalities (Edelstein 1975). Currently the OCD characteristics of alcoholic patients can be quantified by a modified Yale-Brown Obsessive Compulsive Scale (Modell et al. 1992).

Serotonin, a neurotransmitter associated with the pathogenesis of OCD, is affected by the use of codeine, marijuana, morphine, and alcohol, all of which produce hyposerotoninemia.

Codeine abusers have been described as concerned with obsessionality, reviewing the day's events, excessive showering, ordering, arithmomania, checking, cleaning, symmetry, sameness, and inability to switch from one task to another (Senjo 1989). Sometimes the drug awakens the dormant OCD state. A male patient with a childhood history of attention-deficit disorder and a family history of OCD reported OCD symptoms during cocaine intoxication (Satel and McDougle 1991). Subjects actively using cocaine and marijuana were at an increased risk for OCD (Crum and Anthony 1993). It seems that an initiation pattern from alcoholism to marijuana and then to cocaine develops. Drugs thrive in patients with dependent states, and OCD patients find symptom relief and a "push" to make decisions when using drugs (Miller and Gold 1988).

As previously stated, addictions are refractory to treatment, and when they are combined with a major psychiatric illness, the patient prognosis is dimmed. However, patients who are treated for substance abuse and OCD demonstrated greatly reduced OCD symptoms and had higher overall abstinence rates at 12-month follow-up (Fals-Stewart and Schafer 1992).

In morphine addiction, tolerance and dependence correlate with serotonin (Way 1979). Acute alcoholism may cause hyposerotoninemia, functional hypoglycemia, and dehydration (Essman 1981). These biological responses to alcohol suggest that there may be an underlying mechanism that may precipitate OCD in those individuals with a predisposition to OCD. This predisposition to alcoholism may be genetically determined and causes low serotonin brain levels. The finding that selective serotonin reuptake inhibitors (e.g., citalopram, fluoxetine, fluvoxamine, and zimelidine) decrease ethanol intake support this hypothesis (Ferreire and Soares-da-Silva 1991).

We have not found anything in the literature pertaining to specific pharmacological treatment for these dual disorders. In general, we use selective serotonin reuptake inhibitors, beta blockers, and noradrenaline blockers and abstain from using benzodiazepines.

References

Anton RF: New directions in the pharmacotherapy of alcoholism. Psychiatric Annals 25:353–362, 1995

Crum PS, Anthony JC: Cocaine use and other suspected risk factors for obsessive-compulsive disorder: a prospective study with data from the Epidemiologic Catchment Area surveys. Drug Alcohol Depend 31:281–295, 1993

Edelstein EL: Elaborations on the meaning of repetitive behavior in drug dependent personalities. Br J Addict 70:365–373, 1975

Edwards G, Gross M: Alcoholic dependence: provisional description of a clinical syndrome. BMJ 1:1058–1061, 1976

Eisen JL, Rasmussen SA: Coexisting obsessive-compulsive disorder and alcoholism. J Clin Psychiatry 50:96–98, 1989

Essman WB: Drug effects upon aggressive behavior, in Aggression and Violence: A Psychobiological and Clinical Approach. Edited by Valzelli L, Morgese L. Milano, Italy, Saint Vincent, 1981, pp 150–175

Fals-Stewart W, Schafer J: The treatment of substance abusers diagnosed with obsessive-compulsive disorder: an outcome study. J Subst Abuse Treat 9: 365–370, 1992

Ferreire L, Soares-da-Silva P: 5-hydroxytryptamine and alcoholism. Human Psychopharmacology-Clinic Experimental 6:21–24, 1991

Goldstein A: Heroin addiction and the role of methadone in its treatment. Arch Gen Psychiatry 26:291–297, 1972

Himle JA, Hill EM: Alcohol abuse and the anxiety disorders: evidence from the Epidemiologic Catchment Area Survey. Journal of Anxiety Disorders 5: 237–245, 1991

Hoffman JH: Understanding Obsessive-Compulsive Disorder and Addiction. Center City, MN, Hazelden Foundation, 1994, pp 1–16

Levine DG: "Needle freaks": compulsive–self-injection by drug users. Am J Psychiatry 131:297–300, 1974

Miller NS, Gold MS: Cocaine and alcoholism: distinct or part of a spectrum. Psychiatric Annals 18:538–539, 1988

Modell JG, Glaser FB, Mountz JM, et al: Obsessive and compulsive characteristics of alcohol abuse and dependence quantification by a newly developed questionnaire. Alcoholism 162:266–271, 1992

Neziroglu FA, Yaryura-Tobias JA, Lemli JM, et al: Estudio demografico del trastorno obseso-compulsivo. Acta Psiquiatr Psicol Am Lat 40:217–223, 1994

Rieman BC, McNally RJ, Cox WM: The comorbidity of obsessive-compulsive disorder and alcoholism. Journal of Anxiety Disorders 6:105–110, 1992

Rylander G: Psychosis and the pundning and choreiform syndromes in addiction to central stimulant drugs. Psychiatr Neurol Neurochir 75:203–212, 1972

Satel SL, McDougle CJ: Obsessions and compulsions associated with cocaine abuse. Am J Psychiatry 148:947, 1991

Senjo M: Obsessive-compulsive disorder in people that abuse codeine. Acta Psychiatr Scand 79:619–620, 1989

Tien AV, Anthony JC: Epidemiological analysis of alcohol and drug use as risk factors for psychotic experiences. J Nerv Ment Dis 178:473–480, 1990

Way EL: Review and overview of four decades of opiate research, in Neurochemical Mechanism of Opiates and Endorphins. Edited by Loh JJ, Ross DH. New York, Raven, 1979, p 3

Wyatt RJ, Karoum F, Suddth R, et al: The role of dopamine in cocaine use and abuse. Psychiatric Annals 18:531–534, 1988

Chapter 8
Somatic Conditions

I nterpreting functional medical complaints of psychiatric patients presents problems that should be sorted out. Is the complaint a psychological symptom, or is it organic? Consider a patient who complains of depression and has silent pancreatic cancer or patients who complain of irritability and muscular twitches and have a hypocalcemic condition: are such cases manifestations of organic pathology expressed with psychiatric symptoms?

Similarly, a patient may consult a clinician for gastric symptoms from a peptic ulcer, accompanied by an underlying passive-aggressive personality that reaches its utmost expression by affecting the gastric mucosa. Such a case is an example of psychiatric pathology manifested as a gastrointestinal disorder. Then the question is: what is the treatment of choice for all cases? Should clinicians use a pluralistic biopsychological approach?

It is important to understand patients' psychiatric characteristics along with their functional (Hall 1980) and organic medical complaints. Somatic diseases are common in psychiatric illnesses (Koranyi 1980), and psychiatric conditions seem preponderant in general hospitals. Of all inpatients and outpatients treated in the department of internal medicine and orthopedics of the Fukuoka University Hospital, 53.4% had psychiatric symptoms (Nishioka et al. 1990).

Psychiatric comorbidity in somatization disorders shows that the most prevalent comorbidities were major depression (54.6%), generalized anxiety disorder (33.6%), and phobic disorders (31.1%), and risk ratios were highest for panic disorder (16.25%), major depression (9.41%), schizophrenia (7.77%), and obsessive-compulsive disorder (7.04%) (Brown et al. 1990).

In a one-in-six random sample, Australian psychiatrists ($N = 1,154$) participated in a study of treatment of anxiety and somatoform disorders. Supportive psychotherapy, behavioral therapy, anxiolytics, and antidepressants were the most popular treatment choices (Andrews et al. 1987).

The recognition of psychosomatic and somatopsychic medicine facilitates the study of somatoform disorders, which are influenced almost equally by psychological and physical factors. According to Socrates, the body cannot be cured without curing the soul, which is why Hellenic physicians could not cure many diseases, because they ignored humans as an integral unit. Socrates praised the Thracians, because they admitted the importance of healing the soul to heal the body.

For Rof-Carballo (1955), one of the psychosomatic movement's founders, psychosomatic pathology is the crisis of adolescence in psychiatric medicine's maturity. He emphasized that, as in any other growth crisis, the developing discipline of psychosomatic medicine seems clownish, with a fashionable propensity and, at times, emotional rather than logical elements. He further stated that this subdiscipline is the greatest contribution to modern medicine.

We will review several disorders with psychogenic and somatogenic factors and their putative relation to obsessive-compulsive disorder (OCD).

Hypochondriasis

The essential feature of hypochondriasis is preoccupation with having a serious disease based on misinterpreting one or more bodily signs or symptoms (American Psychiatric Association 1994).

The term *hypochondriasis* (from the Greek *hypo*, meaning under, and *chondros*, meaning cartilage) was first used by Galen of Pergamon in the second century, and with only minor modification, the original connotation remains. Furthermore, Galen's original concept of this condition still holds validity. Educated in Greek humoral theory of pathogenesis, he believed hypochondriasis was a form of melancholia (from the Greek *melano*, meaning black, and *cholos*, meaning bile). A great clinician, he connected hypochondriasis and melancholia (i.e., depression) or somatic symptoms with sadness.

Historically, hypochondriasis emerges in the nosological panorama with a symptom cluster of abdominal pain, belching, and flatulence, accompanied by fear and sadness (Fischer-Homberger 1970). A similar clinical description is found in neurasthenia (Weiss and Spurgeon English 1943) (Table 8–1).

By the 17th century, melancholia and hypochondriasis were synonyms. Hypochondriasis was known as the disease of the Western world's middle and affluent class. It was socially accepted and then gradually became fashionable

Table 8–1.   Neurasthenia

Mental symptoms	Physical symptoms
Lack of initiative and ambition	Fatigue, lack of energy
Difficulty in concentration	Headache or dizziness
Feelings of inferiority	Muscular soreness
Pessimism	Fleeting back and chest pain
Suicidal ideas	Anorexia, indigestion or pyrosis
Need to be dependent	Flatulence, constipation or eqigastralgia
Sadness	Some impairment in sexual function
Fearfulness	
Other	

(Idzorek 1975). Throughout the years, it established itself ambiguously in the provinces of internal medicine and neuropsychiatry, competing with other conditions presenting common symptomatology. The age at onset ranges from 30 to 39 in men and from 40 to 49 in women (Kenyon 1964).

Hypochondriacal complaints also are caused by physical illnesses (e.g., thyroid disease, organic brain syndrome, systemic lupus erythematosus, and others) in 15% of cases (Ladee 1966). In a diagnostic clinical study, hypochondriacal patients presented statistically significant complaints of pain compared with a control group. These complaints were mostly identified with psychiatric syndromes and functional somatic syndromes (e.g., fibromyalgia, irritable bowel syndrome, chronic fatigue syndrome, and temporomandibular joint syndrome). Patients considered their physical functioning worse than did control subjects and used more hospitalizations (Noyes et al. 1993). This corroborated previous observations.

Various hypochondriasis scales appear to measure different syndrome features. Fear of disease is associated with anxiety, and a false belief of having a disease (disease conviction) is associated more with somatic symptoms (Kellner et al. 1992).

In assessing life events and hypochondriacal attitudes or concerns, several findings are worth mentioning. Before the onset of hypochondriasis, patients tend to mimic symptoms experienced by other family members (Apley 1959); for example, the somatic symptoms of depressed adults tend to resemble those of their mothers (Kreitman et al. 1965). Family illness also is a precipitating factor (Bianchi 1973), and in depressed patients there is a high incidence of respiratory tract disease (Burns and Nichols 1972). Three correlations of the Life Events Scale with the Illness Attitude Scale

(Kellner 1981) are significant: hypochondriasis, thanatophobia, and bodily preoccupation (Kellner et al. 1983).

In a study of hypochondriasis and OCD, OCD assessment scales were not applicable to hypochondriasis patients. This population had a higher number of patients with panic disorder and agoraphobia (McKay and Neziroglu 1993). For other patients, there is an "OCD-like" form of hypochondriasis (Fallon et al. 1991)

One classification divides hypochondriasis into three core symptoms: 1) fear of a disease; 2) hypochondriac ideation, at times as a nihilistic form in depressive patients; and 3) hypochondriacal ideas without depression but with obsessionality (Prat et al. 1971). This classification indirectly relies on the "hidden presence" of phobia, depression, and obsessions, respectively.

Hypochondriasis also is classified as primary or secondary. Two major studies have been conducted to classify this syndrome. One concluded that hypochondriasis can be a part of other syndromes; that primary and secondary hypochondriasis present similarities in most variables studied; and that for both groups, the main symptoms are located in the head, neck, abdomen, and chest. The course after onset, in rank order, was phasic (43%), fluctuating (28%), worsening (22%), and static (6%) (Kenyon 1964). Another study reached different conclusions as to whether anxiety or depression determined the presence of secondary symptoms (Pilowsky 1970). In primary hypochondriasis, patients complained of musculoskeletal problems and skin care or appearance conditions. The skin symptoms are reminiscent of body dysmorphic disorder. In secondary hypochondriasis, the main symptoms are depersonalization, poor sexual adjustment, and apprehension of becoming ill. These symptoms suggest that histrionic features participate in hypochondriasis configuration.

A more objective assessment used a structured psychiatric interview and a structured hypochondriasis interview. It found a large incidence of illness phobia and fear of dying (Bianchi 1971). This hypochondriasis-phobia correlation seems unclear and is hence controversial in proper diagnosis. However, symptoms overlap, and the vagueness of patients' statements makes it cumbersome to clearly delineate both conditions. There are a variety of alternative classifications that separate hypochondriasis and illness phobia (Bianchi 1971; Leonhard 1968; Marks 1987; Mayou 1976; Pilowsky 1967; Ryle 1947).

Studying hypochondriasis in medical settings provides helpful additional data to delineate this disorder's complexities. A substantial number of medical clinic patients have been identified as problem patients because they challenge medical knowledge. This patient population holds ambivalent feelings and opinions toward the medical profession and is known as the "familiar face" (Kemp 1963), the "crock" (Bender 1964), the "rotating patient" (Lipsitt 1968), and the "hateful patient" (Groves 1978). We expect that patients with hypochondriasis strongly believe in their illnesses, and therefore, they consult general practitioners for treatment (Bridges and Goldberg 1985).

Finally, we should not overlook transient hypochondriacal symptoms in medical students, a traditional malady in any medical school. About 70% of medical students have temporary hypochondriasis (Hunter et al. 1964; Woods et al. 1966).

Hypochondriasis seems to overlap poorly defined nosological boundaries with clinical entities that should be considered for differential diagnosis purposes. These include 1) monosymptomatic delusion, 2) hysteria, 3) conversion hysteria, 4) prodromal schizophrenia, 5) somatization disorder, 6) major depression, 7) obsessive-compulsive disorder, 8) generalized anxiety disorder, 9) somatoform pain disorder, 10) body dysmorphic disorder, and 11) factitious disorders. The common element in these conditions seems to be a faulty perception or an impaired cognition resting on dubious somatic complaints. At first glance, it appears that this is a group of disparate psychiatric disorders; however, on closer examination, most are similar because they involve physical symptoms presumably caused by psychological distress (Turner et al. 1984).

Treatment

Hypochondriasis pharmacotherapy relies on treatment of its most prominent symptoms (depression, obsessive-compulsive symptoms, anxiety). Antidepressants, anxiolytics, or anti–obsessive-compulsive agents are used.

In one sample, psychotherapy or psychoanalysis are used with satisfactory to good results (Ladee 1966). Medication, electroconvulsive therapy, and psychotherapy were selected in uncontrolled studies, with good outcomes in 48% of cases (Kenyon 1964; Pilowsky 1968). Other studies have used medication and psychotherapy, with results indicating improvement in 64% of patients (Kellner et al. 1983). Symptomatic treatment consisting of supportive measures remains the most popular approach to secondary symptoms (Burns 1971; Gelder et al. 1984; Kellner 1986; Lesse 1967; Stenback and Rimon 1964).

Behavioral therapy also is indicated for hypochondriasis treatment based on correlation with phobia (Marks 1981; Salkovskis and Warwick 1986;

Warwick and Salkovskis 1985) and anxiety (Wolpe 1986). In primary hypochondriasis, systematic desensitization, thought stopping, implosion (Kellner 1985), and exposure and response prevention (Warwick and Marks 1988) are used. Cognitive therapy also is used based in the hypothesis that hypochondriasis results from health anxiety (Warwick and Salkovskis 1990).

Hysteria

Hysteria, another 3,000-year-old syndrome, has been changed semantically and reclassified and has undergone conceptual reformulations to explain its pathology.

Charcot et al. widely explored the phenomenology and pathophysiology of this condition (Rof-Carballo 1955). They concluded that hysteria can be cured, appears in a specific constitutional type, and is a psychogenic reaction that tends to simulate and often initiate panic. Classic hysteria presents three major symptoms: 1) mobilization (tonic and clonic movements), 2) immobilization (paralysis), and 3) *la belle indifférence*. Interestingly, patients with hysteria need an audience for their objective symptoms (e.g., Charcot's hysterical arch).

Currently, hysteria is considered a somatization disorder. It is no longer well defined, and its meaning is confusing. This syndrome comprises five diagnoses or interpretations: 1) conversion disorder, 2) Briquet's syndrome, 3) personality disorder, 4) a specific pathological psychodynamic pattern manifesting itself as a personality trait, and 5) a colloquialism used to described undesirable behavior (Chodoff 1974). Hysteria is a different somatopsychic problem from hypochondriasis. However, it is decreasing in the Western world (Merskey 1978), whereas hypochondriasis is increasing in neuropsychiatry and general medicine.

Schizophrenia

Prodromal schizophrenia is multifacetic. Thus, it may start with hypochondriacal manifestations, and this onset may lead to misdiagnosis. In hypochondriasis, false beliefs exist. However, such beliefs seem weaker than the false belief of body dysmorphic disorder and therefore modifiable. In schizophrenia the false belief is strong and rigid and therefore unchangeable (see Chapter 5). Eventually the evolution of the syndrome will determine a final diagnosis.

Comorbidity, the transformation of one condition into a new condition, also is observed in prodromal schizophrenia, hypochondriasis, and OCD and in many stages of the OCD continuum in general.

Monosymptomatic Hypochondriasis

An association between hypochondriasis and paranoid states, or psychosis, has been reported. A classic observation is the presence of a single delusion—for example, infestation with parasites, syphilis, or AIDS. A syndrome representing this symptomatology is monosymptomatic hypochondriacal psychosis (MHP) (Munro 1980). This syndrome is closely related to Marfan's systematized delusions.

This illness has a single delusional system, distinct from the remainder of the personality. The delusion may be accompanied by illusional misperception or, at times, poorly defined hallucinations (Munro and Chmara 1982). Munro and Chmara (1982) developed a diagnostic checklist based on 50 cases. This checklist includes features of the illness, predisposing factors, factors associated with the illness, and additional symptoms. For Munro, MHP is distinct from body dysmorphic disorder because the personality is different (Munro 1978a). This disorder seems to focus on an organ or a limited functional area. Sometimes MHP includes delusion of parasitosis (Munro 1978b; Rapp 1986), worm infestation (Munro 1978c), and alimentary stench (Beary and Cobb 1981; Osman 1991).

In one study, nine females and two males complained of skin disorders, including acne lesions, changes in skin texture and luster, and hair thinning. These changes, if present, were mild and did not justify the severe degree of anxiety that accompanied them. The author described this as dermatological hypochondriasis and associated them with schizophrenia (Zaidens 1950).

Treatment

Treatment for MHP consists of drug and behavior therapy. Few investigations have been done, and the number of patients involved in trials has been minimal. Therefore, it is difficult to conclude what the best treatment is.

Of the drugs administered for MHP, pimozide, a strong dopamine blocker, has been reported as successful (Hamann and Avnstorp 1982; Lyell 1983; Munro 1984, 1988; Munro et al. 1985; Reilly 1975; Reilly and Batchelor 1986; Reilly et al. 1978; Ungvari and Vladar 1984). Pimozide, according to these results, seems to be an excellent drug. The oral pimozide dose ranges from 2 to 12 mg daily. Those prescribing pimozide should consider untoward effects, such as extrapyramidal symptoms, dystonias, and prolongation of the QT segment of the electrocardiogram. Other neuroleptics have been used, with excellent to moderate results: these include fluphenazine (Frithz 1979), flupenthixol, trifluoperazine, and zimeldine. Electroconvulsive therapy also has been used (Reilly and Batchelor 1986).

Antidepressants are the second choice of treatment. A few trials of one to two patients each have been reported, with satisfactory results. The drugs included doxepine or imipramine (Brotman and Jenike 1984), nortriptyline (Pyklo and Sicignan 1985), imipramine (Cashman and Pollock 1983), amoxapine (Tollefson 1985), clomipramine (Fernando 1988; Sondheimer 1988), and fluoxetine (Fishbain and Goldberg 1991). Behavior therapy using primarily exposure in vivo for olfactory delusions had good results (Beary and Cobb 1981).

We have not accumulated enough treatment data to provide good therapeutic strategy to treat such a difficult group of patients. It seems that physical complaints make patients seek help from a general practitioner, who may be as unaware of this condition as the patient.

OCD

The intense preoccupation or worriedness about being ill and seeking continuous medical reassurance is reminiscent of OCD similitude. For hypochondriasis to be an OCD variant, other obsessive-compulsive symptoms must be present (e.g., compulsions and doubting). Therefore, if patients obsess over being ill, compulsively check for physical evidence of disease, and need reassurance because of doubting, it is fair to raise the question of OCD comorbidity. It is common to see a combination of hypochondriasis and OCD symptoms. One study shows that the use of an anti–obsessive-compulsive agent (e.g., fluoxetine) sometimes benefits both conditions.

Bodily concern, worriedness, and *obsessionality about problems related to physical health* are interchangeable terms. Preoccupation with cutaneous problems can be viewed as a body dysperception, hypochondriasis, or OCD (Stein and Hollander 1992). Nonspecific dermatitis caused by compulsive hand washers often are seen in dermatology (Rasmussen 1985). Certain clinical OCD forms rarely come to a psychiatric facility, mostly when symptoms are prominently physical. In a dermatology clinic, patients were screened for OCD. A significant number (15%) had previously undiagnosed OCD. All of them came for treatment of a chronic pruritic condition (Hatch et al. 1992).

Other somatic conditions, such as respiratory tract diseases, had higher life prevalence of panic disorder (47%), OCD (13%), and eating disorder (13%) (Zandbergen et al. 1991). Gastrointestinal disorders also are somatic problems in OCD patients who ignore its presence. They usually seek help from a gastroenterologist. Patient concerns relate to bowel functions, mainly diarrhea and constipation. Irritable bowel pathogenesis certainly relates to chronic severe anxiety and certain forms of OCD, and of course, it is part of the hypochondriasis spectrum. Bowel obsessions respond well to the use of tricyclic antidepressant medication (Jenike et al. 1987).

Conclusion

According to one study, empirical data on the degree of overlap between hypochondriasis and OCD are too limited for definite conclusions (Barsky 1992). The body of information is small, perhaps because most patients do not see their conditions as psychogenic. Therefore, pathogenesis, diagnosis, treatment, and the presence of comorbidity remain relatively unknown owing to a lack of sufficient patients to study.

Somatoform disorders are historically old, encompassing conditions that may be related. One theoretical work on somatization outlines a model of amplifying symptoms. The amplification of normally fluctuating levels of bodily preoccupation and concern reaches a level of sustained intensity, causing psychological impairment and maladaptive behavior (Kirmayer et al. 1994).

References

American Psychiatric Association: Diagnostic and Statistical Manual of Mental Disorders, 4th Edition. Washington, DC, American Psychiatric Association, 1994

Andrews G, Hadzi-Pavlovic D, Psychol M, et al: Views of practicing psychiatrists on the treatment of anxiety and somatoform disorders. Am J Psychiatry 144: 1331–1335, 1987

Apley J: The Child With Abdominal Pains. Oxford, Blackwell, 1959

Barsky AJ: Hypochondriasis and obsessive-compulsive disorder. Psychiatr Clin North Am 15:791–801, 1992

Beary MD, Cobb JP: Solitary psychosis—three cases of monosymptomatic delusion of alimentary stench treated with behavioral psychotherapy. Br J Psychiatry 138:64–66, 1981

Bender D: Reexamination of the crock, in Psychosomatic Medicine. Boston, MA, Little, Brown, 1964

Bianchi GN: The origins of disease phobia. Aust N Z J Psychiatry 5:241–257, 1971

Bianchi GN: Patterns of hypochondriasis: a principal component analysis. Br J Psychiatry 122:542–548, 1973

Bridges KW, Goldberg DP: Somatic presentation of DSM III psychiatric disorders in primary care. J Psychosom Res 29:563–569, 1985

Brotman AW, Jenike MA: Monosymptomatic hypochondriasis treated with tricyclic antidepressants. Am J Psychiatry 141:1608–1609, 1984

Brown FW, Golding JM, Smith GR: Psychiatric comorbidity in primary care somatization disorder. Psychosom Med 52:445–451, 1990

Burns BH: Breathlessness in depression. Br J Psychiatry 119:39–45, 1971

Burns BH, Nichols MA: Factors related to the localisation of symptoms to the chest in depression. Br J Psychiatry 121:405–409, 1972

Cashman FE, Pollock B: Treatment of monosymptomatic hypochondriacal psychosis with imipramine (letter). Can J Psychiatry 28:85, 1983

Chodoff P: The diagnosis of hysteria: an overview. Am J Psychiatry 131:1073–1078, 1974

Fallon BA, Javitch JA, Hollander E, et al: Hypochondriasis and obsessive-compulsive disorder: overlaps in diagnosis and treatment. J Clin Psychiatry 52:457–460, 1991

Fernando N: Monosymptomatic hypochondriases treated with a tricyclic antidepressant. Br J Psychiatry 152:851–852, 1988

Fischer-Homberger E: Hypochondire. Bern, Switzerland, Verlag Hans Huber, 1970

Fishbain DA, Goldberg M: Fluoxetine for obsessive fear of loss of control of malodorous flatulence. Psychosomatics 32:105–107, 1991

Frithz A: Delusions of infestation: treatment by depot injections of neuroleptics. Clin Exp Dermatol 4:485–488, 1979

Gelder M, Gath D, Mayou R: Oxford Textbook of Psychiatry. Oxford, Oxford University Press, 1984

Groves JE: Taking care of the hateful patient. N Engl J Med 298:883–887, 1978

Hall RCW: Medically induced psychiatric disease: an overview, in Psychiatric Preservation of Medical Illness. Somatopsychic Disorders. Edited by Hall RCW. New York, Spectrum Publications, 1980, pp 3–9

Hamann K, Avnstorp C: Delusions of infestation treated by pimozide: a double-blind crossover clinical study. Acta Derm Venereol (Oslo) 62:55–58, 1982

Hatch ML, Paradis C, Friedman S, et al: Obsessive-compulsive disorder in patients with chronic pruritic conditions: case studies and discussion. J Am Acad Dermatol 26:549–551, 1992

Hunter CA, Lohrenz JG, Schwartzman AE: Nosophobia and hypochondriasis in medical students. J Nerv Ment Dis 139:147–152, 1964

Idzorek S: A functional classification of hypochondriasis with specific recommendations for treatment. South Med J 68:1326–1332, 1975

Jenike MA, Vitagliano HL, Rabinowitz J, et al: Bowel obsessions responsive to tricyclic antidepressants in four patients. Am J Psychiatry 144:1347–1348, 1987

Kellner R: Illness Attitude Scales. Abridged manual (mimeographed). Albuquerque, NM, University of New Mexico, 1981

Kellner R: Functional somatic symptoms and hypochondriasis. Arch Gen Psychiatry 42:821–833, 1985

Kellner R: Somatization and Hypochondriases. New York, Praeger, 1986

Kellner R, Pathak D, Romanik R, et al: Life events and hypochondriacal concerns. Psychiatr Med 1:133–141, 1983

Kellner R, Hernandez J, Pathak D: Hypochondriacal fears and beliefs, anxiety, and somatisation. Br J Psychiatry 160:525–532, 1992

Kemp R: The familiar face. Lancet 1:1223–1226, 1963

Kenyon FE: Hypochondriasis: a clinical study. Br J Psychiatry 110:478–488, 1964

Kirmayer LJ, Robbins JM, Paris J: Somatoform disorders: personality and the social matrix of somatic distress. J Abnorm Psychol 103:125–136, 1994

Koranyi EK: Somatic illness in psychiatric patients. Psychosomatics 21:887–891, 1980

Kreitman N, Sainsbury, Pearce K, et al: Hypochondriasis and depression in outpatients at a general hospital. Br J Psychiatry 3:607–615, 1965

Ladee GA: Hypochondriacal Syndromes. New York, Elsevier, 1966

Leonhard K: On the treatment of eideohypochondriac and sensohypochondriac neuroses. Int J Soc Psychiatry 2:123–133, 1968

Lesse S: Hypochondriases and psychiatric disorders masking depression. Am J Psychotherapy 21:607–620, 1967

Lipsitt DR: The "rotating patient": a challenge to psychiatrist. J Geriatr Psychiatry 2:51–61, 1968

Lyell A: Delusions of parasitosis. Br J Dermatol 108:485–499, 1983

Marks IM: Cure and Care of Neuroses. New York, Wiley, 1981

Marks IM: Fears, Phobias, and Rituals. New York, Oxford University Press, 1987

Mayou R: The nature of bodily symptoms. Br J Psychiatry 129:55–60, 1976

McKay D, Neziroglu F: Hypochondriases: common pathways to obsessive-compulsive disorder. Symposium presented at the 27th annual meeting of the Association for Advancement of Behavior Therapy, Atlanta, GA, November 1993

Merskey H: Disorders of conscious awareness: hysterical phenomena. Br J Hosp Med 19:305–309, 1978

Munro A: Monosymptomatic hypochondriacal psychoses: a diagnostic entity which may respond to pimozide. Can Psychiatr Assoc J 23:497–500, 1978a

Munro A: Monosymptomatic hypochondriacal psychosis manifesting as delusions of parasitosis. Arch Dermatol 114:940–943, 1978b

Munro A: Two cases of delusions of warm infestations. Am J Psychiatry 135:234–235, 1978c

Munro A: Monosymptomatic hypochondriacal psychosis. Br J Hosp Med 24:34–38, 1980

Munro A: Pathological jealousy: an excellent response to pimozide. Can Med Assoc J 131:852–853, 1984

Munro A: Monosymptomatic hypochondriacal psychosis. Br J Psychiatry 153:37–40, 1988

Munro A, Chmara J: Monosymptomatic hypochondriacal psychosis: a diagnostic checklist based on 50 cases of the disorder. Can J Psychiatry 27:374–376, 1982

Munro A, O'Brien JV, Ross D: Two cases of "pure" or "primary" erotomania successfully treated with pimozide. Can J Psychiatry 30:619–622, 1985

Nishioka Y, Nishizono M, Yamamoto J: The distinction of mental illness found by DIS among internal and orthopedic patients. Jpn J Psychiatry Neurol 44:33–54, 1990

Noyes R, Kathol R, Fisher M, et al: The validity of DSM-III-R hypochondriases. Arch Gen Psychiatry 50:961–970, 1993

Osman AA: Monosymptomatic hypochondriacal psychosis in developing countries. Br J Psychiatry 159:428–431, 1991

Paykel ES, Myers JK, Dienelt MN, et al: Life events and depression: a controlled study. Arch Gen Psychiatry 21:753–760, 1969

Pilowsky I: Dimensions of hypochondriasis. Br J Psychiatry 113:89–93, 1967

Pilowsky I: The response to treatment in hypochondriacal disorders. Aust N Z J Psychiatry 2:88–94, 1968

Pilowsky I: Primary and secondary hypochondriasis. Acta Psychiatr Scand 46:273–289, 1970

Prat J, Porta A, Vallejo J: Sindromes obsesivoides en psiquiatría, in Patología Obsesiva. Edited by Monserrat-Esteve S, Costa Molinari JM, Ballús C. Málaga, Spain, Graficasa, 1971, pp 314–337

Pyklo T, Sicignan J: Nortriptyline in the treatment of a monosymptomatic delusion. Am J Psychiatry 142:1223, 1985

Rapp MS: Monosymptomatic hypochondriasis (letter). Can J Psychiatry 31:599, 1986

Rasmussen SA: Obsessive-compulsive disorder in dermatologic practice. J Am Acad Dermatol 13:956–957, 1985

Reilly TM: Pimozide in monosymptomatic psychosis. Lancet I:1385–1386, 1975

Reilly TM, Batchelor DH: The presentation and treatment of delusional parasitosis: a dermatological perspective. Int Clin Psychopharmacol 1:340–353, 1986

Reilly TM, Jopling WH, Beard AW: Successful treatment with pimozide of delusional parasitosis. Br J Dermatol 98:457–459, 1978

Rof-Carballo J: Patologia Psicosomatica. Madrid, Spain, Paz Montalvo, 1955

Ryle JA: Nosophobia. Journal of Mental Science 94:1–17, 1947

Salkovskis PM, Warwick HMC: Morbid preoccupations, health anxiety and reassurance: a cognitive behavioral approach to hypochondriasis. Behav Res Ther 24:597–602, 1986

Sondheimer A: Clomipramine treatment of delusional disorder—somatic type. J Am Acad Child Adolesc Psychiatry 27:188–192, 1988

Stein DJ, Hollander E: Dermatology and conditions related to obsessive-compulsive disorder. J Am Acad Dermatol 26:237–242, 1992

Stenback A, Rimon R: Hypochondria and paranoia. Acta Psychiatr Scand 40: 379–385, 1964

Tollefson G: Delusional hypochondriasis, depression, and amoxapine. Am J Psychiatry 142:1518–1519, 1985

Turner SM, Jacob RG, Morrison R: Somatoform and factitious disorders, in Comprehensive Handbook of Psychopathology. Edited by Adams HE, Sutker PB. New York, Plenum, 1984, pp 307–345

Ungvari VG, Vladar K: Pimozid-therapie des Dermatozoenwahns. Dermatol Monatsschr 170:443–447, 1984

Warwick HMC, Marks IM: Behavioral treatment of illness phobia. Br J Psychiatry 152:239–241, 1988

Warwick HMC, Salkovskis PM: Reassurance (letter). BMJ 290:1028, 1985

Warwick HMC, Salkovskis PM: Hypochondriasis. Behav Res Ther 28:105–117, 1990

Weiss E, Spurgeon English O: Psychosomatic Medicine: The Clinical Application of Psychopathology to General Medical Problems. Philadelphia, PA, WB Saunders, 1943

Wolpe J: Individualization: the categorical imperative of behavior therapy practice. J Behav Ther Exp Psychiatry 17:145–153, 1986

Woods SM, Natterson J, Silverman J: Medical student's disease: hypochondriasis in medical education. J Med Educ 41:785–790, 1966

Zaidens SH: Dermatologic hypochondriasis. Psychosom Med 12:250–253, 1950

Zandbergen J, Bright M, Pols H, et al: Higher lifetime prevalence of respiratory diseases in panic disorder? Am J Psychiatry 148:1583–1585, 1991

Chapter 9
Body Dysmorphic Disorder

ody dysmorphic disorder (BDD) typifies the "intellectual re-cycling" of old conditions. Semantic modifications, nosologi-cal changes, technological advancements, and a reconceptualization of BDD make the disorder a palatable subject. This rebirth attracts the interest of researchers and clinicians alike, yielding dividends benefiting diagnosis and treatment outcome. The term *dysmorphia* comes from the Greek dismorfia (*dis*, meaning abnormal or apart, and *morpho*, meaning shape). Herodotus used this word when referring to the myth of the ugliest girl in Sparta; it literally means ugliness related to facial appearance (Philippopoulos 1979).

In 1891, Morselli described for the first time two types of fixed ideas; fear of ugliness and fear of being buried alive. The term *dysmorphophobia,* coined by Morselli, portrayed a subjective feeling of physical deformity that patients believe is noticeable to others, although their appearance is normal. He emphasized the symptom's obsessive nature (doubting of the deformity) and then emphasized the thoughts and sensations that may develop in the body or mind. Morselli believed that both conditions—fear of being deformed and fear of being buried alive—are a type of "rudimentary paranoia" (p. 10) or fixed ideas. First, in describing his dysmorphophobia cases, Morselli seemed to anticipate comorbidity recognition, mentioning three embedded key words: obsessiveness, phobia, and paranoia. Second, he suggested the participation not only of the mind, but also of the body as well by relating the dysperception to a bodily disturbance.

Although the debate continues, the word dysmorphophobia was replaced by dysmorphic, which seems more descriptive and less confusing. In 1987 DSM-III-R adopted the term body dysmorphic disorder in lieu of dysmorphophobia (American Psychiatric Association 1987). In this chapter we use both terms interchangeably.

Currently BDD is considered an intense preoccupation, an obsession, an overvalued idea, or a delusion pertaining to body shape. The complexity of body image concept is a result of the nonspecificity and the sparsity of our knowledge about its meaning. Is BDD a symptom, a syndrome, a disease, part of the obsessive-compulsive disorder (OCD) spectrum, or an aesthetic demand for beauty (Andreasen and Bardach 1977; Birtchnell 1988; de Leon et al. 1989; Neziroglu and Yaryura-Tobias 1993a; Phillips et al. 1993)? These are some of the questions to be addressed in this chapter.

In neuropsychiatry and psychology, authors usually present points of view rather than facts. Here we will provide views and facts spanning about 100 years.

Symptomatology

We will focus on BDD as a disturbance of thought and body image with two major components or primary symptoms: 1) a faulty belief and 2) a bodily dysperception. If patients have a faulty somatosensory mechanism, patients will "feel" the presence of ugliness as a real perceptual input, and therefore they will believe in their ugliness. However, if there is no somatosensory involvement, the patient will have only a disorder of thought.

BDD patients rarely present with gross ugliness features. To the observer, their physical appearance usually goes unnoticed. They are shy, with poor eye contact, and camouflage their ugliness. They may cover their bodies with bulky clothes or wear a hat or sunglasses. Often they consult a clinician for other emotional disturbances because of their embarrassment about their primary problem. It might take them years to decide on a consultation. Some remain homebound for years, withdrawing from the social world. Basically, they are in pain, have exaggerated self-consciousness, feel emotionally unstable, have low self-esteem, and are socioeconomically deprived.

In several studies, almost 90% of the distortion was face related, followed by hair, skin, and eyes (Hollander and Phillips 1993; Neziroglu and Yaryura-Tobias 1993a; Phillips et al. 1993). Another report stated that only 33% of the distortion was face related, followed by the genitals (Hay 1970a). Skin importance does not depend on its coloration or hue degrees, but on clean, pure skin (Zaidens 1950). However, political connotations may force a person to reject his or her skin color, notably if it is not white. Many patients have asked for depigmentation treatment unrelated to the presence of vitiligo. This request was culturally, not politically, determined.

One systematic question we ask of our patients with OCD or its spectrum is whether they engage in self-harm. Patients with facial skin dysmorphia make a point to pick and dig their skin. Severe cases of skin picking and digging may require plastic surgery. We find it perplexing that a person who is obsessively concerned with facial appearance would carry out such drastic measures.

Case 1

Carol, a 30-year-old woman who was single and voluntarily unemployed, had been picking and digging her face for 4 years. She developed BDD at age 15. She was obsessed with the looks of the skin of her face and the shape of her breasts and thighs. Although she was able to finish high school, college became a nightmare, and she requested a leave of absence. She never went back. She withdrew from social contacts and gradually became homebound. As the result of picking, she sustained recurrent infections and ulcerations in her face. The lost of substantial amount of skin tissue required the intervention of a plastic surgeon.

Case 2

The face of John, a 24-year-old law student, was reminiscent of the face of a model. He had the fashionable "looks" to be a model in the advertisement world. Nonetheless, 2 years before we saw him, he left school, moved into an apartment, and refused to go out. His parents had to come once a week to bring groceries, which they left by the door. John would say, "I am ugly, perhaps not that much, but ugly enough to cover my face with a hood. I am alone but I cover my face with a hood. Actually, I don't even look in the mirror. I no longer check my face compulsively in the mirror. When I was 18, I had a nose job. I wish I could sue the surgeon. Look at my nose. I am going to have a second nose job. I can't take my ugliness. This is nothing. My ideal of a beautiful face is almost unreachable." He never gave a satisfactory explanation as to why he left his seclusion. One of our therapists spoke to him through the door for about 3 months. Finally he opened the door. Three months later he came to the Institute. He was placed on an intensive behavioral program 5 days per week for 8 weeks. He also received pimozide 4 mg/day po. After 1 month on pimozide, he developed ipsilateral contractions of the muscles of the right hemithorax (the Pisa syndrome). He recovered on benztropine (Cogentin) and was placed on a combination of benztropine 2 mg/day po and pimozide 3 mg/day po. Six months later he resumed his studies. In addition, he had plastic surgery on his nose. His nose looks the same, but this is not a therapeutic issue, at least for the time being.

Hair is important in determining body image acceptance by others; lack of it symbolizes loss of strength and virility. Although hair is a recognized sexual symbol, one must remember that during the pharaohs' rule in Egypt, a shaved female head was considered sexually attractive. However, hirsutism may affect body perception, as in one case of a man with an aversion to personal body hair on the chest, legs, and arms (Watts 1990). In a 28-patient sample, some complained of facial hair, whereas others complained of hair loss on the scalp. In this sample, dysmorphophobia was accompanied mostly by depression; there were two cases of dementia and two cases of schizophrenia. Moreover, one patient committed suicide, and two patients attempted it (Cotterill 1981). BDD is a serious condition.

Case 3

Jack is a 16-year-old male who came for consultation because of depression, insomnia, irritability, tension, poor school performance, and gradual loss of interest. During our first meeting, I asked him why he didn't remove his baseball cap. He refused to do so, without a satisfactory explanation. I became suspicious. "Look, Jack," I said to him, "I must give you a physical checkup." Finally he agreed, and to my surprise I found myself looking at fresh grafted hair in what used to be a normal hairline. Why did his parents go along with this? What were the criteria used by the plastic surgeon to proceed with surgery? I was unable to come up with a satisfactory explanation except for Jack's need to unnecessarily change his otherwise normal hairline. Although he initially rejected my diagnosis of BDD, he agreed to come for therapy.

Symptom multiplicity is a cumbersome feature that will unavoidably confuse the diagnosis. Symptoms range from obsessions to delusional thinking. Patients with BDD may present obsessionality unrelated to body image. These obsessions are usually mild or moderate, and they generally come and go, whereas body image obsessions are intense and painful and last many hours. Ability to resist is minimal, and attempting to reject the obsession is ineffective. Patients with BDD may combine compulsive mirror checking with magical thinking. These patients wish their ugliness would disappear suddenly by looking at the mirror.

Part of the symptom cohort includes fixed ideas, reference ideas, schizoid traits, self-centered behavior, and severe distress. Andreasen and Bardach (1977) presented a cluster of symptoms that included ideas of reference, anxiety, depression, anger, and hypochondriacal symptoms without psychosis. In a 30–BDD patient sample, 37% complained of tactile sensations, such as facial tightness (Phillips et al. 1993). Tactile sensations may suggest a somatosensory involvement.

Our experience with BDD shows the presence of well-described obsessive-compulsive symptoms. We have not clearly elicited delusional pathology, unless patients' body image distortion and false beliefs can be considered truly psychotic. We observe the thought process to have a strong quality of stubbornness, fixation, or rigidity, making it difficult to modify the patient's body image concept. This quality of the thought process can be described as an overvalued idea.

Patients have minimal insight of their illness, and their judgment remains intact in areas unrelated to their body image problem. Attention span and memory are well preserved, and physical and neurological examinations are normal.

This patient population cannot function because they fear public exposure, and as a consequence they lack social skills. This handicap is compounded by shyness, lack of assertiveness, and low self-esteem. Notably, the presence of social phobia anticipates BDD's onset (Phillips et al. 1993).

Epidemiology

Few epidemiological data are available for BDD, because most reports are single cases or do not include epidemiological information. In one report on 30 BDD patients with multiple psychiatric disorders, the mean consultation age was 33.2 years, and the mean age at BDD onset was 14.8 years; 57% were male, and 83% never married. Of this sample, 57% were unemployed, 37% lived with their parents, and 17% were living in a halfway house (Phillips et al. 1993).

In another report on 13 BDD patients, 11 of whom also had OCD, 62% were male, with a mean age of 24.7 years; the mean age at onset of the disorder was 16 years (Neziroglu and Yaryura-Tobias 1993a). However, this study contained only two patients with a diagnosis of BDD only. Further studies with larger numbers of BDD-only patients are needed.

Differential Diagnosis

The clinician must diagnose an entity that, although known for more than 100 years, remains vague, complex, and elusive. On reviewing mosaic symptomatology, one cannot ignore the many symptoms, either isolated or in clusters, that conform to the core of other neuropsychiatric conditions. Therefore, the possibility of symptom imbrication exists and should be considered when evaluating a patient. Whether BDD is an independent entity remains questionable.

Personality traits and disorders, major affective disorder, psychosis, mono-symptomatic hypochondriasis, and OCD are among the neuropsychiatric disorders to be screened and differentiated from BDD.

Personality Traits and Disorders

Self-consciousness, emotional stability, and self-esteem are three psychological dimensions that are altered in BDD (Rosenberg 1965). Narcissism, schizoid traits, obsessionality (Andreasen and Bardach 1977), conversion hysteria (Dahl 1986), personality disorganization (Fisher 1970), and avoidant and obsessive-compulsive behaviors (Neziroglu et al. 1996) are personality disturbances associated with BDD. Patients with BDD score high in tests that assess hysteroid-obsessoid features, hostility, and personal illness (Hay 1970b). Interestingly, depersonalization does not seem to affect body image (Cappon and Banks 1965).

In eight patients with both BDD and OCD, the Minnesota Multiphasic Personality Inventory (Hathaway and McKinley 1943) yielded these results: 88% had elevated scores in depression; 75%, in psychasthenia; and 8%, in schizophrenia (Neziroglu and Yaryura-Tobias 1993a). These results are similar to patients with OCD only.

It has not been determined what influence personality disorder exerts on the treatment outcome of BDD.

Major Affective Disorder

BDD emotionally and socially disables patients to a degree where they are often severely impaired in functioning. Often their ability to work, go to school, engage in interpersonal relations, and enjoy leisure activities is hampered. Thus, they develop secondary or reactive depression. At times a major depression may coexist with body image disturbances (Fernando 1988; Hardy and Cotterill 1982; Hay 1970a). Patients with major depression may manifest symptoms similar to those seen in BDD, in which they perceive themselves as less physically attractive (Noles et al. 1985). Conversely, BDD patients may exhibit symptoms of major depression; thus, rather than secondary depression, a comorbid major depression is present.

M. B. Stein (1985) reported the case of a 32-year-old woman who had a past history of recurrent depression. However, her main concern was her ugly and unsightly hair. For that reason, she sought continuous assistance from hairdressers but was unhappy with the results. Depression and dissatisfaction with her hair remitted after 3 weeks of treatment with trazodone 600 mg/day po at bedtime. The author proposed the eponym "the Vidal Sasson syndrome" (after a company that manufactures hair products) to identify this clinical entity manifested by depression, with a questionable obsessive-compulsive or monosymptomatic hypochondriacal component affecting body image (M. B. Stein 1985). Often BDD patients' response to their own perception of "ugliness" is depression, and their response to exposing their "ugly" part to others is anxiety.

Psychoses

The differential diagnosis for BDD should include three psychotic processes: schizophrenia, monosymptomatic hypochondriasis, and Capgras's syndrome. These three processes share with BDD thought disturbances and misperceptions. All these conditions have similar thought and perceptual pathology. For instance, the BDD belief system may evolve slowly from doubtfulness to certainty and from an obsessional idea to an overvalued idea or a clear delusional idea. It is like planting the seed of a delusional thought that may or may not grow to full development (forma frustra) (see Chapter 5).

In one classic case, the Wolf-Man of Freud had a fixed idea about his nose shape and penis size and was subsequently diagnosed with infantile neurosis. However, on reviewing the case, a diagnosis of a psychosis seemed more plausible. The patient again underwent analytical therapy; the nose was considered to symbolize the genitals. This idea was reinforced by the patient, who complained of an undersized penis. The patient fully recovered with analysis (Brunswick 1928). Had this patient been seen today, might he have been diagnosed as having BDD?

The overlapping of symptoms in BDD and schizophrenia has been studied throughout the years (Connolly and Gibson 1978; Dietrich 1962; Hay 1970a; Korkina 1959; Vitiello and de Leon 1990). It is claimed that patients with schizophrenia perceive themselves as having a large body (Burton and Adkins 1961), whereas others find their bodies small (Fisher and Seidner 1963).

In Korkina's sample of 41 patients referred to her Moscow Institute, 8 cases had a smell disorder, 33 were dysmorphophobic patients, and 35 were diagnosed as having schizophrenia (Korkina 1959). The eight cases of smell disorder could be considered to be olfactory hallucinations. For Pryse-Phillips (1971), olfactory hallucinations were common findings, as he showed in 99 cases collected during a period of 2 years. The question is whether there are olfactory hallucinations in patients with BDD.

In another 17-patient BDD study, 11 had a severe personality disorder, one had a depressive illness, and five were schizophrenic (Hay 1970b). In this report, patients exhibited at least one of Schneider's first-rank schizophrenia illness symptoms (Schneider 1959).

In one case of a young man who complained of the shape of various body parts, his body image distortion became delusional, accompanied by loss of balance and muscle twitches in the face, limbs, and trunk. After hospitalization, he was diagnosed with subacute sclerosing panencephalitis (Salib 1988). This case demonstrates the existing link between organicity and functionality in the development of psychopathology.

A liaison between Capgras's syndrome and body image distortion also should be considered. Capgras's syndrome consists of the delusional belief that known persons or objects are replaced by impostors or "doubles." Signer and Benson (1987) reported two interesting Capgras's syndrome cases associated with body image dysperception. In the first case a woman complained of a growing penis in lieu of an extirpated enormous uterine fibroid tumor, and she claimed her deceased husband had been replaced by an impostor. In the second case, an obsessional student having auditory hallucinations firmly believed a "physically created" person was growing in his body. These two cases further emphasize the interconnectedness of BDD and what seems to be a multivariate psychopathology (Signer and Benson 1987). Finally, this syndrome may be diagnosed in adolescents also having a "dysmorphic delusion" (Kouranu and Williams 1984).

OCD

Interest has developed in the interface between OCD and BDD. What diagnostic criteria should be used? DSM-IV (American Psychiatric Association 1994) criteria for OCD, BDD, and delusional disorder are too limited to resolve diagnostic hesitations for clinical purposes. These hesitations reasonably arise from the multiple interfaces of BDD emergence.

Anecdotal reports are inconclusive as far as diagnostic accuracy (Tanquary et al. 1992; Vitiello and de Leon 1990). However, in a 13–BDD patient study classified according to DSM-III-R (American Psychiatric Press 1987) criteria, 85% were diagnosed as having OCD (Neziroglu and Yaryura-Tobias 1993a). A review article has suggested that BDD be classified as a form of OCD, not as a somatoform or delusional disorder, and that patients be treated with selective serotonin reuptake inhibitors or pimozide, both of which have proven effective (Filteau et al. 1992).

Again, one theme of concern is to identify the body's boundaries in space. This concern preoccupies students of psychosis and other disorders of the body, such as BDD and anorexia nervosa. One study, in an attempt to clarify body image boundary definiteness and psychopathology, hypothesized that groups with stronger body image boundaries and groups with weaker body image boundaries should be found. Four groups consisting of hysterical patients, paranoid schizophrenic patients, obsessive-compulsive patients, and paranoid schizophrenic patients were examined using the barrier, penetration, and barrier-minus-penetration scores; results were nonsignificant (Vinck and Pierloot 1977). However, it should be mentioned that no BDD patients were included in the sample.

Other illnesses with features similar to OCD, such as anorexia nervosa, social phobia, and disorders associated with cosmetic surgery also have been discussed (Hollander et al. 1992).

Monosymptomatic Hypochondriasis

Similarities between BDD and monosymptomatic hypochondriasis (MSH) have been reported. MSH is characterized by well-defined and circumscribed false beliefs. Three major beliefs have been identified: 1) the belief that their body parts are deformed (as in BDD?); 2) the belief that they emit offensive body odors (olfactory delusional syndrome, also known as MSH [Bishop 1980; Brotman and Jenike 1984; Munro and Chmara 1982]); and 3) delusions of parasitic infestation.

There is not enough clinical evidence to further subclassify this condition. In BDD and MSH, the thought process operates differently. Patients with dysmorphophobia have overvalued ideation, whereas in those with MSH, thinking is always delusional. As seen in various chapters of this book, the pathology of thought follows gradients that are difficult to delineate. Therefore, further analysis of these disorders is needed.

Pathogenesis

Knowledge of the pathogenesis of BDD is still in its rudimentary stages. This lack of knowledge can be attributed to the fact that BDD, although known for more than 100 years, has been ignored for many years as an important psychiatric condition. Perhaps because patients believe they have a physical defect, they consult dermatologists or plastic surgeons rather than psychiatrists or psychologists. BDD patients overlook or ignore the psychiatric components of their illness. They refuse to accept their body as it is.

The concept of BDD pathophysiology may include three major aspects: 1) dynamic, 2) organic, and 3) psychosocial. Does BDD emerge from a philosophical posit, a neurobiological paradigm, or a psychosocial demand?

Dynamic Aspects

In addition to our biopsychological interest in BDD, we have concerns about the patient as a whole. It is our opinion that these patients live a devastated life of isolation and self-destructive behavior that sharply contrasts with a need for a supreme aesthetic endeavor that is illogical. Because false beliefs and dysperceptions are the foundation of the disorder, what role does life dynamics, or "elan vital," play in the lives of these patients?

Humans exist as consciousness, spirit, and essence, three elements of an integrative life that are immanent to us and of temporal permanence. However, Nietzsche remarked that humans are an unfinished product with the capability of transformation, a quality absent in other living organisms. Thus, humans are not integral, but rather incomplete rather than absolute and imperfect rather than perfect. These characteristics are magnified in BDD and also in OCD. Fortunately, humans possess the biopsychosocial plasticity to adapt.

Furthermore, humans have a perennial need to satisfy their narcissism and to believe in their eternity. As de Unamuno (1945) said, "For the Universe we are nothing, but for us we are everything." The dynamics of a patient with BDD conforms to the Unamunian thinking. This is translated in the attitude of the patient who wants to achieve perfect bodily beauty and stop time to reach those goals. This narcissistic belief, expressed by self-centered behavior, also is observable in patients with OCD and in patients with some types of personality disorders (e.g., histrionic, borderline). Within this construct of incompleteness, narcissism, perfectionism, and temporal arrest, the attitudes and behaviors of BDD emerge.

As an object humans exist in space and time, although our self might part from the universal wholeness. Our self may lose its integral harmony; our body may move away from and distance itself from the self. This distancing may cause a dysperception of the body as a whole, as reported in schizophrenia. It is feasible that the same mechanisms are manifested in certain types of BDD. When this occurs, there is a need to be perfect and this may overwhelm and shade any priority from the self. The obsession with body image may fetter humans to pain, provoking aggression; conversely, masochistic traits, guilt, and an addiction to suffering may cause self-destructive behaviors. This pathological balance between body and mind might be encountered when analyzing the dynamics of BDD. Patients with BDD live in conflict with themselves and with the world. This conflict affects socializing, paralyzes school and working activity, and throws the patient into a chronic state of depression and despair.

Organic Aspects

Distinguishing organic from functional aspects in neuropsychiatric diseases is conventional because no evidence has been provided for the idea that psychological activity can exist without neuronal participation. We will accept this premise as truth and review some of the organic symptoms that may lead to BDD.

BDD is manifested in a diversity of ways that can be grouped, as a guideline, for didactic and research purposes. These groupings are 1) primary or secondary neurological disorder, 2) phantom phenomena, 3) negative body concept in the presence of actual physical deformity, and 4) disturbed and negative body concept in the presence of minimal or no actual deformity: a) patients with minimal deformity requesting plastic surgery (dysmorphophobia) and b) other body image manifestations of psychiatric disorders (Lacey and Birtchnell 1986).

The concept of body image can be traced to the 1920s, when neurologists and psychiatrists explored the vast territory of mind and body. It was Head (1920) who started these explorations by describing the brain's faculty to screen weight, shape, size, and form and incorporate these into schemata.

Body dysperception, known in the past as disturbed somatopsyche (Wernicke 1906), has been associated with the interparietal syndrome. This syndrome consists of corporal dysperception, agnosia, and apraxia. Other researchers also have contributed to an understanding of the interparietal syndrome (Angyal 1935, 1936a, 1936b; 1936c). This syndrome relates to schizophrenia and might help explain toxic psychosis (Gurewitch 1932). Toxic psychosis, as seen in mescaline and hashish intoxication, affects the parietal function (Mayer-Gross and Stein 1928). Thus, it is not surprising to find that the pioneering work on body image clinically relates to the schizophrenic process.

Some schizophrenia patients may extend their body image by projecting it into space or report a shrinking of their body image by introjecting space into their bodies (Schilder 1935). This is based on the assumption that schizophrenia patients cannot discriminate between projection and introjection (Ferenczi 1912).

To study the internalized picture a person has of the body's physical appearance, evaluations were made using an adjustable body-distorting mirror (Cardone and Olsen 1969). The results indicated that although patients performed significantly poorer on the body image task, the group also made less accurate perceptual judgments involving similar distortions on a nonbody control task. Because some patients were on chlorpromazine therapy, an additional study was conducted to observe whether chlorpromazine modifies the body image. The results were controversial (Cardone and Olsen 1969).

Of note is another study that examined two related phenomena: 1) the judgment of whether a human body part belongs to the body's right or left half and 2) the imagined spatial transformation is more object-specific than could previously be assumed. This study produced rotatory stimuli that are oriented in space. Results showed that temporal and kinematic properties of imagined spatial transformations are more object-specific than were previously assumed (Parsons 1987). These experiments may help explain the schemata phenomena observable in OCD patients. OCD's schemata is described as the need to carry objects on the body in an equally distributed manner.

Anatomy Correlates

What anatomical connections cast light on our clinical observations in patients with BDD? First, we must remember that when one cerebral cortical area is stimulated, other areas respond. Hence, we infer that the cerebral cortex functions through association pathways. Therefore, knowing the brain's regional functions assists in elucidating the complex neuropsychiatric phenomena of BDD.

The prefrontal cortex connects to the temporal and parietal lobes via the cingulum pathways. Bilateral prefrontal region lesions may cause concentration loss, decreased intellectual performance, and memory and judgment deficits. Lesions in the somatosensory area, which borders the frontal and parietal lobes, causes loss of perception or reception.

Parietal lobe activities include interpretation and integration of information from sensory areas (i.e., somatosensory and visual cortex). Parietal lesions cause sensory ataxia, general awareness loss, apathy or indifference, faulty sensory impulse recognition, and inability to interpret spatial relationships.

Lesions of the striate cortex, or primary visual area, on one side result in a contralateral hemianopsia; lesions in the secondary visual area cause inability to interpret visual impulses.

The temporal lobes receive and interpret auditory information, pattern recognition, and higher visual coordination. The temporal lobe interconnections manage highly integrated activity. Lesions in this region modify normal behaviors and cause dysperceptions (i.e., hallucinations) and seizures. These anatomofunctional correlations are summarized in Table 9–1.

Because the phenomenology of BDD presents abnormal thinking and dysperceptions, we may attempt to associate them with cerebral structures. In other words, BDD pathophysiology may correlate with sensorial, motor,

Table 9–1. Body dysmorphophobia anatomofunctional correlates

Region	Deficit
Visual cortex	Perception
Somatosensory area	Reception-perception
Temporal lobe	Higher visual correlation
Parietal lobe	Interpretation of integration of information
Prefrontal lobe	Judgment

and higher cortical functions. An imbalance in this extensive loop may certainly provoke false beliefs and body dysperception.

One analogue model for the interpretation of BDD misperception is the phantom limb phenomenon. In this phenomenon, patients who have undergone excision of a limb continue to report its presence. For example, patients may try to stand on a missing foot. This false reality may require months to vanish. Although this phenomenon is mostly observed in the limbs, it also has been reported after the loss of other organs, such as the breasts, teeth, penis, or nose. It should be noted that the phenomenon is not experienced in congenital anomalies (Simmel 1961), after amputation during childhood, or during a gradual limb loss, as in leprosy (Simmel 1956).

The question is whether this false perception is cenesthesic or delusional, involving proprioceptive regions, somatosensory perception, or the presence of a neuroma at the amputation stump site. Two meticulous descriptions of phantom delusions have been published (Henderson and Smyth 1948; Riddoch 1941).

We would like to report a case that illustrates the participation of the brain in body image disturbances. A 72-year-old man sustained a left subcortical parietal hematoma that caused body image distortion and phantom limb sensations. The lesion interrupted thalamic tracts to parietal regions and callosal fibers linking parieto-occipital association areas. Certain cerebral function aspects in this patient were reminiscent of "split-brain" disorder (Cambier et al. 1984).

To conclude, the pathogenesis of BDD involves a triad: visual reception, interpretation, and response. This triad operates as follows: seeing; comparing; believing; judging; and finally, behaving accordingly. If the specificity of a brain lesion is the result of a noxa that directly and indirectly affects neuronal interconnections rather than one specific anatomical site, then some BDD forms are a result of organic malfunction.

Social and Psychological Aspects

Is there a single body image or more than one? Does the body image change with aging? It seems that elderly persons with a youthful appearance are more optimistic, more outgoing, and more social (Kligman and Graham 1989). Consistent with physical changes in adulthood, current and ideal ratings of body image become more discrepant in older groups, and more dissatisfaction is found among women (Altabe and Thompson 1993).

Who or what determines the perfect body image? Is it given by aesthetics or cultural demands (Ford et al. 1990)? Is it determined by publicity agencies promoting beautification products? Is it sexually controlled?

Historically, the way the body appears in the mind has preoccupied both sociologists and psychologists. Schilder advanced the idea that body image is a personality construct with perceptual and expressive characteristics (Schilder 1935). Since that time, three factors have been studied to explicate the concept and the consequences of body image: 1) individualization and socialization, 2) personality development, and 3) acceptance and rejection of the body part by the individual or family members.

Aesthetics is the study of beauty and ugliness. How are beauty and ugliness defined? Beauty is perceptually accepted and pleasurable to the senses, causing emotional responses with physiological reactions. Ugliness is perceptually unacceptable and unpleasant to the senses, also causing emotional and physiological responses.

In determining what is beautiful or ugly, two main modifiers—social guidelines and cultural traditions—are strong factors. Human beauty is determined by uniting skin, flesh, and fat, resulting in a geometric composite providing "the looks." Cultural and societal tastes change dynamically. Furthermore, each individual has opinions as to what is beautiful or ugly, and these are unavoidably modified by aging, gender, race, and color. Hedonism, as a pleasurable and likable activity or as the focus of life for many individuals, naturally provides enjoyment and is used advantageously by the cosmetics industry and by commercial plastic surgeons to foster beauty as a major life aim.

The symptoms of BDD seem to have an early onset, typically during adolescence. Adolescents worldwide are concerned with their physical image; their sexual identity; and, most importantly, with the need to be free and independent. However, as years go by, the facial image and the body in general sustain physical changes. Does the body image change with aging? Consistent with physical changes in adulthood, body dissatisfaction is more frequently noted in older groups and among women (Altabe and Thompson 1993).

Ford et al. (1990) questioned who or what determines the perfect body image. We proceed to ask, "What is the influence of the mass media and publicity agencies that promote beautification products?"

The feeling of ugliness elicits repugnance and shame (Munro and Chmara 1982), and patients report being tortured by this concern (Philippopoulos 1979), described as a compulsion (Stekel 1950). Ugliness may determine preference or rejection among family members and may even affect health issues. Studies of mothers' rejection of their children show the preference for better physically endowed children (MacGregor 1951). Beauty and ugliness seem to be the underlying determinants of outcome in health and illness (Czechowicz and Diaz de Chumaceiro 1988). Ugliness is represented by the clown figure, which has accompanying social repercussions, in art and literature; this has been further discussed by Klages and Hartwich (1982).

Undoubtedly, beauty appeals to the senses, and ugliness produces rejection. Advertising plays a preponderant role, communicating that the body must be beautiful. Two main targets are emphasized: 1) improved self-confidence and 2) enhanced sexual attractiveness. This continuous bombardment by conflicting and hidden messages results in considerable ego dissatisfaction. Synthesizing the central conflict, beauty-ugliness is well portrayed by "beauty is good and ugly is not" (Clifford and Bull 1978; Dion et al. 1972).

One conflict is the body image's mental representation in reality and its comparison with others' opinions of one's body image in their reality. Thus, there is a need to maintain a specific body image to better, for example, sexuality (Laufer 1991). In a psychosocial study of a university population's sexual behavior, two variables—sexual attitude and body image perception—were the best predictors for sexual approach/avoidance behavior (Faith and Share 1993).

Considering that one major localization of body image distortion includes secondary sexual organs (e.g., breast or penis), it is not surprising to find body image alterations in individuals with transsexualism or fetishism (Greenacre 1953). Current emphasis in sexual freedom is causing an abnormal rejection of the shape and size of the secondary sexual organs, causing impotence and frigidity as well as body dysmorphia–like symptoms.

The penis is characterized by psychological vulnerability. This disadvantage for male sexual prowess is illustrated in patients with koro, a disorder found in southeast Asia. This disorder consists of a perception of decreasing penis length because of imagined hyperinvolution from intra-abdominal traction. Koro results in acute anxiety reaction, a response that is less common among BDD sufferers, and koro patients fear both a loss of virility and death after penile retraction. In a 2-year follow-up study, patients showed remarkable constancy in their penis length perception (Chowdhury 1989). This seems to suggest that the cognitions in this disorder, which is similar to BDD, are refractory to treatment. This condition is as culturally bound as obesity, anorexia nervosa, and bulimia disorders, which also include body image distortions (Sims 1988).

The silent beauty of the romantic era is gone. Consequently, the upsurge in body image revisionism intrudes on what is a closed subject for those favoring moral and spiritual values. Meanwhile, copulation becomes a sensorial journey of two individuals, with or without an emotional component. This new set of sexual values has created a further deterioration in human behavior in which the body becomes an object of embarrassment. In BDD, there always is a sexual component that should be identifiable.

In women with BDD, early sexual traumatic experiences are a common finding. The clinician must establish a good rapport with the patient before sexual or physical abuse material surface. In general, patients with BDD who have been sexually abused tend to remain homebound.

Case 4

Joan is a 29-year-old single woman who remained homebound for 11 years. Her main symptoms were depression, difficulty swallowing both solid food and liquids, outbursts of anger, and severe displeasure with her body image. At the age of 23, she decided to have psychotherapy, but because she was homebound, therapy was conducted via telephone. She would not allow any visitors in the house. She lived with her parents, who took care of all her needs. As time went by, her symptoms worsened. She decided to move to the basement, a place without any daylight or a window for direct ventilation. Her difficulties in swallowing forced her to drink only one glass of water per day. She lost a considerable amount of weight and became dehydrated. Joan made several telephone contacts with one of the authors (F.N.) and finally agreed to hospitalization after 10 years of hesitation.

On admission, Joan looked extremely pale, thin, and dehydrated. She refused medication out of fear of choking. She underwent an intensive behavior and cognitive therapy program. Eventually she spoke of having been sexually abused by her father. In addition, the father used to masturbate in the living room in front of her. Was that the reason she moved to the basement and refused to see her father? Why didn't Joan move out of the house when she was still functional? Was the phobia that produced the swallowing difficulty the result of forced oral intercourse? Joan resorted to seeing herself as an ugly person in body and soul. Her reality was intact, but the individual and family pathology of this case is extensive.

Bruch's pioneering work in eating disorders called attention to the primary anorectic patient's disturbed body image (Bruch 1962). However, body width misperception in women with eating disorders did not differ from that in a healthy control population (Birtchnell et al. 1987). In another study, females and males with body image distortion but without eating disorders associated weight rather than shape with their misperception (Dolan et al. 1987). In a study comparing heterosexual and homosexual males, homosexuals were more dissatisfied with their weight. They desired an underweight ideal, making them prone to eating disorders (Herzog et al. 1991).

During the growth process, concomitant with assimilating, accommodating, and accepting or rejecting Piaget's scheme, adolescents have a body image disturbance (Simmons and Rosenberg 1973).

Youthful skin, a perfect complexion, and an absence of wrinkles are some features many BDD patients check for routinely in the mirror. This mirror "approval" is not uncommon in thousands of children as they enter adolescence. Skin disorders, such as acne (Koo and Smith 1991; D. J. Stein and Hollander 1992), may cause obsessive and compulsive behaviors. Psoriasis appears in patients who are dissatisfied with their body image and feel unhappy with interpersonal relationships (Hardy 1982).

Cosmetic Surgery

For some, body image is a complex, dynamic psychological concept and refers to the picture of one's body formed in one's mind (Lacey and Birtchnell 1986). However, people generally reject this postulate and vigorously opt for surgical intervention. The Freudian school did not favor cosmetic surgery, claiming that symptom substitution occurs and inappropriately alters the defense mechanisms (Hill and Silver 1950). It is inadvisable to undergo cosmetic surgery if the brain is seriously disorganized and expectations are unrealistic. However, at a 15-year follow-up of six schizophrenic patients and 32 severely neurotic patients, rhinoplasty did not aggravate their mental disturbance (Edgerton et al. 1960). However, these were not BDD patients, and it is hard to determine whether the outcome would have been the same in such patients.

In a study of the rationale for cosmetic nasal surgery, surgery patients had a more accurate perception of their nose size than did control patients. Moreover, in a follow-up from a small number of postsurgical assessments using the same protocol, patients reported a nose size normal for the control group (Jerome 1991). Breast augmentation significantly increased confidence in a group of separated or divorced women, but breast reduction was requested by single or cohabitating women (Birtchnell et al. 1990). Women seeking breast augmentation seem less assertive and less feminine (Beale et al. 1980). Unfortunately, to date there have been no prospective studies looking at the efficacy of plastic surgery among BDD patients. Therefore, it is inconclusive whether surgery is an effective treatment for this group of patients. In our experience, most patients who undergo surgery are not satisfied. In fact, a few have worsened because they were further dissatisfied with their "ugly" part.

Biological Treatment

Biological treatment consists of electroconvulsive therapy (ECT) or pharmacotherapy. The literature on treatment is meager and is further complicated by European (see "Monosymptomatic Hypochondriasis") and North American studies that used different diagnostic criteria. Controlled treatment studies have not been done. We agree with Hollander and colleagues that studies are methodologically and diagnostically confined (Hollander et al. 1992). Therefore, we refer to a few open studies that might help the clinician choose what is currently considered the most suitable pharmacotherapeutic approach. Finally, the trial-and-error approach is always a partial solution.

In one study, 30 BDD patients met DSM-III-R criteria for at least one other psychiatric disorder, particularly mood disorders (93%; $N = 28$). Most patients received many treatments: 28 had pharmacotherapy, 24 underwent insight-oriented therapy, 3 received behavior therapy, and 4 had ECT (Phillips et al. 1993). Thirteen BDD patients diagnosed according to DSM-III-R criteria also had an OCD diagnosis (85%; $N = 11$). Pharmacological treatment consisted of, in order of frequency, clomipramine, pimozide, fluoxetine, and lithium. Some of these patients received behavior therapy combined with drug treatment. Overall, results were good (Neziroglu and Yaryura-Tobias 1993b).

Two dysmorphophobia patients treated with behavior therapy, pimozide, and diazepam had a good response after the addition of phenelzine 45 mg/day po in one case and imipramine 200 mg/day po in another (Marks and Mishan 1988). The authors also prescribed antidepressants to ameliorate depression.

A five–BDD patient group was treated with clomipramine ($n = 4$) or fluoxetine 80 mg/day po ($n = 1$) after a negative trial with imipramine and pimozide; all patients improved greatly (Hollander et al. 1989). In one report, a dysmorphophobia patient (atypical somatoform disorder) who failed to respond to neuroleptics and heterocyclic antidepressants did well with tranylcypromine 10 mg po tid (Jenike 1984). In another report, a patient with skoptic syndrome, an entity manifested by obsessionality with secondary sexual characteristics, was successfully treated with lithium 900 mg/day po (Coleman and Cesnik 1990).

In the international literature on BDD and somatodelusional disorders, two psychotropic medication groups with distinct pharmacological properties and therapeutic indications are mentioned: 1) the selective serotonin reuptake inhibitors and 2) the neuroleptic dopamine blockers.

A serotonergic mechanism to explain this disorder's pathophysiology could be proposed based on favorable responses to the administration of selective serotonin reuptake inhibitors. There are two caveats that challenge this hypothesis. One is the use of pimozide, a potent dopamine reuptake blocker with strong antipsychotic action that stimulates resocialization and encourages the verbalization of delusional symptomatology (Yaryura-Tobias et al. 1974). The other is a report indicating that tryptophan depletion causes an acute exacerbation of BDD (Barr et al. 1992). Controlled studies are needed to compare the efficacy of various pharmacological agents.

Behavior Therapy

Most behavior therapy literature consists of case studies and uncontrolled single-subject designs. Munjack's (1978) early case study focused on a nonpsychotic 27-year-old man who complained of an abnormally red complexion. The patient was taught relaxation training, and a hierarchy was constructed consisting of "criticism about red face" and "scrutiny of his face by others." Clinical improvement was reported with systematic desensitization. Braddock (1982) reported successfully treating a 16-year-old female who complained of a "funny and crinkly nose" and a wrinkled forehead. Seven months after these initial complaints, she was homebound and wanted plastic surgery. A behavioral approach was used in which all references to her forehead and nose were avoided. In addition, she was encouraged to develop social skills and become more assertive, although it does not appear that any formal social skills or assertion training was offered.

Jerome (1987), in discussing the differences between anorexia and dysmorphophobia patients, suggested that both diagnostic groups may benefit from behavior therapy. He indicated that the former group may show clinical improvement after mirror confrontation, because anorectic patients avoid checking their bodies in the mirror, and the latter group may benefit from avoidance of mirror checking. He stated that his hypothesis came from patients who reported themselves much improved after cosmetic surgery, even when no objective change occurred. He noted that dressings after surgery prevented patients from looking at the particular "deformed" body part, thus serving as response prevention.

Marks and Mishan (1988) conducted a pilot study on five chronic BDD patients using exposure and response prevention. Four of the five were treated as inpatients because they lived far away. All five were isolated and avoided social interaction as a result of BDD. Two of the five did not have visible defects but complained of their body smell and resorted to washing. In fact, one patient later developed a psychosis. It is questionable whether these patients had true BDD or perhaps delusional disorder, somatic type. In addition, the efficacy of exposure and response prevention alone may be questioned, because two patients received medication in addition to behavior therapy, and one was later treated for schizophrenia.

Neziroglu and Yaryura-Tobias (1993b) reported on the effect of exposure and response prevention without medication in five BDD patients. Three patients received intensive 90-minute behavior therapy sessions 5 days weekly; two underwent the same treatment once weekly. Four of the five improved on the overvalued idea scale, which assessed the strength of the belief in their deformity, and on the Yale-Brown Obsessive Compulsive Scale modified for BDD, which assessed time occupied by thoughts and spent in activities related to body defect. They concluded that behavior therapy and cognitive therapy were effective BDD treatment modalities.

In another study, Neziroglu and Yaryura-Tobias (1993a) reported on 13 BDD patients who underwent behavioral and psychopharmacological treatment. Treatment consisted of intensive behavior therapy (90-minute sessions, 5 days weekly), weekly or monthly exposure and response prevention sessions, and cognitive therapy. MMPI scores in these patients were similar to those in OCD patients and showed elevated scores on scales 2 (depression), 7 (psychasthenia), and 9 (schizophrenia). Ten patients of 13 had high overvalued ideas, and all but one had moderate to severe depression, as assessed by the Beck Depression Inventory (Beck 1978). On the Yale-Brown Obsessive Compulsive Scale, only one patient scored below severe range (cutoff of 16). Body parts most affected were the nose (46%), hair (38%), and complexion (23%). The authors discussed the medications given but not the response, because the study was not a controlled drug trial. For each patient body part affected, exposure and response prevention target therapy, as well as cognitive therapy, was provided. However, once again treatment outcome was not available because the study's purpose was to acquire demographic information, assess psychological test response, describe BDD patients' symptoms, and illustrate appropriate treatments.

Psychological therapies in addition to behavior therapy were reported. Philippopoulos (1979) wrote a case study of an 18-year-old woman in whom a psychodynamic approach was used. Therapy was conducted two to three times weekly for 1 year. Dreams, fantasies, transference, and free associations were interpreted. The patient recovered, and her gains were maintained for several years. Bloch and Glue (1988) reported on a 20-year-old BDD patient who obsessed about her eyebrows. She was seen weekly for 20 months, and transference issues were raised to explore her underlying feelings of rejection by her father. She improved, with gains maintained 6 months later.

Watts (1990) described a combined behavioral and interpretative approach with one patient. The patient was exposed to his perceived hairy arms, legs, and chest for 15 to 20 minutes; then interpretations were made about body hair's symbolic meaning (e.g., male aggressiveness, the eternal boy, the Peter Pan figure remaining forever free and untrapped in sexual immaturity). The patient improved with a combined approach. The study's limitation is its inability to distinguish which treatment affected the symptoms.

Vitiello and de Leon (1990) reported on a 37-year-old man who thought his face was ugly. He camouflaged it with a full beard and continuously checked his face in mirrors. He received psychodynamic psychotherapy weekly for years, along with an unspecified amount of behavior therapy and pharmacological treatment consisting of benzodiazepines, tricyclic antidepressants, and clomipramine 200 mg/day for 6 months. None of the treatment modalities altered his BDD.

As noted from these studies, behavior therapy outcome research is needed in BDD, as currently available data are limited.

Prognosis

Combining pharmacotherapy with behavior and cognitive therapy might yield the best outcome. Unfortunately, our experience suggests caution when discussing treatment outcome with patients and relatives. Patient prognosis also is guarded in the presence of comorbidity. For instance, the prognosis for patients with BDD and juvenile schizophrenia or BDD and dysmorphophobia is unfavorable (Morozov 1976).

References

Altabe M, Thompson JK: Body image changes during early adulthood. Int J Eat Disord 13:323–328, 1993

American Psychiatric Association: Diagnostic and Statistical Manual of Mental Disorders, 3rd Edition, Revised. Washington, DC, American Psychiatric Association, 1987

American Psychiatric Association: Diagnostic and Statistical Manual of Mental Disorders, 4th Edition. Washington, DC, American Psychiatric Association, 1994

Andreasen NC, Bardach J: Dysmorphophobia: symptom or disease? Am J Psychiatry 134:673–675, 1977

Angyal A: The perceptual basis of somatic delusions in a case of schizophrenia. Archives Neurology and Psychiatry 34:270–279, 1935

Angyal A: Coincidence of the interparietal syndrome and automatic changes of posture in a case of schizophrenia. Archives Neurology and Psychiatry 37:629–637, 1936a

Angyal A: Phenomena resembling Lilliputian hallucinations in schizophrenia. Archives Neurology and Psychiatry 36:34–41, 1936b

Angyal A: The experience of the body-self in schizophrenia. Archives Neurolology and Psychiatry 35:1029–1053, 1936c

Barr LC, Goodan WK, Price LH: Acute exacerbation of body dysmorphic disorder during tryptophan depletion. Am J Psychiatry 149:1406–1407, 1992

Beale S, Lisper H, Palm B: A psychological study of patients seeking augmentation mammoplasty. Br J Psychiatry 136:133–138, 1980

Beck AT: Depression Inventory. Philadelphia, PA, Philadelphia Center for Cognitive Therapy, 1978

Birtchnell SA: Dysmorphophobia—a centenary discussion. Br J Psychiatry 153:41–43, 1988

Birtchnell SA, Dolan BM, Lacey JH: Body image distortion in non–eating disordered women. Int J Eat Disord 6:385–391, 1987

Birtchnell SA, Whitfield P, Lacey JH: Motivational factors in women requesting augmentation and reduction mammoplasty. J Psychosom Res 34:509–514, 1990

Bishop ER: Monosymptomatic hypochondriasis. Psychosomatics 21:731–747, 1980

Bloch S, Glue P: Psychotherapy and dysmorphophobia: a case report. Br J Psychiatry 152:271–274, 1988

Braddock LE: Dysmorphophobia in adolescence: a case report. Br J Psychiatry 140:199–201, 1982

Brotman AW, Jenike MA: Monosymptomatic hypochondriasis treated with tricyclic antidepressants. Am J Psychiatry 143:917–918, 1984

Bruch H: Perceptual and conceptual disturbances in anorexia nervosa. Psychosom Med 24:187–194, 1962

Brunswick RM: A supplement to Freud's "History of an Infantile Neurosis." Int J Psychoanal 9:439–476, 1928

Burton A, Adkins J: Perceived size of self-image body parts in schizophrenia. Arch Gen Psychiatry 5:131–140, 1961

Cambier J, Elghozi D, Graveleau P, et al: Right hemiasomatognosia and sensation of amputation caused by left subcortical lesion. Role of callosal disconnection (in French). Rev Neurol (Paris) 140:256–262, 1984

Cappon D, Banks R: Orientational perception. Arch Gen Psychiatry 13:375–379, 1965

Cardone SS, Olsen RE: Chlorpromazine and body image: effects on chronic schizophrenics. Arch Gen Psychiatry 20:576–582, 1969

Chowdhury AN: Dysmorphic penis image perception: the root of Koro vulnerability. A longitudinal study. Acta Psychiatr Scand 80:518–520, 1989

Clifford B, Bull R: The Psychology of Person Identification. London, Routledge & Kegan Paul, 1978

Coleman E, Cesnik J: Skoptic syndrome: the treatment of an obsessional gender dysphoria with lithium carbonate and psychotherapy. Am J Psychother 44:204–217, 1990

Connolly FH, Gibson M: Dysmorphophobia: a long term study. Br J Psychiatry 132:568–570, 1978

Cotterill JA: Dermatological non-disease: a common and potentially fatal disturbance of cutaneous body image. Br J Dermatol 104:611–619, 1981

Czechowicz H, Diaz de Chumaceiro CL: Psychosomatics of beauty and ugliness: theoretical implications of the systems approach. Clin Dermatol 6:9–14, 1988

Dahl AA: Some aspects of the DSM-III personality disorders illustrated by a consecutive sample of hospitalized patients. Acta Psychiatr Scand 328:61–67, 1986

de Leon J, Bott A, Simpson GM: Dysmorphophobia: body dysmorphic disorder or delusional disorder, somatic symptom? Compr Psychiatry 30:457–472, 1989

de Unamuno M: Del Sentimiento Tragico de la Vida. Buenos Aires, Argentina, Espasa-Calpe, 1945

Dietrich H: Uber Dysmorphophobie. Arch Psychiatr Nervenkr 203:511–518, 1962

Dion K, Berscheid E, Walster E: What is good is beautiful. J Pers Soc Psychol 24:285–290, 1972

Dolan BM, Birtchnell SA, Lacey JH: Body image distortion in non–eating-disordered women and men. J Psychosom Res 31:513–520, 1987

Edgerton MT, Jacobson WE, Meyer E: Surgical-psychiatric study of patients seeking plastic (cosmetic) surgery: Ninety-eight consecutive cases with minimal deformity. Br J Plast Surg 13:136–145, 1960

Faith MS, Share ML: The role of body image in sexually avoidant behavior. Arch Sex Behav 22:345–356, 1993

Ferenczi S: On the definition of introjection, in Final Contributions to the Problems and Methods of Psychoanalysis. New York, Basic Books, 1912, pp 316–318

Fernando N: Monosymptomatic hypochondriasis treated with a tricyclic antidepressant. Br J Psychiatry 152:851–852, 1988

Filteau MJ, Pourcher E, Baruch P, et al: Dysmorphophobia (body dysmorphic disorder) (in French). Can J Psychiatry 37:503–509, 1992

Fisher S: Body Experience in Fantasy and Behaviour. New York, Appleton-Century-Crofts, 1970

Fisher S, Seidner R: Body experiences of schizophrenia, neurotic and normal women. J Nerv Ment Dis 137:252–257, 1963

Ford KA, Dolan BM, Evans C: Cultural factors in the eating disorders: a study of body shape preferences of Arab students. J Psychosom Res 34:501–507, 1990

Greenacre P: Certain relationships between fetishism and faulty development of the body image, in Psychoanalytic Study of the Child. Edited by Eisler R, Hartman H, Freud A, et al. New York, International University Press, 1953, pp 79–98

Gurewitch M: Uber das Interparietale Syndrom Bei Geisterkrank-Heiten. Zeitschrift der Gesellschaft der Neurologie und Psychiatrie 140:593–603, 1932

Hardy GE: Body image disturbance in dysmorphophobia. Br J Psychiatry 141:181–185, 1982

Hardy GE, Cotterill JA: A study of depression and obsessionality in dysmorphophobia and psoriatic patients. Br J Psychiatry 140:19–22, 1982

Hathaway SR, McKinley JC: Minnesota Multiphasic Personality Inventory. Minneapolis, MN, University of Minnesota, 1943

Hay GG: Dysmorphophobia. Br J Psychiatry 116:399–406, 1970a

Hay GG: Psychiatric aspects of cosmetic nasal operations. Br J Psychiatry 116:85–97, 1970b

Head H: Studies in Neurology. London, Oxford, 1920

Henderson WR, Smyth CE: Phantom limb. J Neurol Neurosurg Psychiatry 11:88–112, 1948

Herzog DB, Newman KL, Warshaw M: Body image dissatisfaction in homosexual and heterosexual males. J Nerv Ment Dis 179:356–359, 1991

Hill G, Silver AG: Psychodynamic and aesthetic reasons for plastic surgery. Psychosom Med 12:345–357, 1950

Hollander E, Phillips KA: Body image and experience disorders, in Obsessive-Compulsive–Related Disorders. Edited by Hollander E. Washington, DC, American Psychiatric Press, 1993, pp 17–48

Hollander E, Liebowitz MR, Winchel R, et al: Treatment of body dysmorphic disorder with serotonin reuptake blockers. Am J Psychiatry 146:768–770, 1989

Hollander E, Neville D, Frenkel M, et al: Body dysmorphic disorder: diagnostic issues and related disorders. Psychosomatics 33:156–165, 1992

Jenike MA: A case report of successful treatment of dysmorphophobia with tranyl-cypromine. Am J Psychiatry 141:1463–1464, 1984

Jerome L: Anorexia nervosa or dysmorphophobia. Br J Psychiatry 150:560–561, 1987

Jerome L: Bodysize estimation in characterizing dysmorphic symptoms in patients with body dysmorphic disorder (letter). Can J Psychiatry 36:620, 1991

Klages W, Hartwich P: Die Clowndysmorphophobie. Psychother Psychosom Med Psychol 32:183–187, 1982

Kligman AM, Graham JA: The psychology of appearance in the elderly. Clin Geriatr Med 5:213–222, 1989

Koo JY, Smith LL: Psychologic aspects of acne. Pediatr Dermatol 8:185–188, 1991

Korkina MV: The clinical significance of the syndrome of dysmorphobia and the phenomenological substance of the syndrome of dysmorphobia. Journal of Neuropathology and Psychiatry 8:994–1000, 1959

Kouranu RF, Williams BV: Capgras' syndrome with dysmorphic delusion in an adolescent. Psychosomatics 25:715–717, 1984

Lacey JH, Birtchnell SA: Body image and its disturbance. J Psychosom Res 30:623–631, 1986

Laufer ME: Body image, sexuality and the psychotic core. Int J Psychoanal 72:63–71, 1991

MacGregor F: Some psycho-social problems associated with facial deformities. Am Sociol Rev 16:629–638, 1951

Marks I, Mishan J: Dysmorphophobic avoidance with disturbed bodily perception: a pilot study of exposure therapy. Br J Psychiatry 152:674–678, 1988

Mayer-Gross W, Stein J: Pathologie der Wahrnehmung, in Handbuch der Geisteskrankheit. Edited by Bumke O. Berlin, Germany, Springer, 1928, pp 57–96

Morozov PV: Prognosis of juvenile schizophrenia with dysmorphophobic disorders (according to catamnestic findings) (in Russian). Zh Nevropatol Psikhiatr Im S S Korsakova 76:1358–1366, 1976

Morselli E: Sulla dismorfofobia e sulla tafefobia. (On dysmorphophobia and on phobias.) Bolletinno della Accademia di Genova 6:110–119, 1891

Munro A, Chmara J: Monosymptomatic hypochondriacal psychosis: a diagnostic checklist based on 50 cases of the disorder. Can J Psychiatry 27:374–376, 1982

Munjack DJ: The behavioral treatment of dysmorphobia. J Behav Ther Exp Psychiatry 9:53–56, 1978

Neziroglu F, Yaryura-Tobias JA: Body dysmorphic disorder. Phenomenology and case descriptions. Behavioral Psychotherapy 21:27–36, 1993a

Neziroglu F, Yaryura-Tobias JA: Exposure, response prevention, and cognitive therapy in the treatment of body dysmorphic disorder. Behav Ther 24:431–438, 1993b

Neziroglu F, McKay D, Todaro J: Effect of cognitive behavior therapy on persons with body dysmorphic disorder and comorbid Axis II diagnoses. Behavior Therapy 27:67–77, 1996

Noles SW, Cash TF, Winstead BA: Body image, physical attractiveness and depression. J Consult Clin Psychol 53:88–94, 1985

Parsons LM: Imagined spatial transformation of one's body. J Exp Psychol Gen 116:172–191, 1987

Philippopoulos GS: The analysis of a case of dysmorphophobia. Can J Psychiatry 24:397–401, 1979

Phillips KA, McElroy SL, Keck PE, et al: Body dysmorphic disorder: 30 cases of imagined ugliness. Am J Psychiatry 150:302–308, 1993

Pryse-Phillips W: An olfactory reference syndrome. Acta Psychiatr Scand 47: 484–509, 1971

Riddoch C: Phantom limbs and body shape. Brain 64:197–222, 1941

Rosenberg M: Society and the Adolescent Self-Image. Princeton, NJ, Princeton University Press, 1965

Salib EA: Subacute sclerosing panencephalitis (SSPE) presenting at the age of 21 as a schizophrenia-like state with bizarre dysmorphophobic features. Br J Psychiatry 152:709–710, 1988

Schilder P: The Image and Appearance of the Human Body. London, Paul Kegan, 1935

Schneider K: Clinical Psychopathology. Philadelphia, PA, Grune & Stratton, 1959

Signer SF, Benson FD: Two cases of Capgras symptom with dysmorphic somatic delusions. Psychosomatics 28:327–328, 1987

Simmel ML: Phantoms in patients with leprosy and in elderly digital amputees. Am J Psychol 69:529–545, 1956

Simmel ML: The absence of phantoms for congenitally missing limbs. Am J Psychol 74:467–470, 1961

Simmons RG, Rosenberg F: Disturbance in the self image at adolescence. Am Sociol Rev 38:553–568, 1973

Sims AC: Towards the unification of body image disorders. Br J Psychiatry 153 (suppl 2):51–55, 1988

Stein DJ, Hollander E: Dermatology and conditions related to obsessive-compulsive disorder. J Am Acad Dermatol 26 (pt 1):237–242, 1992

Stein MB: The Vidal Sasson syndrome (letter). N Engl J Med 26:463, 1985

Stekel W: Compulsion and Doubt, Vol 2. London, Peter Nevel, 1950

Tanquary J, Lynch M, Masand P: Obsessive-compulsive disorder in relation to body dysmorphic disorder. Am J Psychiatry 149:1283–1284, 1992

Vinck J, Pierloot R: Body image boundary definiteness and psychopathology. Acta Psychiatr Belg 77:348–359, 1977

Vitiello B, de Leon J: Dysmorphophobia misdiagnosed as obsessive-compulsive disorder. Psychosomatics 31:220–222, 1990

Watts RN: Aversion to personal body hair: a case study in the integration of behavioural and interpretative methods. Br J Med Psychol 63:335–340, 1990

Wernicke EC: Grundiss der Psychiatrie. Leipzig, Germany, F Barth, 1906

Yaryura-Tobias JA, Patito JA, Mizrahi J, et al: The action of pimozide on acute psychosis. Acta Psychiatr Belg 74:421–429, 1974

Zaidens SH: Dermatologic hypochondriasis: a form of schizophrenia. Psychosom Med 12:250–253, 1950

Chapter 10
Eating Disorders

E ating disorders may be divided into three primary areas: anorexia nervosa, bulimia nervosa, and obesity. The relationship between eating disorders and obsessive-compulsive disorder (OCD) must be explored based on the similarities and dissimilarities among the disorders.

For example, could the act of under- or overeating be considered an urge or compulsion? Is the anxiety before bingeing or overeating similar to the anxiety felt by patients with OCD before engaging in compulsions? Once the compulsion is performed, there is a reduction of anxiety. Immediately after the act of bingeing or overeating (or, in the case of anorectic patients, eating minimally), the anxiety is decreased. Often the compulsions of eating disorder patients are preceded by obsessions about food.

Finally, the socioeconomic connotation of food and imbricated appetite disorders arouse biopsychosocial interest. Mecklenburg et al. (1974) used a medical approach to anorexia, attributing it to a hypothalamic dysfunction, as did Lasegue (1873), who was the first to describe it as a disguised obsession. Others have emphasized the social influences or trends that make eating disorders prominent in Western culture, where they are considered "the modern obsessive-compulsive disorder" (Rothenberg 1986).

In this context we introduce eating disorders and their association with OCD. Most of the chapter will be devoted to anorexia nervosa, because it is the eating disorder that has been most compared with OCD.

Primary Anorexia Nervosa

Symptomatology

Primary anorexia nervosa (PAN) is a disorder that is characterized by a refusal to maintain body weight over a minimal weight that is normal for age

185

and height, an intense fear of gaining weight, and body image disturbance. It is called "primary" to differentiate it from the secondary anorexia that is present in other medical conditions (e.g. depression, cancer). This syndrome was first described by Lasegue in 1873 and Gull in 1874. PAN also is known as *pubertal starvation amenorrhea* (Van de Wiele 1977), *eupepsia hysteria* (Gull 1874), and *fat-weight phobia* (Crisp 1967).

Anorectic patients usually display a high degree of maladaptive behavior. They present an important substratum of fear, uncertainty, low frustration tolerance, and dysphoria and are rigid, obsessive, and perfectionistic. These characteristics have been ascribed to them by many researchers (Dally 1969; F. S. DuBois 1949; Kay and Leigh 1954; King 1963; Morgan and Russell 1975; Norris 1979; Palmer and Jones 1939). In addition, these patients exhibit anxiety and depression. In a detailed comorbidity review, depression and obsessive-compulsive features were the most frequently reported symptoms (Rothenberg 1988). Moreover, anorexic patients display constriction, conformity, and obsessionality (Vitousek and Manke 1994). However, a premorbid obsessional personality may be overrepresented (Holden 1990). Overall, PAN's symptomatology very much resembles that of OCD.

Anorectic patients often have disturbed personalities. Patients manifest contentment resembling the "la belle indifference" of hysterical personalities. In fact, Lasegue named this *anorexie hysterique* to aptly indicate that anorexia is the sole object of preoccupation and conversation and is certainly "a disguised obsession."

A rigid personality, inward or outward aggressiveness, hysteroid signs, and obstinacy are common findings. Most important is the mono-obsessive quality of the thought focused on body shape, size, and weight. Food becomes the hate and love object.

The patient is obsessed with his or her body image, seeing it as distorted. This body dysperception establishes a putative connection between PAN and dysmorphophobia. Buvat and Buvat-Herbaut (1978) found dysmorphophobia in 97 of 107 girls and eight of eight boys with PAN.

Another perceptual disturbance is the inability to distinguish obesity from slimness. To prove this, self-perception was measured by a distorting photographic technique (Garfinkel et al. 1977). However, Button et al. (1977) did not find body perception differences between females with PAN and healthy females.

Affective changes—primarily depression during the premorbid or postmorbid stage—were mentioned by Cantwell et al. (1977). At times a noticeable increase in mental and motor activity, resembling excitatory psychomotor activity, surprises the family and the clinician, considering the severity of weight loss. Jogging, gymnastics, and ballet may mask anorexia nervosa cases; in fact, not only may jogging be a better substitute for vomiting or purging, but also it is socially acceptable.

Age at Onset

PAN appears during puberty and OCD during childhood and adolescence. In one study comparing female anorectic patients to nonanorectic OCD patients, the former group was younger and demonstrated obsessive-compulsive symptoms before their eating disorder problems (Kasvikis et al. 1986).

Physical Examination

Patients are usually coerced to come for consultation, and when they do come, they are often emaciated. The presence of physical symptoms may be determined by the individual's constitution and degree of emaciation and chronicity. The skin may appear dry and coarse, with an orange-yellow color of the palms of the hands. The hands may show joint hypertrophy. The oral cavity may exhibit cheilosis, lingual indentation, a white-coated tongue, caries, lingual-occlusal erosion (Hellstrom 1977), and enamel dissolution (Hurst et al. 1977). In doubtful cases in which patients deny being anorectic, an oral examination may yield useful diagnostic clues. Heart examinations may reveal irregularities in conduction, slow pulse, low blood pressure, and bradycardia (Hay and Leonard 1979). Examination of the abdomen may reveal tympanism as a result of bowel distention. With anorectic patients, a physical examination is usually useful.

Laboratory Findings

Laboratory test findings are often not helpful in explaining the ongoing pathological process because the results are caused by severe undernutrition. The alterations in bodily, biochemical, and electrophysiological parameters are not exclusive to PAN but can be found in any other condition involving starvation. Therefore, specific biological parameters are inconclusive for diagnosing PAN.

Sometimes the cachexia produces organic disturbances affecting various bodily systems (e.g., pancreas and liver damage) (Nordgren and Von Scheele 1977) or loss of subcutaneous fat, muscle mass, and gastrointestinal dilation as assessed by radiological laboratory testing (Haller et al. 1977).

Cerebral computed axial tomography scans showed enlargement of cortical sulci and subarachnoid spaces in three of four patients (Enzmann and Lane 1977). An interesting case of reversible cerebral atrophy caused by protein loss and fluid retention was described by Heinz et al. (1977). Correction of the nutritional loss normalized the radiological findings.

Undernourishment may affect the acid-base electrolyte balance, causing a chloride-responsive metabolic alkalosis (Warren and Steinberg 1979). In addition, an imbalance in carbohydrate and thyroid metabolism or a vitamin deficiency may be evident. An abnormal response to a 5-hour oral glucose tolerance test may be found in approximately 63% of patients (Silverman 1974). Hypoglycemia may produce hypokalemia, subsequently causing hypotension, muscle twitches, and atrioventricular conduction disturbances.

Hormonal imbalance consists primarily of a low basal metabolism, a consequence of hypothyroidism. A central inhibition of thyroid function has been postulated by Croxson and Ibbertson (1977). Two cerebro-hormone axes can be heuristically considered to explain the complexities of PAN pathogenesis. The cerebro-thyroid axis, expressed by thyroid-stimulating hormone response to thyrotropin-releasing hormone, may contribute to an understanding of PAN for those who support the concept that eating disorders are a manifestation of depression. The other axis is the hypothalamic-pituitary-adrenal axis. Because the satiety center is located in the hypothalamus, it is acceptable to look for a hypothalamic dysfunction in PAN. The hypothalamic-pituitary-adrenal axis can be studied by means of the dexamethasone suppression test. The dexamethasone suppression test is primarily used for major depression and, to a lesser extent, for OCD (see Chapter 13).

Silverman (1974) reported hypovitaminosis A and hypercarotinemia in 60% of patients.

An anatomo-chemical pathway for PAN and OCD has been postulated. This association implicates the hypothalamus and the serotonergic system (see Chapter 13). In this regard, neurochemical studies of patients with PAN whose weights were restored showed findings comparable with those seen in OCD patients. A blunted response to the partial serotonin agonist *m*-chlorophenylpiperazine and an amelioration of obsessionality and body weight preoccupation were recorded (Kaye et al. 1993). Another study showed elevated cerebrospinal fluid levels of 5-hydroxyindoleacetic acid (Kaye et al. 1993).

Diagnostic Guidelines

The following six guidelines may be used in diagnosing PAN:

1. Onset before age 25.
2. Anorexia, with accompanying weight loss of at least 25% of original body weight.
3. A distorted, implacable attitude toward eating food or toward weight that overrides hunger, admonitions, reassurances, or threats; for example:
   a. Denial of illness and failure to recognize nutritional needs.
   b. Apparent enjoyment of losing weight, with overt manifestations that food refusal is a pleasurable indulgence.
   c. A desirable body image of extreme thinness, with overt evidence that it is rewarding for the patient to achieve and maintain this state.
   d. Unusual hoarding or handling of food.
4. No known medical illness that could account for the anorexia and weight loss.
5. No other known psychiatric disorder, with particular reference to primary affective disorders, schizophrenia, OCD, and phobic neurosis. Even though it may appear phobic or obsessional, food refusal alone does not qualify for obsessive-compulsive or phobic disease.
6. At least two of the following manifestations:
   a. Amenorrhea.
   b. Lanugo (persistence of downy pelage).
   c. Bradycardia (persistent resting pulse rate of 60 beats per minute or less).
   d. Periods of overactivity.
   e. Episodes of bulimia (compulsive overeating).
   f. Vomiting (may be self-induced).

PAN may be divided into typical (the restricting type) and atypical (the binge eating/purging type) forms. Patients with the restricting type do not engage in binge eating or purging during the episode, whereas those with the binge eating/purging type engage in self-induced vomiting or the misuse of laxatives, diuretics, or enemas.

Case 1

A.Z. is a 22-year-old woman who was admitted for the treatment of a depressive syndrome, described as having a peak on awakening. She felt suicidal and mentally and physically exhausted. She was obsessed with food and morbid thoughts she could not reject. She engaged in two main compulsions: double-checking and uncontrollable eating, followed by induced vomiting. The patient's father had alcoholism and was authoritarian and critical toward A.Z. Her mother was soft, vulnerable, and superficial and was quite unable to express her feelings. At the age of 15, A.Z. developed anorexia nervosa after continuous family quarrels. She ate one meal a day and gradually developed a series of eating rituals consisting of food lists, table setting, and food preparation. To comply with her "lipophobia," A.Z. ate a strict fat-free diet, to the point that she would rinse her food before eating it if she suspected any fat "contamination." On examination she presented all the classic physical symptoms of anorexia, including concave abdomen, muscle atrophy, yellow skin in the palms of her hands, lanugo, and amenorrhea. In addition, magnetic resonance imaging showed brain atrophy, a reflection of her hypoproteinemia. She was treated with cyproheptadine until she gained some weight (she weighed 70 pounds on admission). Thereafter she was placed on clomipramine. Her management problems were characterized by her severely abnormal eating habits and vomiting. She displayed manipulative behavior, anger, depression, and procrastination. A strict behavioral protocol and cognitive supportive therapy rounded out the major portions of her treatment. She was discharged 4 months after admission, improved but with a guarded prognosis.

Differential Diagnosis

PAN should first be differentiated from secondary anorexia nervosa. King (1963) identified the following cluster of nine characteristics of PAN:

1. Upbringing by a dominant, restrictive mother and a passive father
2. High intelligence
3. Childhood personality trait of athleticism, obsessionality, dyspepsia, and petty stealing
4. Postpubertal disgust with sexual thought and development, with absence of even minor sexual activity
5. Postpubertal dependence on the mother, irritability, lack of humor, paranoid sensitivity, withdrawal, and marked obsessionality
6. Onset of anorectic illness within the first 7 years after puberty
7. Anorectic illness commencing with anorexia, amenorrhea, or both, with these symptoms preceding other neurotic symptoms
8. Development of bradycardia, downy hair growth, or both during anorectic illness

9. Anorectic illness accompanied by constipation, bulimia, irritability and overactivity, hostility to dependency figures, autistic sexual attitudes, and withdrawal

The differential diagnosis should be established with secondary anorexia nervosa caused by hypophyseal disturbances, such as Simmonds's cachexia, the atypical anorexia nervosa of hypothalamic tumors (Heron and Johnston 1976; White et al. 1977), and gonadal dysgenesis (Kron et al. 1977; Liston and Shershow 1973). Anorectic symptoms resembling those seen in anorexia nervosa may be observed in superior mesenteric artery syndrome (Froese et al. 1978). Young (1975) noticed a relationship between anorexia nervosa and the Kleine-Levin syndrome observed in males: sleep or drowsiness attacks lasting several days, followed by awakening for biological purposes to satisfy hyperphagia. In these patients, mood swings, periods of hyperactivity or lethargy, craving for sweets, and a relationship between sex hormones and the hypothalamus was observed. A mirror image between PAN and Kleine-Levin has been suggested (Labbe 1954).

In general, PAN is an exclusively female syndrome, although a distinct weight phobia syndrome in 10 males was identified by Hasan and Tibbetts (1977). Although there may be possible syndrome variations, PAN in more recent years has seemed to follow a different presentation, appearing as a multifaceted process, thereby concealing other neuropsychiatric conditions linked to psychosocial variables. One variable is strong social factors demanding slimness, imposed on personalities that need pleasing and are conditioned to follow current trends. Another is self-destructive behavior, represented by a conscious wish to die by self-starvation as a response to the inability to cope with life. These two variables should be elicited during diagnostic examination.

Anorexia Nervosa and OCD

Evidence suggests that PAN, compulsive eating, and bulimia manifest prominent obsessive-compulsive features. Researchers have systematically looked into the clinical overlap of OCD and eating disorders, with one study comparing such patients with a healthy population (Pigott et al. 1991) and another studying OCD and eating disorders during adolescence (Rothenberg 1990). The monothematic symptoms of eating disorders are food obsessionality and distortion of body image. Selecting, buying, preparing, and eating food becomes a sequential, ritualistic behavior.

Several authors have indicated a close similarity between anorexia nervosa and OCD (Luyckx and Van den Bosh de Aguilar 1972; Maxmen et al. 1974; Rahman et al. 1939). Some have suggested that anorexia be renamed *anorexia nervosa with cachexia* (F. S. DuBois 1949), and others have reported on the high incidence of obsessional traits (Dally 1969; Kay and Leigh 1954; King 1963; Morgan and Russell 1975; Norris 1979). Inclusion of anorexia nervosa in the OCD spectrum is based on the prominent presence of obsessive-compulsive symptoms (Cantwell et al. 1977; Clancy and Norris 1961; Hau et al. 1979; Rothenberg 1988; Rowland 1970; Strober 1980; Yaryura-Tobias and Neziroglu 1983). These symptoms include an urge to eat, an urge not to eat, and rituals surrounding food preparation and the process of eating. Unless these urges are satisfied and rituals performed, patients feel anxious. In addition, patients spend most of their time obsessing about food. Even in the absence of obsessions and compulsions centering around food, many other obsessive-compulsive symptoms have been noted (Solyom et al. 1982).

One study found significantly elevated scores on the Yale-Brown Obsessive Compulsive Scale; these scores were similar to the scores reported for OCD patients (Kaye et al. 1993). In a comparative study of PAN and OCD patients, both groups obtained similarly high obsessive symptom and trait scores on the Leyton Obsessional Inventory (Solyom et al. 1982), corroborating comparable results (Smart et al. 1976).

Obsessive-compulsive characteristics also have been mentioned in Bruch's (1973) work, where meticulosity, rigidity, perfectionism, and food obsessions were noted in this population. Halmi (1974) found that 54% of normal weight patients, compared with 23% of obese patients, had obsessive-compulsive symptoms.

Other personality aspects of the anorexia nervosa patient include perfectionism, high goals, and high expectations of life. Ushakov (1971) and Bruch (1973) spoke about the illness' meticulosity. The need to steal was reported by King (1963). Anorexia in patients who steal food may be rooted in kleptomania, also a compulsive act.

The personality of parents and relatives not only may have hereditary significance for elucidating the syndrome's etiology, but also a psychological impact on the patient's learned behavior. In 56 families with anorexia nervosa, an unusually high incidence of phobic avoidance and obsessive character traits was present (Kalucy et al. 1977). Crisp et al. (1974) noticed high levels of obsessionality in fathers of anorectic patients, combined with high levels of anxiety and depression associated with their daughters.

Eating is a ritual, starting with the selection, purchase, and cooking of food, followed by the ornamentation of the dish and setting the table. This eating ritual is to secure mastery or control where dependency may not be needed (Galdston 1974). Furthermore, patients may count their mouthfuls or their chewing movements or have good and bad thoughts while eating. Eating binges are reported in which food is swallowed rapidly, almost without mastication. This behavior is typical of hyperphagia. Occasionally, because of an irresistible compulsion, frozen food is devoured without thawing.

Hypothalamic dysfunction is indicated by gonadal dysfunction and thyroid disturbances (Katz et al. 1977; Mecklenburg et al. 1974). Although PAN is seen almost exclusively in females, it has been described in males (Bruch 1971).

An unusual syndrome, somatogenic asthenia leading to vomiting, has been described. The vomiting reaction becomes fixated and is either voluntary or involuntary, leading to limitation of food intake to prevent vomiting. Additional symptoms are depression, reference ideas, and eventually emaciation. This syndrome is known as the *vomitophobic syndrome* (Korkina et al. 1977).

A case of PAN and Tourette's syndrome has been reported by Yaryura-Tobias (1979). In a group of 51 adolescents with PAN, several had autistic behavior patterns, and two females had Tourette's syndrome with obsessive-compulsive traits and social interaction problems. One of three boys with anorexia nervosa had Asperger syndrome. An underlying trait might be common to Asperger syndrome (Gillberg and Rastam 1992). Anorexia nervosa's biochemical aspects remain veiled, although increased dopamine activity has been suggested by Barry and Klawans (1976). However, laboratory findings are difficult to interpret, because they may result from malnutrition and starvation.

Therapy

Treatment of anorexia nervosa encompasses different psychotherapy modes. Behavioral techniques and family therapy have been used. Family lunch therapy sessions were introduced by Rosman et al. (1975). Various pharmacological agents have been used for symptom relief or general treatment of this syndrome including substances with anabolic properties, such as insulin, chlorpromazine, or steroids. Some tricyclic drugs, mainly those blocking the action of serotonin uptake, have been successful, such as amitriptyline (Needleman and Waber 1977) and clomipramine (López Ibor and López Ibor Alino 1971). We had positive experience with clomipramine in doses of

250 mg/day. One patient's weight went from 87 to 160 pounds 4 months after clomipramine was initiated. The availability of selective serotonin reuptake inhibitors widened the scope of therapies for obsessive-compulsive spectrum disorders in general.

One other substance that appears to be beneficial is cyproheptadine, a drug with antihistaminic, antiserotonin, and anabolic action (Goldberg et al. 1979). However, a double-blind study showed that cyproheptadine was not better than placebo (Vigersky and Loriaux 1977). Our experience indicates that it may be useful in patients with low weight who cannot tolerate tricyclic antidepressants. The addition of thyroid medication can be a useful adjuvant.

One problem in evaluating drug efficacy in anorexia nervosa is vomiting and use of laxatives, both of which may jeopardize drug absorption. In extreme cases, psychosurgery has been attempted. D'Andrea et al. (1974) reported success in patients with anorexia nervosa and obsessive symptomatology after a stereotactic thalamotomy was performed.

Prognosis

The prognosis for patients with PAN is dependent on illness length, symptom severity, and treatment availability and response. A poor predictor is the association of PAN with OCD (Halmi et al. 1973). Korkina et al. (1977) found a more favorable prognosis in psychasthenic patients than in patients with hysterical traits. Of 100 female anorectic patients, 48% with the following characteristics had good outcomes: shorter illness duration, older age at onset, lower weight, bulimia, vomiting, anxiety while eating near others, and poor parental relationship (Hau et al. 1979). The mortality rate is between 7% and 21% (A. DuBois et al. 1979).

Bulimia Nervosa

Symptomatology

Bulimia nervosa (BN) refers to episodic eating binges characterized by eating large quantities of food within a discrete period of time and experiencing a lack of control over eating during the episode. Self-induced vomiting; use of laxatives, diuretics, enemas, or other medications; fasting; or excessive exercise are used to compensate for the overeating and subsequent weight gain. The binge eating seems impulsive. The lifetime prevalence of BN is about 2.5% (Whitaker et al. 1990). Among OCD patients (N = 62), the lifetime prevalence for anorexia, bulimia, or both was 12.9% (N = 8), and an additional 17.7% (N = 11) met subthreshold criteria for either anorexia or bulimia (Rubenstein et al. 1992).

In 500 patients with BN, four clinical subtypes were found. These subtypes were 1) overt bulimia (8.9%), 2) obsessive-ritualistic bulimia (2%), 3) sexually evocative bulimia (2.9%), and 4) masochistic bulimia (4.9%) (Hall et al. 1992). The remaining 81.3% of patients had primary BN.

The personality characteristics of bulimic patients are similar to those of anorectic patients in terms of obsessionality, perfectionism, and a need to be accepted. Patients become obsessed with food, body weight, and appearance. They spend inordinate amounts of time obsessing about food even during nonbingeing episodes. Their days may revolve around what and where they will eat. They may report an urge to eat that is uncontrollable. This urge becomes so strong that they will overcome all obstacles to prevent eating (i.e., locking the refrigerator, not having food readily available, locking up the kitchen, separating their food from that of other family members). There is anxiety buildup preceding the binge episode, followed by revulsion, guilt, and depression. To undo the binge eating, some patients purge or use various medications. Others exercise excessively, almost compulsively. Often weight fluctuation is noted in binge eaters.

Age at Onset

BN usually begins during adolescence. The precipitating factors seem to be sociocultural, and with a higher incidence in upper classes.

Bulimia Nervosa and OCD

BN may be associated with other eating disorders, anxiety, major depression, or OCD, and therefore its course, treatment, and outcome may be dependent on variables introduced by these neuropsychiatric entities. Of these conditions, depression and OCD appear to play a significant role in the clinical development of BN. In one study comparing BN patients with OCD patients, scores for both groups on the Minnesota Multiphasic Personality Inventory (Hathaway and McKinley 1943) did not differ significantly (Bulik et al. 1992).

Eating disorders start during adolescence, an age bracket during which OCD also appears. However, late onset among elderly individuals has been reported (Cosford and Arnold 1992). In elderly persons, multifactorial causes such as depression and OCD seem to precipitate an eating disorder. Body appearance and psychiatric comorbidity (OCD, depression, substance abuse, and personality disorder) are precipitating factors that will aid the clinician in arriving at a correct diagnosis and treatment (Kennedy and Garfinkel 1992). Social pressure may cause frustration, followed by depression if the slim figure desired is not attained by the adolescent. In addition, obsessive preoccupation with weight, food, and looks is a contributory factor to consider when planning a treatment program. Although the centrality of obsessive-compulsive symptomatology is not accepted in BN dynamics, a trend is evident. OCD symptoms supersede the depressive pattern (Rothenberg 1990).

Obesity

There is little information about obesity and its relationship to OCD. We question whether obesity is a single entity. In a group of obese individuals who were enrolled in an Optifast (food substitute) program, some patients were more likely to exhibit obsessive-compulsive eating behavior patterns than others (Mount and Neziroglu 1990). An eating obsessive-compulsive questionnaire was devised for this study to assess the degree of food obsessionality. Those patients who scored high on the questionnaire responded better to a behavior therapy program consisting of exposure and response prevention (ERP) than they did to stimulus control. ERP treatment is used in OCD, whereas stimulus control is the common treatment for obesity. In stimulus control, individuals are taught how to avoid events or situations that evoke eating behavior. In ERP, individuals are taught to expose themselves to food and learn how to resist their urge to eat. More studies are needed to determine the similarities and dissimilarities between obesity and OCD.

References

Barry VC, Klawans, HL: On the role of dopamine in the pathophysiology of anorexia nervosa. J Neural Transm 38:107–122, 1976

Bruch H: Anorexia nervosa in the male. Psychosom Med 33:31–47, 1971

Bruch H: Eating Disorders. New York, Basic Books, 1973

Bulik CM, Beidel DC, Duchmann E, et al: Comparative psychopathology of women with bulimia nervosa and obsessive-compulsive disorder. Compr Psychiatry 33:262–268, 1992

Button EJ, Fransella F, Slade P: A reappraisal of body perception disturbances in anorexia nervosa. Psychol Med 7:235–243, 1977

Buvat J, Buvat-Herbaut M: Dysperception of body image and dysmorphophobias in mental anorexia. A propos of 114 cases involving both sexes. I. Altered mechanism of perception in mental anorexia. Ann Med Psychol (Paris) 136:547–561, 1978

Cantwell DP, Sturzenberger S, Burroughs JL, et al: Anorexia nervosa. An affective disorder? Arch Gen Psychiatry 34:1087–1093, 1977

Clancy J, Norris A: Differentiating variables: obsessive-compulsive neurosis and anorexia nervosa. Am J Psychiatry 118:58–60, 1961

Cosford PA, Arnold E: Eating disorders in later life: a review. International Journal of Geriatric Psychiatry 7:491–498, 1992

Crisp AH: The possible significance of some behavioral correlates of weight and carbohydrate intake. J Psychosom Res 11:117–131, 1967

Crisp AH, Harding B, McGuinness B: Anorexia nervosa psychoneurotic characteristics of parents: relationship to prognosis. A quantitative study. J Psychosom Res 18:167–173, 1974

Croxson MS, Ibbertson HK: Low serum triiodothyronine (T3) and hypothyroidism in anorexia nervosa J Clin Endocrinol Metab 44:167–174, 1977

Dally P: Chemistry of Psychiatric Disorders. London, Logos Press, 1969

D'Andrea F, DeDevitiis E, Megna G, et al: Remissione de anoressia mentale resistente ad altre terapie in seguito a talamolisi sterotassica. (Remission of mental anorexia following stereotaxic thalamolysis previously resistant to other therapies). Riv Patol Nerv Ment 95:579–590, 1974

DuBois A, Gross HA, Ebert MH, et al: Altered gastric emptying and secretion in primary anorexia nervosa. Gastroenterology 77:319–323, 1979

DuBois FS: Compulsion neurosis with cachexia (anorexia nervosa). Am J Psychiatry 106:107–115, 1949

Enzmann DR, Lane B: Cranial computed tomography finding in anorexia nervosa. J Comput Assist Tomogr 1:410–414, 1977

Froese AP, Szmuilowicz J, Bailey JD: The superior-mesenteric artery syndrome: cause of complication of anorexia nervosa? Can Psychiatr Assoc J 23:325–327, 1978

Galdston R: Mind over matter: observation of 50 patients hospitalized with anorexia nervosa. J Child Psychol Psychiatry 13:246–264, 1974

Garfinkel PE, Moldofsky H, Garner DM: Prognosis in anorexia nervosa as influenced by clinical features, treatment, and self perception. Can Med Assoc J 117:1041–1045, 1977

Gillberg C, Rastam M: Do some cases of anorexia nervosa reflect underlying autistic-like conditions? Behavioral Neurology 5:27–32, 1992

Goldberg SC, Halmi KA, Eckert ED, et al: Cyproheptadine in anorexia nervosa. Br J Psychiatry 134:67–70, 1979

Gull WW: Anorexia nervosa. Trans Clin Soc (London) 7:265–266, 1874

Hall RC, Blakey RE, Hall AK: Bulimia nervosa. Four uncommon types. Psychsomatics 33:428–436, 1992

Haller JO, Slovis TL, Baker DH, et al: Anorexia nervosa—the paucity of radiologic findings in more than fifty patients. Pediatr Radiol 5:145–147, 1977

Halmi KA: Comparison of demographic and clinical features in patient groups with different ages and weights at onset of anorexia nervosa. J Nerv Ment Dis 158: 222–225, 1974

Halmi KA, Broland G, Loney J: Prognosis in anorexia nervosa. Ann Intern Med 78:907–909, 1973

Hasan MK, Tibbetts RW: Primary anorexia nervosa (weight phobia) in males. Postgrad Med J 53:146–151, 1977

Hathaway SR, McKinley JC: Minnesota Multiphasic Personality Inventory. Minneapolis, MN, University of Minnesota, 1943.

Hau LK, Crisp AH, Harding B: Outcome of anorexia nervosa (letter). Lancet 1:125, 1979

Hay GG, Leonard JC: Anorexia nervosa in males. Lancet 2:574–575, 1979

Heinz ER, Martinez J, Haenggeli A: Reversibility of cerebral atrophy in anorexia nervosa and Cushing's syndrome. J Comput Assist Tomogr 1:415–418, 1977

Hellstrom I: Oral complication in anorexia nervosa. Scand J Dent Res 85:71–86, 1977

Heron GB, Johnston DA: Hypothalamic tumor presenting as anorexia nervosa. Am J Psychiatry Q 34:600–622, 1976

Holden NL: Is anorexia nervosa an obsessive-compulsive disorder? Br J Psychiatry 157:1–5, 1990

Hurst PS, Lacey LH, Crisp AH: Teeth, vomiting and diet: a study of the dental characteristics of seventeen anorexia nervosa patients. Postgrad Med J 53:298–305, 1977

Kalucy RS, Crisp AH, Harding B: A study of 56 families with anorexia nervosa. Br J Med Psychol 50:381–395, 1977

Kasvikis YG, Tsakiris F, Marks IM, et al: Past history of anorexia nervosa in women with obsessive-compulsive disorder. Int J Eat Disord 5:1069–1075, 1986

Katz JL, Boyar RM, Raffwarg H, et al: LHRH responsiveness in anorexia nervosa: intactness despite prepubertal cucadiar LH patter. Psychosom Med 39: 241–251, 1977

Kay DWK, Leigh D: Natural history, treatment and prognosis of anorexia nervosa based on a study of 38 patients. J Ment Sci 100:411–431, 1954

Kaye WH, Weltzin TE, Hsu LKG: Is anorexia nervosa related to obsessive compulsive disorder and/or altered serotonin activity? Presented at First International Obsessive-Compulsive Disorder Congress, Capri, Italy, March 1993

Kennedy SH, Garfinkel PE: Advances in diagnosis and treatment of anorexia nervosa and bulimia nervosa. Can J Psychiatry 37:309–315, 1992

King A: Primary and secondary anorexia nervosa syndromes. Br J Psychiatry 109: 470–479, 1963

Korkina MV, Marilov VV, Tsuril'ko MA: Atypical forms of anorexia nervosa. Zh Neuropatol Psikhiatr 77:429–432, 1977

Kron L, Katz JL, Gorzynski, et al: Anorexia nervosa and gonadal dysgenesis. Further evidence of a relationship. Arch Gen Psychiatry 34:332–335, 1977

Labbe PLA: L'anorexie mentale. Acta Psychiatre Belg 52:164–174, 1954

Lasegue C: On hysterical anorexia. Med Timis and Gaz 2:265–266, 367–368, 1873

Liston EH, Shershow LW: Concurrence of anorexia nervosa and gonadal dysgenesis. Arch Gen Psychiatry 29:834–836, 1973

López Ibor JJ, López Ibor Alino JJ: The pharmacological treatment of obsessive neurosis, anorexia nervosa, delusions of reference, and the Kleine-Levin syndrome. Arch Fac Me (Madrid) 20:2–10, 1971

Luyckx A, Van den Bosh de Aguilar M: Anorexia mentale. Psychother Psychosom (Paris) 21:1–6, 1972

Maxmen JS, Silberfarb PM, Ferrell RB: Anorexia nervosa, practical initial management in a general hospital. JAMA 229:801–803, 1974

Mecklenburg RS, Loriaux DL, Thompson RH: Hypothalamic dysfunction in patients with anorexia nervosa. Medicine (Baltimore) 53:147–159, 1974

Morgan HG, Russell GFM: Value of family background and clinical features as predictors of long-term outcome in anorexia nervosa: four-year follow-up study of 41 patients. Psychol Med 5:355–371, 1975

Mount R, Neziroglu F, Taylor CJ: An obsessive compulsive view of obesity and its treatment. J Clin Psychol 46:68–78, 1990

Needleman HL, Waber D: The use of amitripyline in anorexia nervosa, in Anorexia Nervosa. Edited by Vigersky RA. New York, Raven, 1977

Nordgren L, Von Scheele C: Hepatic and pancreatic dysfunction in anorexia nervosa: a report of two cases. Biol Psychiatry 12:681–686, 1977

Norris DL: Clinical diagnostic criteria for primary anorexia nervosa. S Afr Med J 56:987–993, 1979

Palmer HD, Jones MS: Anorexia nervosa as a manifestation of compulsive neurosis: a study of psychogenic factors. Arch Neurol Psychiatry 41:856–860, 1939

Pigott TA, Pato MT, L'Heureux F, et al: A controlled comparison of adjuvant lithium carbonate or thyroid hormone in clomipramine treated patients with obsessive-compulsive disorder. J Clin Psychopharmacol 11:242–248, 1991

Rahman L, Richardsen HB, Ripley HS: Anorexia nervosa with psychiatric observations. Psychosom Med 1:335–365, 1939

Rosman BL, Minuchin S, Liebman R: Family lunch sessions: an introduction to family therapy in anorexia nervosa. Am J Orthopsychiatry 45:846–853, 1975

Rothenberg A: Eating disorder as a modern obsessive-compulsive syndrome. Psychiatry 49:45–53, 1986

Rothenberg A: Differential diagnosis of anorexia nervosa and depressive illness: a review of 11 studies. Compr Psychiatry 29:427–432, 1988

Rothenberg A: Adolescence and eating disorder: the obsessive-compulsive syndrome. Psychiatr Clin North Am 13:469–488, 1990

Rowland C Jr: Anorexia nervosa: a survey of the literature and review of 30 cases. Int Psychiatry Clin 7:37–137, 1970

Rubenstein CS, Pigott TA, L'Heureux F: A preliminary investigation of the lifetime prevalence of anorexia and bulimia nervosa in patients with obsessive-compulsive disorder. J Clin Psychiatry 53:309–314, 1992

Silverman JA: Anorexia nervosa: clinical observations in a successful treatment plan. J Pediatr 84:68–73, 1974

Smart DE, Beumont PJV, George GCW: Some personality characteristics of patients with anorexia nervosa. Br J Psychiatry 128:57–60, 1976

Solyom L, Freeman RJ, Miles JE: A comparative psychometric study of anorexia nervosa and obsessive neurosis. Can J Psychiatry 27:282–286, 1982

Strober M: Personality and symptomatological features in young, nonchronic anorexia nervosa patients. J Psychosom Res 24:353–359, 1980

Ushakov GK: Anorexia nervosa, in Modern Perspectives in Adolescent Psychiatry. Edited by Howells JG. Edinburgh, Scotland, Oliver & Boyd, 1971, pp 274–289

Van de Wiele RL: Anorexia nervosa and the hypothalamus. Hosp Pract 12:45–51, 1977

Vigersky RA, Loriaux DL: The effect of cyproheptadine in anorexia nervosa. A double-blind trial, in Anorexia Nervosa. Edited by Vigersky RA. New York, Raven, 1977, pp 349–356

Vitousek K, Manke F: Personality variables and disorders in anorexia nervosa and bulimia nervosa. Journal of Abnormal Pathology 103:137–147, 1994

Warren SE, Steinberg SM: Acid based and electrolyte disturbances in anorexia nervosa. Am J Psychiatry 136:415–418, 1979

Whitaker A, Johnson J, Shaffer D, et al: Uncommon troubles in young people: prevalence estimates of selected psychiatric disorders in a nonreferred adolescent population. Arch Gen Psychiatry 47:487–496, 1990

White JH, Kelly P, Dormon K: Clinical picture of a typical anorexia nervosa associated with hypothalamic tumor. Am J Psychiatry 134:323–325, 1977

Yaryura-Tobias JA: Gilles de la Tourette's disease: interactions with other neuropsychiatric disorders. Acta Psychiatr Scand 59:9–16, 1979

Yaryura-Tobias JA, Neziroglu FA: Complex obsessive-compulsive disorders, in Obsessive-Compulsive Disorders: Pathogenesis, Diagnosis, Treatment. Edited by Yaryura-Tobias JA, Neziroglu JA. New York, Marcel Dekker, 1983, pp 91–103

Young JK: A possible neuroendocrine basis of two clinical: anorexia nervosa and the Kleine-Levin syndrome. Physio-Psychol 3:322–330, 1975

Chapter 11
Self-Mutilation

S
elf-mutilation is inflicting bodily injuries because of cultural phenomena or mental disturbances. In both ancient and modern times, certain cultural groups have engaged in self-mutilative practices for aesthetic reasons or as part of religious penitence or a costume.

Most social mutilations involve skin and other soft anatomical structures; for example, perforating the nasal cartilage, as seen in certain African and American Indian tribes; perforating the earlobe, which is widespread; circumcising the penis or clitoris; and scarring the skin are still practiced. The Middle Eastern custom of skin tattooing in the dorsal area of the hand and body tattooing by sailors, by (although to a lesser degree) soldiers and members of drug subcultures, and recently as a fashion trend are different expressions of a need to participate in a social rite offering a sense of belonging.

Bone mutilation takes place among the Padaung, a Burma tribe that elongates their women's necks, regarded as a sign of beauty, by placing steel coils around the neck (Keshishian 1979), and among the Chinese by bandaging female feet. Prehistoric maxillodental mutilation has been reported by Verger-Pratoucy (1970). Dental mutilation was performed by inhabitants of the Peotihuacan culture (Fastlicht 1968), African blacks (Weyers 1969), the people of pre-Hispanic Mexico (Noguez 1970), and by Peru's primitive people (Vasquez Soto 1967). Flagellation was practiced by mystics and religious groups; the Shiites of Iran whip their backs with chains; Catholics from Southern Italy scratch their skin with broken glass; and cloistered monks, nuns, and religious penitents use cilices made out of haircloth or iron spikes.

Whether social mutilation relates to obsessive-compulsive behavior has not been determined. However, the obsessive-compulsive traits present in particular ethnic social environments, including the rituals and ceremonies of a mutilative procedure, warrant further research.

From a medical viewpoint, self-mutilation should be considered a symptom rather than a syndrome, because it has been reported in schizophrenic adults, schizophrenic children (Green 1967), apparently normal infants (DeLissovoy 1961; Kravitz 1960), children and adults (Berkson and Davenport 1962), in obsessionality (Gardner and Gardner 1975), and in schizophrenic and retarded children (Frankel and Simmons 1976).

Self-Mutilation in Children

Self-mutilation in children is characterized by head banging and biting of the nails, hands, knuckles, oral mucosa, and finger cuticles. According to Frankel and Simmons (1976), epidemiological evidence strongly supports the contention that self-injurious behavior is learned in low-functioning children as a coercive alternative for obtaining adult attention. In studies using punishment, some evidence is offered for conditional reinforcement and discriminative stimulus pain control in maintaining this behavior. Modification of self-destructive behavior by the use of electric shocks (aversive conditioning) has been successfully reported in many documented studies (Wilbur et al. 1974).

Self-Mutilation in Violent Individuals

Bach-Y-Rita (1974) reported that 37% of 22 habitually violent patient inmates had scars resulting from self-inflicted wounds. Most sensed little or no pain when they cut themselves. Some patients expressed the urge to cut themselves to relieve tension; others induced self-mutilation to obtain gains. Currently no definite correlation between obsessive-compulsive disorders (OCDs) and the self-mutilation of violent individuals has been established.

Complex OCDs

Compulsive-Orectic-Mutilative Syndrome

We isolated a new clinical entity characterized by obsessions, compulsions, aggressive behavior, self-mutilation, insomnia, sexual disorder, family discordance, and elevated pain threshold (Yaryura-Tobias and Neziroglu 1978; Yaryura-Tobias et al. 1995). The *compulsive-orectic-mutilative syndrome* (COMS) appears to affect only females, who usually consult at an advanced stage of the illness.

The syndrome comprises two clinical phases:

1. The *pubertal,* or *early phase,* is characterized by anorexia. During this phase, the patient refuses to eat and has an urge or compulsion to avoid food or a compulsion to vomit. There are symptoms of dysmenorrhea or amenorrhea, loss of more than 20% of body weight, and the presence of lanugo. During this stage, the diagnosis is primary anorexia nervosa. Unfortunately, obsessive-compulsive symptoms go unnoticed, perhaps because the physician is confronted with anorexia and severe weight loss.

2. A *postpubertal,* or *late phase,* occurs after normalization of the appetite and menstruation. This phase is signaled by aggressive behavior and self-mutilation.

Throughout these two phases, the common denominator is obsessive-compulsive symptomatology.

Psychological testing reveals a high IQ, with a discrepancy between verbal (higher) and performance (lower) IQ scores. Patients' aggressive behavior is explosive, uncontrollable, and verbally or physically directed toward others, objects, or themselves. The self-mutilation is generally ritualistic, meticulously performed, and painless. The act's description may imply ecstasy or depersonalization, suggesting a hysteroid component.

In the late phase, normalization of the menstrual cycle often initiates the acts of self-harm. Thus, a hormonal factor may mediate the mechanisms of this syndrome.

Physical areas of mutilation include the skin, oral and vaginal mucosa, cornea, and hair. The skin is usually slashed in symmetric straight lines, avoiding the ventral wrist areas, elbows, and forearms, where vessels are less protected. The laceration materials may be razor blades, broken glass, or scissors. If possible, the patient avoids showing the wounds and requesting medical treatment. This may distinguish the act from an hysterical act needing public witnesses. In our 30-patient population, physical examination did not reveal abnormalities, except in two patients with coarse, yellow-orange skin; hypertrophic hand articulations; and high plasma carotene levels (a primary anorexia nervosa finding). In this group, routine blood chemistry tests did not reveal any anomalies except for hyperuricemia in one patient. Abnormal 5-hour glucose tolerance tests (60%) and nonspecific abnormal electroencephalographic changes (40%) were reported (Yaryura-Tobias and Neziroglu, unpublished data, September 1980).

A differential diagnosis should be made with primary anorexia nervosa. A compulsive-oretic-mutilative and Tourette's syndrome interface has been reported in one case (Yaryura-Tobias 1979). Several clinical entities that share some common features with the syndrome also have been reported. In a sample of 24 self-mutilation patients, 15 were reported to have symptoms of compulsive overeating, severe anorexia, or periods of both, along with dysmenorrhea (Rosenthal et al. 1972).

Mental Retardation

There is a paucity of research in mental retardation and OCD. In mental retardation, OCD's intellectual component is generally absent, and no ego dystonic components and doubting can be found. In one study of 283 mildly to profoundly retarded patients, 10 (3.5%) showed compulsive behavior that was significant enough to cause daily dysfunction (Vitiello et al. 1989). The authors emphasized the externally observable compulsive activity components. Compulsive behavior in mentally retarded patients is essentially motoric, because there are no cues enabling clinicians to look for ideational compulsions. Therefore, clinicians are limited in assessing the intensity and severity of this comorbidity. In addition to compulsive behaviors, other repetitive behaviors can be established.

Our experience with mental retardation and OCD is mostly limited to Cornelia de Lange syndrome and Lesch-Nyhan syndrome (Lesch and Nyhan 1964), both of which have self-mutilation as an important component.

Psychotropic drugs control compulsions, self-mutilation, and aggression. Many patients are affected with an arrest in neural development, and therefore, therapeutic strategies should include small deossification. Consideration of drug interactions also is important. The therapeutic strategy is symptom control. The use of clomipramine and selective serotonin reuptake inhibitors for compulsions, lithium or carbamazepine for aggression, clonazepam for anxiety, and neuroleptic agents for grafted schizophrenia (profschizophrenia) will help manage the pathology's severity. Behavior therapy may help provide structure for patients with management problems, whether at home, group home residence, or school.

Prader-Willi Syndrome

Prader-Willi syndrome is characterized by infantile hypotony, hypogonadism, obesity, mental deficiency, short stature, characteristic facial features, small hands, and an interstitial deletion of chromosome 15q11–13 in one-half of patients. These characteristics are generally conceded as defining this clinical entity (Holm et al. 1993). Prader-Willi syndrome presents six interesting features to neuropsychiatrists: 1) hyperphagia, 2) self-mutilation, 3) temper tantrums, 4) severe aggression, 5) obsessive-compulsive features, and 6) resistance to change.

A behavioral study in 35 adolescents with Prader-Willi syndrome indicated a substantial number of behaviors, notably compulsive and anxious behaviors (Whitman and Accardo 1987). Four major symptoms are 1) stealing food, 2) hoarding food, 3) temper outbursts, and 4) skin picking. The authors described skin picking as a possible variant of the OCD spectrum (Warnock and Kastenbaum 1992). Our experience with five Prader-Willi syndrome patients with severe mutilation pointed to a two-step ritual: the patient first picks the skin and then digs into it, causing severe excoriation and ulcerations with irreparable tissue loss, leaving large scars.

Neuroendocrine Prader-Willi syndrome studies concentrate on growth hormone, growth, insulin, and melatonin. Such studies have indicated that a deficiency in growth hormone may result in the short stature noted in these patients (Angulo and Castro-Magana 1991). In five Prader-Willi syndrome patients, significant insulin-release activity may have indicated hypothalamic involvement (Lautala et al. 1986). One clinical factor definitely correlated with hypothalamic pathology is hyperphagia, a symptom with no satiation point.

Melatonin circadian rhythm has been measured to study whether melatonin mediates the impairment of gonadotropin secretion in Prader-Willi syndrome. Melatonin plasma levels in Prader-Willi syndrome patients were the same as those in the control group (Willig et al. 1986). Because hypopigmentation is another Prader-Willi syndrome characteristic, the immunoreactive β-melanocyte-stimulating hormone was measured in plasma. Results indicated no difference between patients with hypopigmentation and those with healthy skin (Butler and Jenkins 1987).

Patients seem to prefer sweets, and the preference for certain foods is cognitively influenced (R. L. Taylor and Caldwell 1985). In spite of an increase in insulin-release activity, diabetes mellitus was reported in three patients with poor adrenal medullary response (Sareen et al. 1975). We conclude that a faulty carbohydrate metabolism may reinforce the concept of a hypothalamic involvement in Prader-Willi syndrome but may not modify the behavior. In fact, a correlation between sucrose ingestion and behavioral changes was examined in seven Prader-Willi syndrome patients. Results showed that of 162 test correlations performed, only 8 were significant, the number expected by chance (P. L. Otto et al. 1982).

If Prader-Willi syndrome is accepted as a metabolic disorder, psychopharmacokinetic studies should be performed based on evidence that neuroleptic agents and appetite suppressant drugs are inadvisable (Tu et al. 1992).

Psychotropic agents should be considered for treatment of Prader-Willi syndrome when severe symptoms disrupt patients' lives. Behavioral problems and skin picking are usually controlled by the administration of fluoxetine (Dech and Budow 1991; Warnock and Kastenbaum 1992) or fluoxetine with naltrexone (Benjamin and Biuot-Smith 1993). The administration of fenfluramine improved food-related behavior, produced weight loss, and decreased aggressive behavior (Selikowitz et al. 1990). Our experience favors using fluoxetine first and then clomipramine, both of which are drugs of choice for self-harm. For aggression, we prefer carbamazepine.

Prader-Willi syndrome is a "missing footprint" in outlining a more comprehensive OCD spectrum model that encompasses hypothalamic conditions. The following may support this: 1) hyperphagia, 2) disturbance of the carbohydrate metabolism, 3) obsessive-compulsive behavior, 4) self-mutilation, 5) aggressive behavior, 6) altered balance of the hypothalamic-pituitary-adrenal axis, and 7) good response to strong selective serotonin reuptake inhibitors.

Lesch-Nyhan Syndrome

In 1964 Lesch and Nyhan described a syndrome in two brothers, ages 5 and 8 years, who had hyperuricemia, self-mutilation, choreoathetosis, and mental retardation. The self-mutilation was compulsive and consisted of biting the oral mucosa and fingers until amputation. The Lesch-Nyhan syndrome seems to be an X-linked, inborn error of purine metabolism that has been traced to the complete absence or marked reduction of activity of the enzyme hypoxanthine phosphoribosyltransferase. Genetic heterogeneity within the patient group was individualized (McDonald and Kelley 1971). Genetic studies also assist in individualizing and preventing this syndrome by prenatal diagnosis (Boyle et al. 1970; Singh et al. 1976) or by detecting females who are heterozygous for the Lesch-Nyhan mutation (Felix and DeMars 1971).

Japanese research has shown that the administration of 5-hydroxytryptophan (5-HTP) curtails self-mutilation (Mizuno and Yugari 1975; Mizuno et al. 1970). Because of the efficacy of 5-HTP, Mizuno and co-workers advanced the hypothesis that this self-harm is caused by a cerebral monoamine imbalance—notably, serotonin. Two variations of the syndrome, one without abnormal hypoxanthine phosphoribosyltransferase (Etienne et al. 1973) and one with normal intelligence (Scherzer and Ilson 1969), have been reported.

Although this syndrome has been described as occurring exclusively in males, two female cases have been reported (Bazelon et al. 1968).

We examined five cases—in three males and two females—in which the three males had the classic clinical syndrome characteristics (hyperuricemia, choreoathetosis, mental retardation, and self-mutilation), whereas the two females did not have choreoathetosis. All five patients had fathers who had gout. Clomipramine successfully controlled the self-harm. Behavioral techniques for controlling or reducing self-biting have been described by several authors (L. Anderson et al. 1977; Dizmang and Cheatham 1970; Duker 1971).

Cornelia de Lange Syndrome

In 1933 Cornelia de Lange described a clinical entity characterized by micromelia and clinodactyly, low birth weight, and retardation of growth and mental development. An additional feature is compulsive self-mutilation (Bryson et al. 1971). Two cases of compulsive self-mutilative behavior, a feature of Cornelia de Lange syndrome, were reported by Shear et al. (1971). The authors stated that self-mutilation, although only occasionally observed in retarded children, creates a serious management problem. Early recognition calls for prompt intervention and effective early management. Finally, self-harm may represent a distinctive feature of this disorder, suggesting a correlation between organicity and human behavior.

Trichotillomania

Trichotillomania is the intentional removal of hair from the scalp, eyebrows, eyelashes, beard, auxiliary area, or pubic area. It may be accompanied by tricophagia (the ingestion of hair). The DSM-IV diagnostic criteria include recurrent failure to resist impulses to pull, resulting in noticeable hair loss; increasing tension before pulling out hair, followed by a sense of relief after the act is completed; and absence of preexisting skin inflammation, delusions, or hallucinations (American Psychiatric Association 1994). It is categorized under impulse disorders, although its diagnostic criteria fit an obsessive-compulsive model.

The term *trichotillomania* was coined by a French dermatologist, Hallopeau (1889), to connote a hair-pulling compulsion. Until the 1950s most of the reports appeared in dermatology journals, as few studies appeared in the psychiatric and psychological literature.

No epidemiological studies of trichotillomania have been done. Some researchers have reported an extremely low incidence (F. W. Anderson and Dean 1956; Krishnan et al. 1985; Mannino and Delgado 1969; Schachter 1961), whereas others estimate a high occurrence, approximately 1 in every 200 persons by the age of 18 years (Azrin and Nunn 1977; Christenson et al. 1991a; Greenberg and Sarner 1965; Tynes and Winstead 1992). It is noted predominantly in females and occurs more commonly in children than in adults. Men may be able to hide their hair pulling better by masking it as male pattern baldness and shaving their mustaches and beards. When it occurs later in life, during adulthood, it is associated with more psychopathology. Age at onset is frequently between 5 and 12 or early childhood to adolescence (Greenberg and Sarner 1965; Muller 1987). The scalp is the most frequent hair-pulling site, followed by the eyebrows, eyelashes, pubic area, face, trunk, and extremities.

The question is whether trichotillomania is a syndrome on its own, a form of OCD, or a symptom observed in various disorders. It can be present as a major mental retardation symptom (Kanner 1950), in schizophrenia (Butterworth 1972), in borderline personality disorder (Greenberg and Sarner 1965), and in depression (Krishnan et al. 1984). Some researchers have suggested that it might be a form of OCD (Jenike 1990; Philippopoulos 1961; Primeau and Fontaine 1987; Swedo et al. 1989; Tynes et al. 1990), whereas others have stated that it is not an OCD variant (Christenson et al. 1991b; Stanley et al. 1992; Winchel et al. 1992). To explore a possible relationship between trichotillomania and OCD, 65 of 69 first-degree relatives of 16 female probands with severe chronic trichotillomania were compared with two control groups, one with OCD and one with trichotillomania (Lenane et al. 1992). Three of 16 trichotillomania probands had at least one first-degree relative with a lifetime OCD history, and there was an age-correlated rate of 6.4% of first-degree relatives with OCD. No relative in the normal control group met OCD criteria. The authors concluded that the higher OCD rate in trichotillomania families suggests that trichotillomania is an OCD spectrum disorder along with other pathological grooming behaviors. Other researchers have postulated that it is a separate syndrome (Delgado and Mannino

1969; Greenberg and Sarner 1965), similar to other maladaptive habits such as thumb sucking, nail biting, and nose picking (Azrin et al. 1980).

The disorder usually has exacerbation and remission periods and in most cases is chronic (Christenson et al. 1991b; Krishnan et al. 1985). According to some authors, there appears to be both a remitting and a chronic form, which are related to age at onset and sex distribution, with older females being more susceptible to the chronic form (Swedo and Rapoport 1991). Some researchers have emphasized the disturbed family relations in trichotilloma-nia patients' families (Adam and Kashani 1990; Krishnan et al. 1985; Muller 1987; Slagle and Martin 1991). These authors have reported poor marital relations; family tension; and faulty mother-child interaction patterns characterized by ambivalence, hostility, and separation anxiety. It often develops in the context of family psychosocial stress (e.g., child or mother hospitalizations, the additional stress from moving to a new house) or with developmental problems such as sibling rivalry, inability of a younger child to focus activities or play, or school problems in an older child (Oranje et al. 1986). Also, it often accompanies poor peer relationships and academic problems (Delgado and Mannino 1969; Mannino and Delgado 1969).

The tactile sensations and pleasure derived from pulling one's hair could contribute to its maintenance. Of 60 hair pulling patients, 48 reported oral behaviors such as chewing or biting the ends (33%), rubbing hair around the mouth (25%), and licking (8%) and eating the hair (10%) (Christenson et al. 1991a). Several patients described gratification from removing specific hair types, such as gray or coarse hair, or intact hair roots. We observed patients who enjoy the sensation of rubbing hair around the mouth area. Severe cases— patients who are almost completely bald—sometimes pull to develop scabs and then pick them. Some save the scabs, and a compulsive hoarding quality ensues. Most patients (80%) report being sometimes completely aware of pulling their hair and other times experiencing incomplete awareness, 15% report always being aware, and only a small percentage (5%) report having no awareness. Hair pulling frequently occurs while subjects are engaged in sedentary activities (e.g., watching TV, reading, talking on the telephone, lying in bed, driving, writing, or doing paperwork). Patients who score high in sedentary activities usually have a history of major depression, and those with high negative affect scores have a high lifetime prevalence rate of OCD, other anxiety disorders, current and past depression, and obsessive-compulsive personality disorders (Christenson et al. 1993). Stanley et al.

(1992) suggests the high level of pleasure experienced during hair pulling by patients with trichotillomania differentiates them from OCD patients who experience no pleasure during compulsion performance. Other differentiating factors reported by these researchers are fewer obsessions and compulsions as well as lower anxiety levels and depression in patients with trichotillomania compared with OCD patients.

Treatment

Psychological treatment. Despite the poor prognosis, certain psychotherapeutic approaches have demonstrated positive results. Hypnosis is successful in treating habit disorders in highly hypnotizable individuals (Glaski 1981; Rowen 1981; Spiegel and Spiegel 1978) and also with less hypnotizable individuals when combined with restricted environmental stimulation therapy (Barabasz 1987). Restricted environmental stimulation has individuals practice self-hypnosis in an isolated room with no stimulation. Under these circumstances, individuals are hypnotized through self-induction and change any maladaptive habits such as hair pulling. Few case history reports using psychoanalysis or family or group therapy have reported a successful outcome (Lantz et al. 1980; Monroe and Abse 1963; Philippopoulos 1961; Robinowitz 1979). Most earlier studies do not describe the treatment used, but they do indicate a poor prognosis for trichotillomania (Friman et al. 1984; K. Otto and Rambach 1964).

Behavior therapy. Behavior therapy has been more encouraging. Perhaps behaviorists deal with a less disturbed population than do psychoanalysts. The former deal primarily with hair pulling as the patient's major symptom (Azrin et al. 1980), whereas the latter treat individuals with greater psychopathological abnormalities, including family, marital, and interpersonal relationship difficulties.

The first reported behavioral intervention for trichotillomania consisted of self-monitoring paired with response chain interruption, whereby patients monitored their hair-pulling attempts and then told their hands to stop (J. G. Taylor 1963). Other interventions are counting and recording hair pulls (Saper 1971), denial of privileges and applying eye drops to stop pulling (Epstein and Peterson 1973), aversive self-stimulation with a rubber band (Mastellone 1974; Mathew and Kumaraiah 1988; Stevens 1984), and punishment via sit-ups whenever a pull attempt is made (MacNeil and Thomas 1976). Except for Saper's study (1971), at the end of treatment, patients reported hair-pulling rates of 0%. In a 3-year-old child, trichotillomania was treated indirectly by targeting thumb sucking as the behavior to change (Knell and Moore 1988). The parents punished thumb sucking by applying a bad-tasting substance to the thumb. This resulted in eliminating both hair pulling and thumb sucking.

Unfortunately, deriving conclusive evidence from these reports is difficult because of the small number of patients who participated in the various treatment modalities (i.e., one or two patients).

To increase the validity of self-report data and the treatment effects of self-monitoring as described earlier, several investigators added other objective measurements, such as having patients count the number of pulled hairs (Bayer 1972; Stabler and Warren 1974; Wolfsohn and Barling 1978), measure their hair length (Anthony 1978), or both (McLaughlin and Nay 1975). Others combined self-monitoring, hair counting, and measuring hair length with token reinforcement (Wolfsohn and Barling 1978), self-denial of privileges (Cordle and Long 1980), and behavioral contracting (Stabler and Warren 1974). The addition of these techniques increased treatment success rate.

In addition to self-monitoring, other behavior therapies have been applied. Moderate to positive improvement has resulted from covert desensitization (Levine 1976); attention reflection and response prevention by cutting hair close to the scalp (Massong et al. 1980); attention-reflection combined with punishment (Altman et al. 1982); facial screening (covering the patient's face and hair with a soft cloth when he or she attempted to pull) (Barmann and Vitali 1982); and a multiple-component treatment package consisting of self-monitoring, hair collection, goal setting, relaxation, and stimulus control (Bornstein and Rychtarik 1978). The last of these researchers introduced a new dependent measure: size of bald spots.

The most successful self-management treatment in the remediation of hair pulling is habit reversal. This treatment includes 13 components: 1) competing response training, 2) habit awareness training, 3) identifying response precursors (e.g., face touching, hair straightening), 4) identifying situations where the habit is likely to occur (e.g., watching TV, studying, being alone), 5) relaxation training, 6) response prevention training (e.g., practicing the competing reaction for 3 minutes, such as grasping or clenching fists when a habit response precursor or a situation that makes the habit likely to occur exists), 7) habit interruption (grasping or clenching to interrupt hair pulling), 8) positive attention/overcorrection (practice positive hair care, such as combing or brushing hair after pulling), 9) practicing motor responses that

compete with the habit in front of a mirror, 10) self-monitoring, 11) solicita-
tion of social support (e.g., significant others encourage the patient to stop hair
pulling), 12) habit inconvenience review, and 13) display of improvement (i.e.,
have the patient approach situations that were previously avoided). Habit reversal was first introduced as a generally effective treatment for nervous habits
by Azrin and Nunn (1973) and was later tested against negative practice in
34 hair pulling patients (Azrin et al. 1980). Results indicated 90% less hair
pulling with habit reversal compared with 50% less pulling with negative practice. Other researchers have found similarly encouraging results with habit
reversal in four patients with a 6-month positive follow-up (Rosenbaum and
Allyon 1981) and with habit reversal combined with positive self-statements in
one patient (Ottens 1981). When competing response training was compared
with relaxation training in a 14-year-old nail biting and hair pulling patient,
habit reversal decreased the incidence of both habits to zero (DeLuca and
Holborn 1984). Results were maintained 2 years later.

Most of the cases previously described were not severe—in other words,
no bald spots were noted. In a recalcitrant case of trichotillomania, a modified version of habit reversal (daily telephone calls for 3 weeks by therapist
and, no self-monitoring) was used successfully. Gains were attained at posttreatment and at 1-year follow-up (Tarnowski et al. 1987). These authors
used erosion estimates and serial photographing to obtain reliable and valid
improvement assessment. With this method, bald spots are measured and
photographed periodically. This technique results in a more accurate estimate of improvement and gives more visual and direct patient feedback. In
another recalcitrant case of hair and eyelash pulling, a plethora of techniques
were used, including self-monitoring, relaxation, positive self-images with
hair and lashes, response cost (recording a list of time, place, and conditions
where pulling occurs), supportive therapy with family conflict, looking at
bald spots in the mirror after each pull, wearing petroleum jelly on the eyelashes, using jangling bracelets and/or perfume on the fingers to increase
awareness of pulling, and wearing false eyelashes (McLaughlin and Nay 1975).
By combining these techniques, a positive outcome was achieved. Our
trichotillomania population varies from those who lose hair patches to those
who are completely bald, with and without scabs. Many techniques were
used including replicating tactile sensations via usage of koosh balls, plastic
bubble wrappers to pop, yarn, habit reversal, and exposure and response
prevention. Emphasis is on the last. As with severe OCD, the patient with

severe trichotillomania responds best to intensive treatment consisting of at least three weekly sessions.

To date, behavior therapy has been applied to mild and moderate cases of trichotillomania. More controlled experimental designs with objective measurements are needed, especially with more severe and complex cases of trichotillomania.

Pharmacological treatment.   The pharmacological literature review reveals a paucity of studies consisting mostly of single-case reports. Childers (1958) used chlorpromazine successfully in two psychotic women with trichotillomania who had been institutionalized for several years. Krishnan et al. (1984) used isocarboxazid to successfully treat a 32-year-old man who had had trichotillomania for several years and depression for 2 months. Snyder (1980) used amitriptyline to successfully treat a woman with OCD and trichotillomania. Imipramine (Sachdeva and Sidhu 1987), trazodone (Sunkureddi and Markovitz 1993), and fluoxetine (Koran et al. 1992; Primeau and Fontaine 1987; Swedo et al. 1989) have been effective in some studies but not in others (Christenson et al. 1991a). In a 13-year-old girl treated for OCD and trichotillomania, OCD responded to fluoxetine and clomipramine, but these drugs had minimal effect on trichotillomania (Graae et al. 1992). In an open 16-week trial, 12 patients treated with fluoxetine improved significantly, demonstrating a 34% improvement at posttreatment (Winchel et al. 1992). The efficacy of fluoxetine, in doses up to 80 mg/day, was investigated in an 18-week placebo-controlled, double-blind crossover study (Christenson et al. 1991a). The fluoxetine and placebo treatment phases consisted of 6-week trials of each agent, separated by a 5-week washout period. Fifteen of 21 chronic hair pulling patients who completed the study did not demonstrate any change in weekly ratings of hair pulling, the urge to pull, or the estimated amount pulled weekly. Thus, the authors concluded that fluoxetine does not have any short-term effect on trichotillomania. In one study of drug-resistant patients, a low dose of pimozide was added to selective serotonin reuptake inhibitors (Stein and Hollander 1992). In six of seven patients, the pimozide augmentation improved hair pulling.

In another controlled, double-blind crossover study, clomipramine was found to be superior to desipramine (Swedo et al. 1989). In 12 of 13 patients, symptoms significantly improved while taking clomipramine, and three patients had total remission. For those patients who received clomipramine first, there was a discernible clinical deterioration during subsequent desipramine treatment. The authors concluded that because OCD patients were excluded from the study, clomipramine and desipramine were equally effective antidepressant and anxiolytic agents, and the reduction in hair pulling was the result of clomipramine's specific antitrichotillomanic effect. They further speculated that trichotillomania may be related to OCD based on previous studies indicating clomipramine's efficacy in treating OCD (Yaryura-Tobias and Neziroglu 1975; Yaryura-Tobias et al. 1976). Yaryura-Tobias and co-workers suggested that perhaps trichotillomania should be classified as a form of OCD rather than as an impulse control disorder.

Swedo et al. (1991) used positron-emission tomography and 18-F-fluorodeoxyglucose to study resting cerebral glucose metabolism in 10 adult women with trichotillomania and 20 age-matched female control patients. As a group, the patients with trichotillomania showed significantly increased global glucose metabolic rates and normalized right and left cerebellar and right superior parietal glucose metabolic rates. Contrary to expectations, this pattern differed from that in their OCD population. Also, clomipramine-induced improvement negatively correlates with anterior cingulate and orbital frontal metabolism in patients with trichotillomania, but not in OCD patients.

Conclusion

Baer (1992) stated that there were at least two important differences between OCD and trichotillomania:

1. OCD patients provide a logical explanation of their behavior, whereas patients with trichotillomania rarely justify their hair pulling.
2. Response prevention in OCD patients leads eventually to anxiety reduction, whereas in trichotillomania patients, it leads to anxiety increase.

Similarly, Stanley et al. (1992) reported that trichotillomania patients experienced significantly greater pleasure during hair pulling than OCD patients experienced during performance of ritualistic behaviors. Also, trichotillomania patients have fewer associated obsessive-compulsive symptoms, as well as less depression and anxiety, than OCD patients.

It is difficult to reach any conclusions based on these studies. It appears that some patients with trichotillomania may indeed have OCD, whereas others with the same behavior may not. It seems that classification of tricho-tillomania as an OCD variant depends on the phenomenology reported by the patient. Patients who experience hair pulling as an irresistible urge with accompanying anxiety elevation, followed by a reduction in anxiety after pulling, may have an OCD variant. Probably within this patient subset are those 15% of patients who are aware of their urges and behaviors, similar to OCD patients who are aware of their compulsions. Within this group, the act is purposeful and reduces anxiety. This patient population responded to clomipramine in Swedo et al.'s (1989) study. Those patients who are mostly unaware of pulling and experience it as pleasurable probably have a bad habit that may respond to habit reversal.

References

Adam BS, Kashani JH: Trichotillomania in children and adolescents: review of the literature and case report. Child Psychiatry Hum Dev 20:159–163, 1990

Altman K, Grahs S, Friman P: Treatment of unobserved trichotillomania by attention reflection and punishment of an apparent covariant. J Behav Ther Exp Psychiatry 13:337–340, 1982

American Psychiatric Association: Diagnostic and Statistical Manual of Mental Disorders, 4th Edition. Washington, DC, American Psychiatric Association, 1994

Anderson FW, Dean HC: Some aspects of child guidance and clinical intake policy and practices. A study of 500 cases at the Los Angeles Child Guidance Clinics. Los Angeles, Public Health Monograph No. 42, 1956, pp 1–14

Anderson L, Dances J, Alpert M, et al: Punishment learning and self-mutilation in Lesch-Nyhan disease. Nature 265:461–463, 1977

Angulo M, Castro-Magana M: Growth hormone evaluation and treatment in Prader-Willi syndrome. Journal of Pediatric Edocrinology 4:167–173, 1991

Anthony WZ: Brief intervention in a case of childhood trichotillomania by self-monitoring. J Behav Ther Exp Psychiatry 9:173–175, 1978

Azrin NH, Nunn RG: Habit reversal: a method of eliminating nervous habits and tics. Behav Res Ther 11:619–628, 1973

Azrin NH, Nunn RG: Habit Control in a Day. New York, Simon & Schuster, 1977

Azrin NH, Nunn RG, Frantz SE: Treatment of hairpulling (trichotillomania): a comparative study of habit reversal and negative practice training. J Behav Ther Exp Psychiatry 11:13–20, 1980

Bach-Y-Rita G: Habitual violence and self-mutilation. Am J Psychiatry 131:9–13, 1974

Baer L: Behavior therapy for obsessive-compulsive disorder and trichotillomania. Implications for Tourette syndrome, in Advances in Neurology. Edited by Chase TN, Friedhoff AJ, Cohen DJ. New York, Raven, 1992, pp 333–340

Barabasz M: Trichotillomania: a new treatment. Int J Clin Exp Hypn 37:146–154, 1987

Barmann BC, Vitali DL: Facial screenings to eliminate trichotillomania in developmentally disabled persons. Behavior Therapy 13:735–742, 1982

Bayer CA: Self-monitoring and mild aversion treatment of trichotillomania. J Behav Ther Exp Psychiatry 3:139–141, 1972

Bazelon K, Stevens H, Davis M, et al: Mental retardation, self mutilation, and hyperuricemia in females. Trans Am Neurol Assoc 93:113–115, 1968

Benjamin E, Biuot-Smith T: Natrexone and fluoxetine in Prader-Willi syndrome. J Am Acad Child Adolesc Psychiatry 32:870–873, 1993

Berkson G, Davenport RK: Stereotyped movements of mental defectives: I. Initial survey. Am J Ment Defic 66:849–852, 1962

Bornstein PH, Rychtarik RG: Multi-component behavioral treatment of trichotillomania: a case study. Behav Res Ther 16:217–220, 1978

Boyle JA, Rawio KO, Astrin KH, et al: Lesch Nyhan syndrome: preventive control by prenatal diagnosis. Science 169:688–689, 1970

Bryson Y, Sakati N, Nyhan L, et al: Self mutilative behavior in the Cornelia de Lange syndrome. Am J Ment Def 76:319–324, 1971

Butler MG, Jenkins BB: Sister chromatid exchange analysis in the Prader-Labhart-Willi syndrome. Am J Med Genet 28:821–827, 1987

Butterworth T: Discussion. Arch Dermatol 105:539–540, 1972

Childers RT: Report of 2 cases of trichotillomania of longstanding duration and their response to chlorpromazine. J Clin Exp Psychopathol 19:140–144, 1958

Christenson GA, Mackenzie TB, Mitchell JE, et al: A placebo controlled, double blind crossover study of fluoxetine in trichotillomania. Am J Psychiatry 148:1566–1571, 1991a

Christenson GA, Mackenzie TB, Mitchell JE: Characteristics of 60 adult chronic hairpullers. Am J Psychiatry 148:365–370, 1991b

Christenson GA, Ristvedt SL, Mackenzie TB: Identification of trichotillomania cue profiles. Behav Res Ther 31:315–320, 1993

Cordle CJ, Long CC: The use of operant self-control procedures in the treatment of compulsive hairpulling. J Behav Ther Exp Psychiatry 11:127–130, 1980

Dech B, Budow L: The use of fluoxetine in an adolescent with Prader-Willi syndrome. J Am Acad Child Adolesc Psychiatry 30:298–302, 1991

de Lange C: Sur un type nouveau de degeneration (typus amstelodamensis). Arch Med Enfants 36:713–719, 1933

Delgado RA, Mannino FV: Some observations on trichotillomania in children. J Am Acad Child Psychiatry 81:229–246, 1969

DeLissovoy V: Headbanging in early childhood: a study of incidence. J Pediatr 58:803–805, 1961

DeLuca RV, Holborn SW: A comparison of relaxation training and competing response training to eliminate hairpulling and nail biting. J Behav Ther Exp Psychiatry 15:67–70, 1984

Dizmang LH, Cheatham CF: The Lesch Nyhan syndrome. Am J Psychiatry 127: 671–677, 1970

Duker P: Behavior control of self mutilation in a Lesch Nyham patient. J Ment Defic Res 19:11–15, 1971

Epstein LH, Peterson GL: The control of undesired behavior by self-imposed contingencies. Behavior Therapy 4:91–95, 1973

Etienne JC, Chanpanie JP, Pascalis G, et al: Encephalopathie hypercosmique avec auto mutilations. Rev Rhum Ed Fr 40:265–270, 1973

Fastlicht S: Medicine in the Teotihaucan culture I. Pre-Cortes dental mutilations in Teotihuacan and its relation to other cultures. Gac Med Mex 98:351–358, 1968

Felix JS, DeMars R: Detection of females heterozygous for the Lesch-Nyhan mutation by 8 aza-guanine moistent growth of fibero plants. J Lab Clin Med 77: 596–604, 1971

Frankel F, Simmons JQ: Self-injurious behavior in schizophrenic and retarded children. Am J Ment Defic 80:512–522, 1976

Friman PC, Finney JW, Christopherson ER: Behavioral treatment of trichotillomania: an evaluative review. Behavior Therapy 15:249–265, 1984

Gardner AR, Gardner AJ: Self-mutilation, obsessionality, and narcissism. Br J Psychiatry 127:127–132, 1975

Glaski T: The adjunctive use of hypnosis in the treatment of trichotillomania. Am J Clin Hypn 23:198–201, 1981

Graae F, Gitow A, Piacentini J, et al: Response of obsessive-compulsive disorder and trichotillomania to serotonin reuptake blockers. Am J Psychiatry 149: 149–150, 1992

Green AH: Self-mutilation in schizophrenic children. Arch Gen Psychiatry 17: 234–244, 1967

Greenberg HR, Sarner CA: Trichotillomania—a review. Compr Psychiatry 26:123–128, 1965

Hallopeau M: Alopecie par grattage (trichomanie ou trichotillomanie). Ann Dermatol Venereol 10:440–441, 1889

Holm VA, Cassidy SB, Butler MG, et al: Prader-Willi syndrome: consensus diagnostic criteria. Pediatrics 91:398–402, 1993

Jenike MA: Psychotherapy of obsessive-compulsive personality disorder, in Obsessive-Compulsive Disorders: Theory and Management, 2nd Edition. Edited by Jenike MA, Baer L, Minichiello WE. Chicago IL, Mosby-Year Book, 1990, pp 295–305

Kanner L: Child Psychiatry. Springfield, IL, Charles C Thomas, 1950

Keshighian JM: Anatomy of a Burmese beauty secret. National Geographic 155: 798–801, 1979

Knell SM, Moore DJ: Childhood trichotillomania treated indirectly by punishing thumb sucking. J Behav Ther Exp Psychiatry 19:305–310, 1988

Koran LM, Ringold A, Hewlett M: Fluoxetine for trichotillomania: an open clinical trial. Psychopharmacol Bull 28:145–149, 1992

Kravitz H: Headbanging in infants and children. Dis Nerv Syst 21:203–205, 1960

Krishnan RR, Davidson J, Miller R: MAO inhibitor therapy in trichotillomania associated with depression: case report. J Clin Psychiatry 45:267–268, 1984

Krishnan RR, Davidson JRT, Guarjuardo C: Trichotillomania—a review. Compr Psychiatry 26:123–128, 1985

Lantz JE, Early JP, Pillow WE: Family aspects of trichotillomania. J Psychiatr Nurs 8:32–37, 1980

Lautala P, Knip M, Akerblom HK, et al: Serum insulin-releasing activity and the Prader-Willi syndrome. Acta Endocrinol Suppl (Copenh) 279:416–421, 1986

Lenane MC, Swedo SE, Rapoport JL, et al: Rates of obsessive-compulsive disorder in first degree relatives of patients with trichotillomania: a research note. J Child Psychol Psychiatry 33:925–933, 1992

Lesch M, Nyhan WL: A familial disorder of uric acid metabolism and central nervous system function. Am J Med 36:561–570, 1964

Levine BA: Treatment of trichotillomania by covert sensitization. Behav Ther Exp Psychiatry 7:75–76, 1976

MacNeil J, Thomas MR: Treatment of obsessive-compulsive hair pulling (trichotillomania) by behavioral and cognitive contingency manipulation. J Behav Ther Exp Psychiatry 7:391–392, 1976

Mannino FV, Delgado RA: Trichotillomania in children: a review. Am J Psychiatry 126:505–511, 1969

Massong SR, Edwards RP, Range-Sitton L, et al: A case of trichotillomania in a three-year-old boy treated by response prevention. J Behav Ther Exp Psychiatry 11:223–225, 1980

Mastellone M: Aversion therapy: a new use for the old rubber band. J Behav Ther Exp Psychiatry 5:311–312, 1974

Mathew A, Kumaraiah V: Behavioral intervention in the treatment of trichotillomania. Indian J Pediatr 55:451–453, 1988

McDonald JA, Kelley WN: Lesch-Nyhan syndrome: altered kinetic properties of mutant enzyme. Science 171:689–691, 1971

McLaughlin JG, Nay WR: Treatment of trichotillomania using positive covariants and response cost: a case report. Behavior Therapy 6:87–91, 1975

Mizuno T, Yugari Y: Prophylactic effect of L-5-hydroxytryptophan on self-mutilation in the Lesch-Nyhan syndrome. Neuropadiatrie 6:13–23, 1975

Mizuno T, Segawa M, Kurumada T, et al: Clinical and therapeutic aspects of the Lesch-Nyhan syndrome in Japanese children. Neuropadiatrie 2:38–52, 1970

Monroe JT, Abse DW: Psychopathology of trichotillomania and trichophagy. Psychiatry 26:95–103, 1963

Muller SA: Trichotillomania. Dermatol Clin 5:595–601, 1987

Noguez X: Basic bibliography on dental mutilations in Prehispanic Mexico. ADM 27:516–526, 1970

Oranje AP, Peereboom-Wynia JD, De Raeymaecker DM: Trichotillomania in childhood. J Am Acad Dermatol 15:614–619, 1986

Ottens AJ: Multifaceted treatment of compulsive hairpulling. J Behav Ther Exp Psychiatry 12:77–80, 1981

Otto K, Rambach H: Neurotic trichotillomania in childhood. Psychiatr Neurol Med Psychol 16:265–269, 1964

Otto PL, Sulzbacher SI, Worthington-Roberts BS: Sucrose-induced behavior changes of persons with Prader-Willi syndrome. Am J Ment Defic 86:335–341, 1982

Philippopoulos GS: A case of trichotillomania (hairpulling). Acta Psychother Psychosom 9:304–312, 1961

Primeau F, Fontaine R: Obsessive disorder with self mutilation: a subgroup responsive to pharmacotherapy. Can J Psychiatry 32:699–701, 1987

Robinowitz CB: Habit disorders, in Basic Handbook of Child Psychiatry. Edited by Noshpuitz J. New York, Basic Books, 1979, pp 703–705

Rosenbaum MS, Allyon T: The habit reversal technique in treating trichotillomania. Behavior Therapy 12:473–481, 1981

Rosenthal RJ, Renzlen C, Wallsh R, et al: Wrist cutting syndrome: the meaning of a gesture. Am J Psychiatry 128:1363–1368, 1972

Rowen R: Hypnotic age regression in the treatment of a self destructive habit: trichotillomania. Am J Clin Hypn 23:195–197, 1981

Sachdeva JS, Sidhu BS: Trichotillomania associated with depression. J Indian Med Assoc 85:151–152, 1987

Saper B: A report on behavior therapy with outpatient clinic patients. Psychiatr Q 45:209–215, 1971

Sareen C, Ruvalcab RH, Kelley VC: Some aspects of carbohydrate metabolism in Prader-Willi syndrome. Anesthesiology 43:590–592, 1975

Schachter VM: Trichotillomania in children. Prax Kinderpsychol Kinderpsychiatr 10:120–124, 1961

Scherzer AL, Ilson JB: Normal intelligence in the Lesch-Nyhan syndrome. Pediatrics 44:116–120, 1969

Selikowitz M, Suman J, Pendergast A, et al: Fenfluramine in Prader-Willi syndrome: a double blind, placebo controlled trial. Arch Dis Child 65:112–114, 1990

Shear SC, Nyhan WL, Kirman BH, et al: Self-mutilation behavior as a feature of the De Lange syndrome. J Pediatr 78:506–509, 1971

Singh S, Willers I, Goedde HW: A rapid micromethod for prenatal diagnosis for Lesch-Nyhan syndrome. Clin Genet 10:12–15, 1976

Slagle DA, Martin TA: Trichotillomania. Am Fam Physician 43:2019–2024, 1991

Snyder S: Trichotillomania treated with amitriptyline. J Nerv Ment Dis 168: 505–507, 1980

Spiegel H, Spiegel D: Trance and Treatment: Clinical Uses of Hypnosis. New York, Basic Books, 1978

Stabler B, Warren AA: Behavioral contracting in treating trichotillomania: case note. Exp Psychiatry 7:391–392, 1974

Stanley MA, Swann AC, Bowers TC, et al: A comparison of clinical features in trichotillomania and obsessive-compulsive disorder. Behav Res Ther 30:39–44, 1992

Stein DJ, Hollander E: Low-dose pimozide augmentation of serotonin reuptake blockers in the treatment of trichotillomania. J Clin Psychiatry 53:123–126, 1992

Stevens MJ: Behavioral treatment of trichotillomania. Psychol Rep 55:987–990, 1984

Sunkureddi K, Markovitz P: Trazodone treatment of obsessive-compulsive disorder and trichotillomania. Am J Psychiatry 150:523–524, 1993

Swedo SE, Rapoport JL: Trichotillomania (annotation). J Child Psychol Psychiatry 32:401–409, 1991

Swedo SE, Leonard HL, Rapoport JL, et al: A double-blind comparison of clomipramine and desipramine in the treatment of trichotillomania (hair pulling). N Engl J Med 321:497–501, 1989

Swedo SE, Rapoport JL, Leonard HL, et al: Regional cerebral glucose metabolism of women with trichotillomania. Arch Gen Psychiatry 48:828–833, 1991

Tarnowski KJ, Rosen LA, McGrath ML, et al: A modified habit reversal procedure in a recalcitrant case of trichotillomania. Behav Ther Exp Psychiatry 18:157–163, 1987

Taylor JG: A behavioral interpretation of obsessive compulsive neurosis. Behav Res Ther 1:237–244, 1963

Taylor RL, Caldwell ML: Type and strength of food preferences of individuals with Prader-Willi syndrome. J Ment Defic Res 29:109–112, 1985

Tu JB, Hartridge GC, Izawa J: Psychopharmacogenetic aspects of Prader-Willi syndrome. J Am Acad Child Adolesc Psychiatry 31:1137–1140, 1992

Tynes LL, Winstead DK: Behavioral aspects of trichotillomania. J La State Med Soc 144:459–463, 1992

Tynes LL, White K, Steketee GS: Toward a new nosology of obsessive-compulsive disorder. Compr Psychiatry 31:465–480, 1990

Vasquez Soto FR: Preliminary survey of dental mutilation in primitive people of Peru. Odontologia 15:129–146, 1967

Verger-Pratoucy JC: Prehistoric maxillo-dental mutilations. Bull Group Int Rech Sci Stomatol 13:310–333, 1970

Vitiello B, Spreat S, Behar D: Obsessive-compulsive disorder in mentally retarded patients. J Nerv Ment Dis 177:232–236, 1989

Warnock JK, Kastenbaum T: Pharmacologic treatment of severe skin-picking behavior in Prader-Willi syndrome. Two case reports. Arch Dermatol 128:1623–1625, 1992

Weyers H: Ritual tooth mutilation in African Negroes. Zahnarztl Mitt 59:904–909, 1969

Whitman BV, Accardo P: Emotional symptoms in Prader-Willi syndrome adolescents. Am J Med Genet 28:897–905, 1987

Wilbur RL, Chandler PJ, Carpenter BL: Modification of self-mutilative behavior by aversive conditioning. Behavioral Engineering 1:14–25, 1974

Willig RP, Braun W, Commentz JC, et al: Circadian fluctuation of plasma melatonin in Prader Willi's syndrome and obesity. Acta Endocrinol Suppl 279:411–415, 1986

Winchel RM, Jones JS, Stanley B, et al: Clinical characteristics of trichotillomania and its response to fluoxetine. J Clin Psychiatry 53:304–308, 1992

Wolfsohn D, Barling J: From external to self-control: behavioral treatment of trichotillomania in an eleven-year-old girl. Psychol Rep 42:1171–1174, 1978

Yaryura-Tobias JA: Gilles de la Tourette's disease: interactions with other neuropsychiatric disorders. Acta Psychiatr Scand 59:9–16, 1979

Yaryura-Tobias JA, Neziroglu FA: The action of chlorimipramine in obsessive-compulsive neurosis: a pilot study. Curr Ther Res 17:111–116, 1975

Yaryura-Tobias JA, Neziroglu F: Compulsions aggression, and self-mutilation: A hypothalamic disorder? J Orthomolecular Psychiatry 7:114–117, 1978

Yaryura-Tobias JA, Neziroglu F, Bergman L: Chlorimipramine for obsessive-compulsive neurosis: an organic approach. Curr Ther Res 20:541–548, 1976

Yaryura-Tobias JA, Neziroglu FA, Kaplan S: Self-mutilation, anorexia, and dysmenorrhea in obsessive compulsive disorder. International Journal of Eating Disorders 17:33–38, 1995

Chapter 12
Neurological Disorders

W
e selected subsets of several neurological disorders with obsessive and compulsive phenomena. These entities may manifest
organic pathology, psychological characteristics, and the pharmacological responses associated with obsessive-compulsive disorder (OCD).
By analogy, we may extract information helpful to construct hypotheses on
OCD's etiology and pathology and design pharmacological compounds suitable for treating this intriguing disease.

Organic pathology includes anatomical lesions affecting primarily the basal
ganglia and its connections with cerebral regions controlling higher cortical
centers. As a consequence, movement abnormalities, hyperkinesis in children, excitatory behaviors, and OCD symptoms seem to merge into new nosological variants. Of note, much of the motor pathology follows the onset of
psychiatric pathology (Table 12–1).

After a peak, the psychiatric symptoms—notably OCD—wax and wane
and the motor pathology predominates. Medications affecting the cathe-
cholaminergic and indolaminergic pathways are the chosen therapeutic tools.

In 1896 Gadelius of Sweden compared obsessions with suggestibility and
contrast thinking. For him, every idea had a counter-idea, like an echo,
a "mirror image" or reflection. Gadelius postulated an organic lesion with
cortical and subcortical damage (Gadelius 1896/1959). Nevertheless. as
Freudian ideas slowly replaced the neurological core of neuropsychiatry,
a splitting of the two disciplines ensued.

The dichotomy of the brain and the mind is a philosophical, not a scientific, concept. A unitarian approach states that the mind operates through
neural mechanisms subjected to the laws of genetics, physiology, and the
presence of noxa. Philosophy, psychiatry, and neuroscience contradict themselves when trying to explain human experience and behavior (Hundert 1990).
Unfortunately, when explicating mind and body, we must use an organ, the
brain, as both observer and observed, adding an unavoidable bias element.
Fortunately, the current "divorce" between neurology and psychiatry is in
the process of reconciliation, and we may witness their rejoining.

Table 12–1.   Motor activity in OCD spectrum

Tics
Echolalia
Echokinesis
Dyskinesias
Grimacing
Repetitive motions
Palilalia
Increased hyperexcitability
Self-harm
Retracing
Grooming
Catatonia
Freezing

Structural Lesions

Brain damage produces a complex symptomatology as a consequence of affecting many functional brain areas. The main brain damage symptoms are 1) an impairment in abstract thinking; 2) an inability to grasp situations as a result of an emotional response; 3) a fear of danger; 4) a fear to perform tasks; 5) an urge to release tension, leading to rapid responses without deliberation; and 6) an inability to find proper words as a result of the impairment in abstract thinking.

Goldstein (1951) has described the fundamental conditions pertaining to brain organicity: the catastrophic condition, defined as the patient's state in failure situations, and the ordered condition, specified as the state in the success situation. Brain damage may cause personality disorders, impairment in the thought process, motor dysfunction, and emotional changes. Personality changes may cause or precipitate anancastic thinking and behavior, irritability, mental or physical hyperkinesis, or other changes as consequence of an increase in concrete thinking. These changes in personality following brain damage should be separated from symptoms caused by other factors: (1) disturbances of learned or inborn patterns, (2) catastrophic conditions, and (3) the expression of protective mechanisms, to avoid catastrophes (Goldstein 1951).

The presence of obsessive-compulsive symptoms after a head injury is infrequent, yet such an injury should not be ruled out. An in-depth anamnesis may yield unexpected results, and cerebral imaging may corroborate clinical findings.

OCD as a head injury complication has been reported in several extensive reviews, notably in studies of war injuries (Achte 1958; Denny-Brown 1942a, 1942b) or in clinical studies (Croisile et al. 1989; Hillbom 1960; Lishman 1968; Mapother 1937; McKeon et al. 1984).

Cerebral tumors also may produce OCD symptoms. Of 58 patients with brain tumors, 25 were diagnosed with a mental illness. Of these 25, one patient had a left frontal tumor and obsessional illness manifestations (Minski 1933). A 36-year-old woman developed OCD after a nonmalignant tumor of the right parietal vertex was removed. This patient responded to behavior therapy (Paradis et al. 1992).

In a study of 100 patients with temporal lobe lesions, psychiatric manifestations occurred paroxysmally and nonparoxysmally. Paroxysmal symptoms included automatism and olfactory hallucinatory phenomena. Automatism occurred in 48 patients. Odors were usually described as unpleasant or as an "unbearable stench" (Mulder and Daly 1952). Similar olfactory delusions have been described in patients with monosymptomatic hypochondriac delusion and in patients with OCD or body dysmorphic disorder who complained of obsessions of the smell (see Chapters 8 and 9).

In a study by Yaryura-Tobias and Neziroglu (1991), nine OCD patients (mean age, 56 years) had brain lesions that were confirmed by magnetic resonance imaging. The neuroradiological findings showed brain atrophy ($n = 9$), enlarged ventricle-to-brain ratio ($n = 2$), cerebellar atrophy ($n = 2$), multiple infarcts of the internal capsule ($n = 1$), multiple infarcts of the right parietal lobe and both occipital lobes ($n = 1$), as well as basal ganglia ($n = 1$) In this study, four clinical symptoms were characteristic of a cerebral lesion: 1) patient indifference to his or her OCD, 2) concrete thinking, 3) a low level of arousal, and 4) minimal emotional expression. The lesions were tumoral, vascular, or both.

Sometimes tumors cause epileptic attacks leading to transient feelings of compulsion. Such was the case in two patients with glioblastoma. One had a tumor in the right frontoparietal region; the other had a tumor in the left frontal region (Ward 1988). Cerebrovascular accidents, including stroke (Beckson and Cummings 1991) and cerebral infarction, may present OCD symptomatology. Such accidents include arterial hypertension, arteriosclerosis, aneurysm, or diabetes.

Neurological Soft Signs

Neurological soft signs indicate abnormal sensory or motor performance without confirming anatomical location or the presence of neurological lesions represented by gross neurological signs. These signs are unspecific and point to disorders of dominance, speech, right-left orientation, gait, motor coordination, balance, stereognosis graphestesia, tactile symmetry, pronation-supination, and thumb opposition.

One study of 40 medication-free OCD patients compared with 20 healthy control patients found significantly more abnormalities in fine motor coordination and visuospatial function, as well as more involuntary and mirror movements, in the OCD group. Moreover, soft signs correlated with the severity of OCD. An excess of findings on the left side of the body and abnormalities in cube drawings suggested right hemispheric dysfunction in an OCD subgroup (Hollander et al. 1990).

In another study, 20 OCD patients were compared with a group of phobia patients and a group of healthy control patients. OCD patients showed a higher global incidence of soft neurological signs, especially more alterations in movement coordination in the upper extremities and balance, with a trend toward more anomalies in dominance-laterality (Conde López et al. 1990).

A third study compared 39 OCD patients (14 medication free, 13 receiving clomipramine, and 12 receiving fluoxetine) with a group of patients with seasonal affective disorder ($N = 13$), a group with anxiety disorders ($N = 10$), and 43 healthy volunteers. OCD patients scored significantly higher in the total number of involuntary movements.

More studies are needed. The modest number of subjects examined and the small quantity of published studies indicate the preliminary nature of the observations and the need for larger samples.

Epilepsies

Epilepsies are classified according to the type of recurrent seizures produced by excessive paroxysmal neuronal discharge in different brain parts. The discharge either increases excitatory synaptic bombardment or reduces the inhibitory discharge. In addition, seizure disorders may be manifested by behavioral pathology (Turner 1907).

There are three main types of epilepsy:

1. Centerencephalic
   a. Grand mal
   b. Petit mal
2. Focal
   a. Jacksonian
   b. Temporal lobe
   c. Other focal
   d. Frontal
   e. Midtemporal
   f. Occipital
3. Other petit mal variants
   a. Hypothalamic (14-per-second and 6-per-second positive spiking)

This anatomical classification indicates the universal location of seizure disorders within the cerebral content. Therefore, it is not surprising to find clinical correlations between seizure disorders and OCD because OCD symptoms also are widely distributed in the brain. Some authors believe in a relationship between certain forms of epilepsy and authentic obsessive illnesses (Ciani and Vella 1965; Fuchs 1927; Garmany 1947; Jahrreiss 1926; Majluf 1951; Reda 1966).

In centerencephalic and temporal epilepsies, there are three forms of symptom presentation: 1) a psychic aura preceding the ictal episode, 2) an episode occurring as an isolated phenomenon, and 3) a continuous state of obsessiveness (Cabaleiro Goas and Perez Villamil 1966).

Seizure and OCD associations have been reported in complex stereotyped automatism, epileptic personality, scrupulosity syndrome, Tourette's syndrome, organic orderliness, and moral hypertrophy.

The complex stereotyped automatism of focal seizures is characterized by loss of consciousness, amnesia, and behavioral changes. These changes resemble obsessive-compulsive symptoms; examples include playing with buttons, buttoning and unbuttoning a coat, repetitive verbal phrasing, lip smacking, touching, and hanging of clothes in order and disorder. Some of these motor behaviors also may be observed in Tourette's syndrome patients.

The epileptic personality, a diagnosis rejected previously by the North American School of Neuropsychiatry, reflects the similarities between seizure disorders and OCD. The epileptic personality comprises slowness to act and to react, perseveration, circumstantiality, adhesiveness or "glue-iness" (i.e., the patient will not leave people alone), rigid emotional attitudes, and hyperresponsiveness to external factors. Other epileptic personality traits are self-centeredness, hypochondriasis, fixed ideas or strong opinions, panic attacks, fear, anxiety, phobias, rituals, and aggressive behavior. This array of symptoms and behaviors conforms to part of the phenomenological OCD spectrum.

It is noteworthy that scrupulosity, perfectionism, meticulosity, and perseveration are shared by anancastic and epileptic personalities. Scrupulosity syndrome is characterized by excessive concern with right and wrong, cautiousness, preciseness, and hesitation.

Vocalization and speech-related symptoms include compulsive laughter (Roubicek 1946), iterative speech, echolalia, and stuttering similar to Tourette's syndrome.

Patients with seizures or OCD are interested in keeping graphs of their illnesses and making notes and checklists. For example, in temporal lobe epilepsy, there is a concern with moral issues (moral hypertrophy), religiosity, changes in sexual conduct, and hypergraphia (Kligman and Goldberg 1975). Hypergraphia is a tendency toward extensive and, in some cases, compulsive writing. In many instances, we have observed children who are unable to stop writing, going outside the margins of the paper and onto the desk, giving a sense of automatic behavior. This phenomenon has been described by Waxman and Geschwind (1974). They considered these changes of theoretical interest because they provide an example of a behavioral symptom associated with an organic dysfunction at a specific anatomical location.

Patients with seizures sometimes display Goldstein's (1951) organic orderliness, which is much like the orderliness of obsessive-compulsive patients.

Compulsive suicide attempts in psychomotor epilepsy have been described in three cases of psychomotor epilepsy with a temporal focus (Anastassopoulos and Kokkini 1969). The interictal suicide attempts were compulsive, but fortunately patients were restrained in time. Additional symptoms were aggressive behavior, bulimia, hypersexuality, and a hypomanic state, subsequently followed by anorexia and depression. The authors suggested that this sequential course occurred as a result of undetermined factors and was unrelated to changes in the location of the existing lesion. This clinical description not only points to a hypothalamic dysfunction, but also illustrates the OCD continuum and its spectrum.

In children the organic association between obsessive-compulsive symptoms and seizures presents some interesting observations. In Heubner-Hester disease, which is characterized by digestive acid metabolic disturbances, obsessive activities before eating are commonly observed. The ictal and interictal manifestations of limbic epilepsy in childhood included obsessive-compulsive behavior such as hissing, forced thinking, compulsions, and phobias (Glaser et al. 1968).

There is scant information about OCD onset in seizure disorder patients. It seems that seizure disorders precede OCD onset. One patient with a temporal lobe seizure disorder and another with grand mal seizure disorder developed OCD shortly after the onset of their seizures (Kettl and Marks 1986). Similar to the cyclic obsessional condition (Slater and Roth 1972), obsessional doubting appears during the interictal phases (Crichton-Browne 1895; Turner 1907). Jelliffe (1932) noticed compulsions in epileptic patients.

The relationship between OCDs and abnormal electroencephalography (EEG) epileptiform patterns was established by Cabaleiro Goas (1969), Pacella (1944), Reda (1966), and Rockwell and Simons (1947). According to Seva Diaz (1964), 54% of obsessive patients had abnormal EEG epileptiform patterns, whereas Rojo Sierra (1970; cited by Sanchez Planell [1971]), indicated that the percentage of epileptiform patients experiencing obsessive-compulsive symptoms was approximately 38%. We have observed that 25% of 250 patients with OCD presented abnormal, unspecific EEG tracings but with a trend toward paroxysmal activity (Yaryura-Tobias and Neziroglu 1983), as previously reported by Cabaleiro Goas (1969). We also observed 10 epileptic patients who had concomitant obsessive-compulsive symptomatology (Yaryura-Tobias and Neziroglu 1983). In contrast, others have been unable to find a robust incidence of OCD in epilepsy. Ingram (1960) found a low incidence of abnormal EEG patterns in obsessive-compulsive patients. Research done on the ictal and interictal psychiatric manifestations in epilepsy does not mention obsessive-compulsive symptomatology (Flor-Henry 1972). Moreover, Esser (1938), Follin (1941), and Yde et al. (1941) showed that epileptic patients were more susceptible to paranoid psychosis. Similar findings were reported by Dongier (1960) after analyzing the clinical, psychiatric, and interictal data for 516 epileptic patients with psychotic episodes. Studies done by Hill (1953) and Pond (1957) reported repeated intrusions of abnormal ideas and emotions into the consciousness as part of the psychotic syndrome in epileptic patients.

The suggested relationship between OCDs and epilepsy is still uncertain, primarily because the research on OCD pathology has been directed toward dynamic interpretations. Currently, there is enough evidence to associate OCD and the epileptic syndrome. Moreover, just as we speak of "nuclear epilepsies," we may be able to speak of "nuclear OCDs" that can be anatomically and biochemically explained.

Extrapyramidal Disorders

Extrapyramidal disorders are characterized by abnormal involuntary movements, alterations in muscle tone, and disturbances in body posture. These disorders may be accompanied by changes in affect and the presence of psychotic or obsessive-compulsive symptoms.

The major clinical states include parkinsonism, chorea, athetosis, dystonia, and hemiballismus. The pathological substratum of extrapyramidal disorders includes anatomical and biochemical lesions of the basal ganglia. Pathology also may comprise vascular disorders, infections, and brain trauma. We will describe only disorders where obsessive-compulsive symptoms are observed.

Abnormal Involuntary Movements

A number of entities, although not related etiologically, have choreiform movements; these include acute chorea (Sydenham's chorea), hereditary chorea (Huntington's disease), and senile chorea.

Chorea refers to brief, distal, rapid, explosive movements that at first appear purposeful and coordinated but on closer inspection are aimless and uncoordinated. These movements appear in the head, face, trunk, and upper and lower limbs and are accentuated by environmental stimulation and stress, like any other abnormal or involuntary movement. Additional symptoms are grimacing, difficult speech, and chewing and swallowing movements.

Acute chorea usually appears during childhood, between 5 and 15 years of age. Multiple noxic agents appear to be responsible. Acute chorea has been reported during epidemic encephalitis or in encephalopathies accompanying exanthema, pertussis, or diphtheria. It also has been reported as a consequence of hypoglycemia, hyperthyroidism, systemic lupus erythematosus, carbon monoxide poisoning, vascular diseases, tumors, and degenerative processes of the basal ganglia. The closest relationship seems to be with rheumatic fever.

The psychiatric manifestations of chorea range from neurosis to psychosis. As early as 1894, Osler described compulsive symptoms in choreic patients. A high prevalence of OCD has been observed in acute (Sydenham's) chorea (Swedo et al. 1989). Psychological symptoms in children with Sydenham's chorea include increased emotional lability, irritability, hyperactivity, distractibility, age-regressed behavior, and obsessive-compulsive symptoms (Swedo et al. 1993). In Swedo et al.'s (1993) study, the OCD symptoms had a sudden onset preceding the movement disorder and usually disappeared before the cessation of the choreic movement. This acute onset of symptoms is unusual for OCD, which is characterized by a gradual onset. This gradual onset may be caused by the presence of an anatomobiochemical lesion. Anecdotal reports using magnetic resonance imagery and positron-emission tomography have suggested basal ganglia involvement in chorea, which may correlate with similar findings in OCD (Goldman et al. 1993; Kienzle et al. 1991). Of note is that cognitive function in patients with Sydenham's chorea differs from the impaired cognition seen in OCD patients. Perhaps intellectual activity in all of these disorders and in OCD may not be as strongly related as clinicians would like to prove.

In Huntington's chorea (hereditary chorea), obsessive-compulsive symptoms have been reported in two patients who presented repetitive, stereotyped, complex egodystonic behaviors (Cummings and Cunningham 1992). At times, choreic symptoms have a waxing and waning characteristic similar to that seen in Tourette's syndrome.

Blepharospasm (Bihari et al. 1992a) and spasmodic torticollis also present obsessive-compulsive characteristics (Bihari et al. 1992b; Shulze and Stephan 1987).

Other Extrapyramidal Disorders

Other extrapyramidal disorders include tics, athetosis, dystonia musculorum deformans (distortion dystonia), spasmodic torticollis, and hemiballismus. These syndromes are characterized by involuntary movements and, in some of these entities, behavioral changes related to obsessive-compulsive symptomatology.

Parkinson's Disease

This disease, described by Parkinson in 1817, presents neurological, autonomic nervous system, and psychiatric symptoms. It is characterized by tremor, muscle rigidity, and loss of postural reflexes. The autonomic nervous system shows changes in glucose metabolism, excessive perspiration, sebum secretion, and sexual impotence. Psychiatric manifestations include anxiety, depression, psychosis, psychomotor retardation, and obsessive-compulsive symptoms.

Furthermore, administration of levodopa for treatment of Parkinson's disease causes psychiatric side effects, inducing depression and overtly psychotic episodes (Yaryura-Tobias et al. 1972). Obsessive-compulsive symptoms have been observed as a side effect of levodopa administration to Parkinson's patients (Anden et al. 1970) and after its discontinuation (Sacks 1977).

Parkinsonian patients may have an obsessive-compulsive personality that decreases in intensity once the illness becomes manifest. Paralysis agitans frequently begins between ages 50 and 65, a period when obsessive-compulsive symptoms in true OCD diminish. Neuropsychological abnormalities in Parkinson's disease have been reported to be similar to obsessive slowness and may precede the appearance of motor symptoms in many patients (Lees 1989). Finally, obsessive-compulsive symptomatology may be observed in neuroleptic-induced parkinsonism.

Encephalitis

Encephalitis was the first neuropsychiatric disorder studied as both a mental and a motor disorder (Ward 1986). The variety of its clinical symptoms produced theories of neuropsychiatric disorders that anticipated modern neuropsychiatry.

Encephalitis is a psychomotor disorder characterized by headaches, fever, vomiting, a decrease in conscious activity, seizures, and increased intracranial pressure. At times meningeal irritation is present. There are multiple etiological factors, onset may be rapid or gradual, and outcome varies from recovery to death.

The phenomenology of encephalitis indicates that motor symptoms predominate over mental aberrations. Its motor symptoms include seizures, echolalia, palilalia, logoclonia, coprolalia, praxis, parakinesia, and dyskinesia, with dyskinesia mostly represented by oculogyric crises.

A good description of the psychiatric symptoms can be found in the extensive literature pertaining to epidemic encephalitis (encephalitis lethargica, or von Economo's disease). This entity appeared as a pandemia lasting from

1915 to 1926, and it caused devastating effects worldwide. Because psychiatric symptoms are present in this neurological disease, von Economo (1931) emphasized the significance of this illness, which offered unexpected insight into the psychological and physiological mysteries of the mental mechanism. The illness has three stages:

1. In the acute stage, patients are febrile, usually somnolent, and occasionally have hyperkinesis and ocular palsies. Recovery after the acute stage may last several days to a month. There ensues an interval of 3 days to 40 years in which numerous patients, although appearing well, have many complaints.
2. During the second stage, the pseudopsychoneurotic stage, the psychiatric symptoms unfold. Psychotic features, phobias, and obsessive-compulsive manifestations are observed. During this phase, patients may show personality changes, aggressive behavior, and hyperactivity.
3. The third stage is the development of Parkinson's disease along with decreasing psychiatric symptoms.

The first study of the psychiatric symptoms of encephalitis was by Mayer-Gross and Steiner (1921). Their patients presented iterative tendencies, doubting, compulsions, and arithmomania. Similar symptoms were described by Goldflam (1922), Hermann (1922), Burger and Mayer-Gross (1928), and Steiner (1930) and an excellent review was done by Stern (1927). Motor compulsions, represented by wrinkling, spitting, snapping of the fingers, an urge to avoid stepping on cracks in the sidewalk, touching doors, as well as symptoms of psychosis, have been described by Hendricks (1927).

In studying postencephalitic oculogyric crisis, Ewald (1924), and later Chlopicki (1931), de Boor (1949), Falkeiwicz and Rothfeld (1925), Flacha and Palisa (1936), Hohman (1925), Sarro (1932), Schilder (1938), and Storring (1930), described psychiatric symptoms similar to those observed in encephalitis. These symptoms were iterative behavior, arithmomania, and uncontrollable compulsions. During the intervals of improvement, a remission of OCD was observed. Stengel (1931) described a female patient who presented abnormal motor behavior and a cyclic disorder manifested with phobias and obsessions.

Hendricks (1927) recognized the far-reaching theoretical importance of these behavioral syndromes:

> In the study of this disease, we find a common meeting ground for those who are convinced that all psychiatric disorders are essentially changes in either

the structure of physicochemical function of cellular units, and those who contend that the nature of psychological processes is a unique biological mechanism. (p. 990)

Jelliffe (1932) published a monograph on the subject comprising a summary of the work of 100 authors who had presented more than 200 cases up to 1931. He believed the oculogyric crisis is accompanied by obsessive-compulsive phenomena. Years later, other authors emphasized the symptoms of palilalia, paligraphia, bradyphrenia, and obsessional syndromes (Allert and Meyer 1958; Lambertet et al. 1966; Parsons 1977; Schwab et al. 1951).

Childhood encephalitis. Sometimes childhood encephalitis is misdiagnosed as a flu-like state, or grippe, consisting of fever, photophobia, severe headaches, and vomiting. This episode lasts about 3 days and is followed by a silent period of days, weeks, or years. Then behavioral changes consisting of symptoms comparable with those seen in the hyperkinetic syndrome—notably, motor and mental hyperactivity, easy distractibility, inability to concentrate, and short attention span—ensue. Occasionally, disruptive behavior at home and school as well as poor academic performance complete the picture. About half of these children develop parkinsonism during adulthood, which gradually subdues their behavior. Similar gross behavior disturbance may occur in older children and adolescents and usually persists in adult life.

According to Slater and Roth (1972), the immature child's brain reacts to encephalitis differently from the brain of a fully grown individual. Children go through periods in which overt activity and aggressiveness usually develop into malicious, intractable behavioral patterns.

In adolescents with acute encephalitis, the syndrome is usually manifested by hyperactivity with behavioral abnormalities. Milder symptoms of hyperkinesis, tics, yawning, coughing, sniffing, peculiar breathing abnormalities, and repetitive movements are frequently seen in young encephalitic patients, but crises are rarely seen in children.

Some comments on subacute encephalitis. Acute and subacute encephalitis are not rare in clinical practice; manifestations include fever, headache, vomiting, drowsiness, motor dysphasia, visual field defect, increased reflexes, purposeless repetitive movement, nystagmus, ataxia, facial weakness, deafness, and convulsions (Gostling 1967). In addition, psychiatric disturbances ranging from psychosis to consciousness clouding, delirium, or coma also are seen. Psychiatric manifestations may be the first symptoms indicating later onset of the disease.

A survey of subacute encephalitis cases was conducted in 1970 by Himmelhoch et al. The subacute nature of the illness was determined when more than 2 weeks elapsed between the onset of symptoms and the maximum development of illness. In 100 cases, only 8 filled this criterion; all had prominent behavioral features, such as phobias and excessive ruminations, gradually manifested over a 2- to 6-month period.

In contrast, the subacute leukoencephalitis of Van Bogaert (1945) and the inclusion encephalitis of Dawson (1933, 1934) present psychiatric symptoms (Brain et al. 1943; Corsellis 1951; Glaser et al. 1968) resembling catatonic schizophrenia (Malamud et al. 1950) or depressive illness (Van Bogaert 1945) but not OCD.

One other aspect to consider is the connection of chorea with tic and compulsive utterances (Creak and Guttmann 1935) or with neuropsychiatric disorders overlapping symptoms such as hyperkinetic encephalitis and Tourette's syndrome.

Some comments on postencephalitic parkinsonism. The psychiatric symptoms of postencephalitic parkinsonism are identical to those found in other forms of encephalitis. In addition to the neurological symptoms, hypothalamic involvement, indicated by weight increase, sexual impotence, episodes of flushing, and polyuria, has been observed. In many cases oculogyric crises develop concurrently with psychiatric symptoms such as obsessions and motor compulsions. A need to associate the oculogyric crisis with some incessantly reiterated work or thought, obscenities, or a meaningless sequence of word associations or syllables has been reported.

Impairment of volitional control is manifested by involuntary movements, and the rigidity shackling the patient is expressed in the obsessive-compulsive symptoms. This close association between compulsive thought and motor behavior features, and their derivation from regions in the upper brain stem or hypothalamus, may offer theoretical implications in the pathogenesis of OCD. Moreover, organic lesions and the hopeless character of the disability may seriously affect the patient's personality. The patient's life becomes egocentrically restricted, monotonous, and stereotyped. The mood may or may not be depleted. If the patient is severely depressed, he or she may commit compulsive suicide (Harris and Cooper 1937).

According to Skoog (1959), primary OCD can be distinguished from an encephalitic process with obsessive-compulsive symptomatology by the fact that in the latter, the obsessions and compulsions are primitive, stereotypical, methodical, and nonintellectual. These clinical features fit the symptomatology of a histochemical or organic lesion.

Gaston et al. (1967) summarized the relationship between the brain and obsessions with the following classification:

1. Obsessions and extrapyramidal disorders
   a. Encephalitic pathology
   b. Choreiform syndromes and tics
   c. Drug-induced extrapyramidalism
2. Obsessive phenomena and brain injury
3. Obsessive phenomena and epilepsy

Tourette's Syndrome

The natural history of Tourette's syndrome permits a chronological analysis of events aimed at understanding the association between mental and motor pathology in several entities, including Tourette's syndrome.

In 1810 Bouteille reported a pseudo-choreic state accompanied by twitches and facial grimacing. In 1825 Itard described a female who at age 7 had had sudden involuntary movements, utterances, and coprolalia. Trousseau described similar conditions and later encouraged Tourette to announce his clinical observations (Trousseau 1873). In 1878 a condition characterized by involuntary jumping and echolalia also was reported (Beard 1878). A similar syndrome described in Malaysia was referred to as *latah* or *myriachit* in Siberia (Hammond 1884). By 1885 de la Tourette had defined and named this clinical entity. In 1886 the syndrome was known as *"la maladie des tics convulsifs"* (Guinon 1886).

Finally, obsessions, compulsions, and abnormal movements were described in studies on demonology, possession, and witchcraft (Sprenger and Kramer 1486/1975). Janet, who extensively described obsessive-compulsive neurosis, was working in La Salpetriere at the time Tourette outlined his syndrome. Interestingly, both Janet and Tourette were asked to make differential diagnoses between psychiatric clinical entities and demon possession (Oesterreich 1974).

The classic description of this syndrome includes multiple abnormal movements (tics), imitative behavior (echolalia), and obscene verbalizations (coprolalia). Other features were gradually incorporated including obsessions, compulsions, aggressive behavior, and self-mutilation.

This syndrome has obsessive-compulsive symptoms as a major component (Yaryura-Tobias 1975; Yaryura-Tobias and Neziroglu 1977). We also argue the nature of the involuntary movement as to whether a tic can be controlled, because of the discovery that motor and thalamic regions discharge prior to movements (Evarts 1971). This makes our proposal more acceptable because a patient may think the motor compulsion and then proceed to twitch. Therefore, a Tourette's syndrome patient may present voluntary or compulsive jerks. A partial corroboration might be found in the association between the premonitory sensory and mental "just-right phenomena" of OCD and Tourette's syndrome. For most patients, action is preceded by an urge to tic or to perform a mental task (Leckman and Chittenden 1990).

Tourette's syndrome and OCD are comorbid (Yaryura-Tobias and Neziroglu 1977); Tourette's syndrome is a neuropsychiatric condition rather than an isolated neurological syndrome.

Many studies investigating the OCD–Tourette's syndrome relation have been published (Abuzzahab and Anderson 1976; Cath et al. 1992; Damjanovic et al. 1992; Frankel et al. 1986; Hollander et al. 1989; Pitman et al. 1987; Singer and Walkup 1991; Steingard and Dillon-Stout 1992). One study evaluating the OCD and Tourette's association, although admitting that there was clinical evidence of such an association, failed to confirm it (Shapiro and Shapiro 1992). However, in another study examining the connection between Tourette's syndrome and OCD, the apparent high rate of tics and Tourette's syndrome in patients and their relatives was consistent with the hypothesis that in some cases, OCD and Tourette's syndrome may be alternative manifestations of the same pathology (Leonard et al. 1992).

One report stated that patients with OCD–Tourette's syndrome comorbidity have significantly more violent behavior, symmetrical obsessions, touching, counting, and self-harm. Patients with OCD only were more obsessed with dirt, germs, and cleanliness. The compulsions of patients with comorbidity arose spontaneously, whereas OCD patients' compulsions were preceded by cognitions (George et al. 1993).

Symptomatology.　Usually the onset of Tourette's syndrome is in childhood. It is initially manifested by facial tics such as blinking, squinting, grimacing, and twitching. At times, it begins with obsessive-compulsive symptoms. Unfortunately, because children engage in a normal amount of obsessive-compulsive behavior, it may go unnoticed.

With the disease's progression, the tics follow a cephalocaudal distribution, and movements of the neck, truck (especially the diaphragm), and extremities eventually appear. The tics wax and wane, cease during sleep and sexual activity, decrease when attention increases, and increase during viral or microbial infections or fever.

Tourette's syndrome presents both obsessive-compulsive and phobic symptomatology (Faux 1966; Milman 1975). In addition to this symptomatology, a significant degree of aggressive behavior has been noted (Ascher 1948; Borak and Osetowska 1976; de la Tourette 1885; Gonce and Barbeau 1977; Moldofsky et al. 1974; Seignot 1961; Shapiro and Shapiro 1974). Aggression has been reported in 40%–75% of patients with Tourette's syndrome (Van Woert et al. 1976; Yaryura-Tobias and Neziroglu 1977; Yaryura-Tobias et al. 1981). A similar incidence of aggression (65%) was found in a population of 100 true OCD patients (Yaryura-Tobias et al. 1980). In another study, a high incidence of depression, hostility, and obsessionality was reported, and aggression, hostility, and obsessionality were related (Robertson et al. 1988).

Hyperactive behavior should be investigated when Tourette's syndrome is suspected (Pushkov 1985). Our experience indicates that 25% of OCD patients present a history of hyperactivity. This finding is corroborated by observations indicating a high incidence of OCD and attention-deficit disorder with Tourette's syndrome (Como and Kurlan 1991).

A case of triple comorbidity involving schizophrenia, OCD, and Tourette's syndrome has been reported in a 26-year-old woman (Escobar and Bernardo 1993).

Epidemiology.   Sexual distribution indicates a male-to-female ratio of 3:1 (Challas and Braver 1967; Fernando 1967; Kelman 1965; Morphew and Sim 1969; Shapiro et al. 1978; Yaryura-Tobias and Neziroglu 1977). These findings are consistent with the normal sex distribution of childhood tics (Ford and Beyer 1974). In one study, the presence of tics in family members was reported in 10 of 15 patients (Moldofsky et al. 1974). Of 24 patients diagnosed with Tourette's syndrome, three had siblings with the same syndrome, and 31% of blood relatives manifested obsessive-compulsive symptoms, including Tourette's syndrome (Yaryura-Tobias and Neziroglu 1977).

Tourette's syndrome is apparently a genetic disorder with autosomal dominant transmission (Pauls and Leckman 1986; Taylor et al. 1991; van de Wetering and Heutink 1993). There is strong evidence that OCD also is familial (i.e., runs in the family but may be learned; not necessarily hereditary) and genetic (Pauls 1992; Pauls et al. 1986, 1991; Walkup et al. 1988).

Finally, it has been suggested that there may be genetic subtypes of OCD and agoraphobia with panic attacks as a result of partial expression of the Tourette's syndrome gene (Comings and Comings 1987).

Pathogenesis. It appears that Tourette's syndrome, like OCDs, may actually be a hyposerotonergic condition. With this in mind, we measured plasma free and total tryptophan, whole blood serotonin, and 24-hour urinary 5-hydroxyindoleacetic acid in 26 Tourette's syndrome patients and 13 control patients. Results indicated a trend toward lower values of serotonin in the patient population ($P < .10$) (Yaryura-Tobias et al. 1981).

Cohen et al. (1979) revealed a significant reduction in both homovanillic acid and 5-hydroxyindoleacetic acid metabolites in the cerebral spinal fluid of 10 Tourette's syndrome patients, suggesting a reduction in both dopamine and serotonin levels in Tourette's syndrome patients. Methoxyhydroxyphenylglycol, the primary metabolite of brain norepinephrine, was elevated in one severe case. This patient was treated with clonidine, a pharmacological agent that inhibits norepinephrine, primarily in the locus ceruleus, with remarkable efficacy. Clonidine also helped two other young boys with Tourette's syndrome. The fact that clonidine inhibits serotonergic nuclei in the midbrain raphe further implicates the role of serotonin in Tourette's syndrome.

Laboratory findings. Because Tourette's syndrome may present a history of hyperkinesia, impulsiveness, and incoordination, electroencephalograms have been studied. Nonspecific abnormal EEG patterns have been found in 33%–61% of the patients studied (Lucas and Rodin 1973; Shapiro et al. 1978; Yaryura-Tobias and Neziroglu 1977). When compared with control patients, which revealed that 5%–15% of the population has abnormal EEGs (Kiloh et al. 1972), Tourette's syndrome patients show at least two to six times as many EEG abnormalities. This high percentage of abnormal EEGs in Tourette's syndrome patients suggests an organic pathology in a great number of them.

In our investigation, computerized tomography scans were performed on 11 patients. Of these, two were abnormal. One showed an enlargement of the left lateral ventricle, the other, cortical atrophy (Yaryura-Tobias and Neziroglu 1977).

In 1970 Snyder et al. put forward a dopamine hypothesis. This hypothesis was followed by the studies of Meyerhoff and Snyder (1973), who suggested a norepinephrine theory, and Yaryura-Tobias (1975), who proposed a serotonergic hypothesis. Miller (1975) used chlorophenyl γ-aminobutyric acid to treat this syndrome. Preliminary reports indicated a decrease in tic symptomatology, but there have been no conclusive results.

Van Woert et al. (1976), based on the self-mutilative behavior of some patients, postulated an analogy with the Lesch-Nyhan syndrome, proposing a genetic disorder of purine metabolism. However, Moldofsky et al. (1974) measured the enzyme used for purine metabolism, hypoxanthine phosphoribosyltransferase, with negative results.

Evarts (1971) hypothesized that the psychomotor symptoms of Tourette's syndrome patients consist of two components also present in OCD: ideational and motor. Thus, the involuntary movement in Tourette's syndrome could be thought a priori, with its ideation becoming an urge to perform the movement. This theory further asserts that patients may think their movements first. Cerebral anatomical studies in Tourette's syndrome patients have not yielded specific and conclusive pathology (Balthasar 1957; Bing 1925; Bjarsch 1972; Dolmierski and Klossowna 1958; Fisarova and Kule 1967; Tabarka and Ticha 1975). The same could be said of the results of computerized tomography of the brain in 10 Tourette's syndrome patients (Yaryura-Tobias 1981) or the available electroencephalographic data. Another antidopaminergic agent, pimozide, has also been incorporated, with relative therapeutic efficacy, to treat Tourette's (Shapiro et al. 1989).

Obsessive-compulsive symptoms and the urge to make tic movements seem to place Tourette's syndrome within the group of OCDs. The extent to which OCD and Tourette's syndrome are associated requires further studies. One question is how to pharmacologically treat both OCD and Tourette's syndrome— as comorbid conditions or as a continuum (King et al. 1992)? There is a paucity of studies of the use of antiobsessional drugs in children and adolescents, the age group comprising the bulk of Tourette's syndrome patients.

Treatment.   Most psychological therapies have been used in attempts to treat Tourette's syndrome. In 1907 Meige and Feindel used a mirror to teach their patients to control tics; this approach resembles what is currently considered behavior therapy. Results of behavioral techniques have been equivocal (Browning and Stover 1971; Frederick 1971; Rosen and Wesner 1973; Sand and Carlson 1973; Thomas et al. 1971; Yates 1958, 1970). As the various psychotherapeutic techniques for controlling Tourette's syndrome failed, other treatment forms more closely related to a medical model were applied. These techniques span every facet of early 20th century medicine, with some of them—to our current knowledge—acting as a placebo.

With modern medicine and breakthroughs in drug therapy, new therapeutic modes became popular, among them phenothiazines (Eisenberg et al. 1959; Levy and Ascher 1968; Lucas 1964; Mesnikoff 1959; Polites et al. 1965). Currently the available Tourette's medications are haloperidol, clomipramine, fluoxetine, the selective serotonin reuptake inhibitors, clonidine, pimozide, and clonazepam.

Haloperidol, a butyrophenone with potent dopaminergic blocking activity, was used for the first time by Seignot (1961). Until quite recently, haloperidol was the preferred treatment (Abuzzahab and Anderson 1976; Shapiro et al. 1978; Tapia 1969). Tapia (1969) used haloperidol successfully on two girls with both tics and clear obsessive-compulsive symptoms. Tapia speculated that haloperidol seemed effective against the ruminative concern that brings tics, Tourette's syndrome, obsessive-compulsive thoughts, and perhaps forms of stuttering.

Haloperidol and phenothiazines may produce cognitive impairment in children with Tourette's syndrome, thereby creating a major treatment limitation. Symptoms such as decreased motivation, concentration, memory, and attention are common (Shapiro et al. 1978). Complete reversibility of these side effects occurs with decreased dosage or after discontinuation of the medication.

The efficacy of neuroleptics in Tourette's syndrome may come partly from neuromuscular side effects manifested during treatment. For instance, muscle rigidity may prevent Tourette's syndrome patients from performing body tics. This theory is supported by the relatively low effectiveness of haloperidol on coprolalia, obsessions, and tic compulsions. Prescribing antiparkinsonism medication to counteract the neurological side effects of neuroleptics may add to the preexistent pathology.

Based on the obsessive-compulsive nature of the illness, we used clomipramine in two patients (Yaryura-Tobias 1975) and later in 15 patients in a 6-month double-blind placebo-controlled study (Yaryura-Tobias and Neziroglu 1977). Clomipramine was administered in doses ranging from 25 to 350 mg (main dose = 133.33 mg). Results indicated that clomipramine reduced symptoms in 80% of patients. In other studies, three patients with Tourette's syndrome and obsessive-compulsive and phobic symptoms (Ciprian-Ollivier 1980) and one patient with OCD and Tourette's syndrome (Donahoe et al. 1991) responded to clomipramine therapy. In contrast, Caine et al. (1980) reported negative results using clomipramine or desipramine. In this study, the short term of each treatment (4 weeks) and the lower daily medication dosage (up to 150 mg) may explain the disparity.

A trial of fluoxetine (Como and Kurlan 1991) and a trial of fluvoxamine and pimozide (Delgado et al. 1990) yielded favorable results.

Knowledge of the efficacy of selective serotonin reuptake inhibitors is limited by the small number of trials and participants.

Clonidine has been used as a substitute for neuroleptics to avoid side effects. Its efficacy was not superior to that of neuroleptics (Erenberg 1988) but was better than placebo (Leckman et al. 1991) and produced improvement in patients previously treated with haloperidol (Cohen et al. 1980).

The use of benzodiazepines for treatment of Tourette's syndrome has been sparse, and results have been inconclusive (Hewlett 1993). Another benzodiazepine, clonazepam, has been reported to partially relieve Tourette's symptoms (Gonce and Barbeau 1977).

Secondary symptoms, such as aggression and self-harm, should be addressed. The administration of L-5-hydroxytryptophan combined with carbidopa was successful in one Tourette's syndrome patient who had self-induced abrasions of the oral mucosa, guttural utterances, and jerks (Van Woert et al. 1977).

The risks of side effects should be evaluated before neuroleptic drugs are prescribed. The main side effects are extrapyramidal symptoms, abnormal movements, anticholinergic symptoms, disorder of the appetite, cognitive impairment, depression, and fears leading to phobic behaviors. The use of medication in children should be carefully considered and closely monitored (Cohen et al. 1992).

Conclusion

So far, evidence indicates that Tourette's syndrome has psychiatric and neurological symptoms that overlap with those seen in other syndromes that may be similar in their clinical characteristics. For example, involuntary movements in general belong to many clinical entities, but tics belong to fewer clinical entities. Thus, narrowing down the possible differential diagnoses facilitates proper diagnosis. Differential diagnosis should include chorea, transient tics of childhood, and other syndromes with voluntary movements where the incipient symptomatology may not allow for gross diagnosis. Essential diagnostic symptoms of Tourette's syndrome ought to include coprolalia, imitative phenomena, compulsive symptomatology, and aggressive behavior.

References

Abuzzahab FS, Anderson FO (eds): Gilles de la Tourette's syndrome: International Registry, Vol 1. St Paul, MN, Mason Publishing, 1976

Achte KA: On compulsive neuroses of brain injured. Acta Psychiatr Neurol Scand 1:88–89, 1958

Allert ML, Meyer JR: Anankastisches Syndrom als Encephalitis. Nervenarzt 29: 116–120, 1958

Anastassopoulos G, Kokkini D: Suicidal attempts in psychomotor epilepsy. Behav Neuropsychiatry 1:11–20, 1969

Anden NE, Carlsson A, Kerstell J, et al: Oral L-dopa treatment of parkinsonism. Acta Med Scand 187:247–255, 1970

Ascher E: Psychodynamic considerations in Gilles de la Tourette's disease. Am J Psychiatry 105:267–276, 1948

Balthasar J: Uber das Anatomische Substrat der Generalisierten Tic Krankheit (maladie des tics, Gilles de la Tourette). Arch Psychiatr Nervenkr 195: 531–549, 1957

Beard GM: Experiments with the jumpers of jumping Frenchmen of Maine. J Nerv Ment Dis 7:487–490, 1878

Beckson M, Cummings JL: Neuropsychiatric aspects of stroke. International Journal of Psychiatry In Medicine 21:1–15, 1991

Bihari K, Pigott TA, Hill JL, et al: Blepharospasm and obsessive-compulsive disorder. J Nerv Ment Dis 180:130–132, 1992a

Bihari K, Pigott TA, Hill JL: Obsessive-compulsive characteristics in patients with idiopathic spasmodic torticollis. Psychiatry Res 42:267–272, 1992b

Bing R: Uber lokale muskelspasmen und Tics. Schweiz Med Wochenschr 55: 993–1000, 1925

Bjarsch H: Beitrag zur Problematik der Touretteschen Krankheit. Nervenarzt 43: 94–97, 1972

Borak W, Osetowska E: Gilles de la Tourette's disease with congenital vascular malformation and secondary encephalopathy, in Gilles de la Tourette's Syndrome: International Registry, Vol 1. Edited by Abuzzahab FS, Anderson FO. St Paul, MN, Mason Publishing, 1976, pp 81–87

Bouteille EM: Traite des Chorees. Paris, Vincard, 1810

Brain WR, Greenfield JB, Russell DS: Discussion on recent experiences of acute encephalomyelitis and allied conditions. Proc R Soc Med 36:319–327, 1943

Browning RM, Stover DO: Behavior Modification in Child Treatment. Chicago, IL, Aldine-Atherton, 1971

Burger H, Mayer-Gross W: Uber Zwangssymptome Encephalitis Lethargica und uber die Struktur der Zwangserscheinungen Uberhaupt. Zeitschrift für die Gesamte Zeitschrift der Neurologie und Psychiatrie 116:645–686, 1928

Cabaleiro Goas M: El sindrome obsesivo de etiologia epileptica en ninos y pre-adolescentes. Arch Neurobiol (Madr) 32:521–534, 1969

Cabaleiro Goas M, Perez Villamil J: Las Obsesiones y las Fobias, in Temas Psiquiatricos. Madrid, Paz Montalvo, 1966

Caine ED, Polinsky RJ, Ebert MH, et al: Trial of chlorimipramine and desipramine for Gilles de la Tourette syndrome. Ann Neurol 5:305–306, 1979

Cath DC, Hoogduin CA, van de Wetering BJ: Tourette syndrome and obsessive-compulsive disorder. Adv Neurol 58:33–41, 1992

Challas G, Braver W: Tourette's disease: relief of symptoms with R1625. Am J Psychiatry 120:283–284, 1967

Chlopicki W: Uber Anfallweise Auftretende Zwangserscheinungen im Verlaufe von Parkinson Nach Epidemic Encephalitis. Archiven Fortschrifte der Psychiatrie 93:1–27, 1931

Ciani N, Vella G: Epilepsia ed obsessioni. Quaderro di Chirurgia 8:6–10, 1965

Ciprian-Ollivier J: Three cases of Gilles de la Tourette's syndrome. Treatment with chlorimipramine: a preliminary report. Journal of the Academy of Orthomolecular Psychiatry 9:116–120, 1980

Cohen DJ, Shaywitz BA, Young JG, et al: Central biogenic amine metabolism in children with the syndrome of chronic multiple tics of Gilles de la Tourette. Norepinephrine, serotonin, and dopamine. J Am Acad Child Psychiatry 18: 320–341, 1979

Cohen DJ, Detlor J, Young JG, et al: Clonidine ameliorates Gilles de la Tourette syndrome. Arch Gen Psychiatry 37:1350–1357, 1980

Cohen DJ, Riddle MA, Leckman JF: Pharmacotherapy of Tourette's syndrome and associated disorders. Psychiatr Clin North Am 15:109–129, 1992

Comings DE, Comings BG: Hereditary agoraphobia and obsessive-compulsive behaviour in relatives of patients with Gilles de la Tourette's syndrome. Br J Psychiatry 151:195–199, 1987

Como PG, Kurlan R: An open-label trial of fluoxetine for obsessive-compulsive disorder in Gilles de la Tourette's syndrome. Neurology 41:872–874, 1991

Conde López V, de la Gándara Martín JJ, Blanco Lozano ML, et al: Minor neurological signs in obsessive-compulsive disorders (in Spanish). Actas Luso Esp Neurol Psiquiatr Cienc Afines 18:143–164, 1990

Corsellis JAN: Subacute sclerosing leuco-encephalitis: a clinical and pathological report of two cases. Journal of Mental Science 97:570–583, 1951

Creak M, Guttmann E: Chorea, tics and compulsive utterances. Journal of Mental Science 81:834–839, 1935

Crichton-Browne J: Dreamers and mental states. Lancet 2:1–3, 1895

Croisile B, Tournaire C, Confavreux C, et al: Bilateral damage to the head of the caudate nuclei. Ann Neurol 25:313–314, 1989

Cummings JL, Cunningham K: Obsessive-compulsive disorder in Huntington's disease. Biol Psychiatry 31:263–270, 1992

Damjanovic A, Kostic VS, Sternic N: Gilles de la Tourette's syndrome. Srp Arh Celok Lek 120:197–202, 1992

Dawson JR: Cellular inclusions in cerebral lesions of lethargic encephalitis. Am J Pathol 9:7–15, 1933

Dawson JR: Cellular inclusions in cerebral lesions of epidemic encephalitis. Archives of Neurology and Psychiatry (Chicago) 31:685, 1934 de Boor W: Die Lehre von Zwang Sammelbericht uber die Jahre 1918 bis 1947. Fortschr Neurol 17:49–85, 1949

de la Tourette G: Etude d'une affection nerveuse caracterisee par de l'incoordination motrice accompagnee de coprolalie. Arch Neurologiques Paris 9: 19–42, 1885

Delgado PL, Goodman WK, Price LH, et al: Fluvoxamine/pimozide treatment of concurrent Tourette's and obsessive-compulsive disorder. Br J Psychiatry 157:762–765, 1990

Denny-Brown D: The sequelae of war head injuries. N Engl J Med 227:771–780, 1942a

Denny-Brown D: The sequelae of war head injuries (concluded). N Engl J Med 227:813–821, 1942b

Dolmierski R, Klossowna M: O Chorobie Gilles de la Tourette's. Neurol Neurochir Psychiatr Pol 8:639–646, 1958

Donahoe DH, Meador M, Fortune T, et al: Tourette's syndrome and treatment with clomipramine hydrochloride. West Virginia Medical Journal 87:468–470, 1991

Dongier M: Statistical study of clinical and electroencephalographic manifestations of 536 psychotic episodes occurring in 516 epileptics between clinical seizures. Epilepsia (Amsterdam) 1:117–142, 1960

Eisenberg L, Ascher E, Kanner L: A clinical study of Gilles de la Tourette's disease (maladie des tics) in children. Am J Psychiatry 115:715–723, 1959

Erenberg G: Pharmacologic therapy of tics in childhood. Psychiatric Annals 18: 399–408, 1988

Escobar R, Bernardo M: Schizophrenia, obsessive-compulsive disorder, and Tourette's syndrome: a case of triple comorbidity (letter). J Neuropsychiatr Clin Neurosci 5:108, 1993

Esser PH: Die Epileptiformen Anfalle der Schizophrenen und die' Differential diagnostichen Schwierigkeiten im Grenzgebiet von Epilepsie und Schizophrenie. Zbl ges Nevrol Psychiat 16:1–24, 1938

Evarts EV: Activity of thalamic and cortical neurons in relation to learned movement in the monkey. Int J Neurol 8:321–326, 1971

Ewald G: Schanuanfaelle als Postenzephalitische Stoerungen. Schrift fur Psychiatrie und Neurologie 57:222–224, 1924

Falkeiwicz T, Rothfeld T: Uber Zwangsbewegungen und Zwangschauen bei Epidemic Encephalitis. Deuzsche Zeitschrift fur Nervenkrankheit 85:269–281, 1925

Faux EJ: Gilles de la Tourette's syndrome. Arch Gen Psychiatry 14:139–142, 1966

Fernando SJM: Gilles de la Tourette's syndrome. Br J Psychiatry 113:607–617, 1967

Fisarova M, Kule J: Syndrom Gilles de la Tourette. Ceskolovenská Psychiatrie 63: 231–235, 1967

Flacha A, Palisa G: Zur Psychopathologie des Zeiterlebens im Postencephalitic Bickkrampf. Z Ges Neurol Psychiat 154:599–620, 1936

Flor-Henry P: Ictal and interictal psychiatric manifestations in epilepsy, specific or non-specific. A critical review of some of the evidence. Epilepsia 13:773–783, 1972

Follin S: Epilepsies et Psychoses Discordantes. Paris, France, Université de Paris Ecole de Medicine, Thesis, 1941

Ford RB, Beyer EC: Tic de Gilles de la Tourette: case report and brief discussion. J S C Med Assoc 70:1–3, 1974

Frankel M, Cummings JL, Robertson MM, et al: Obsessions and compulsions in Gilles de la Tourette's syndrome. Neurology 36:378–382, 1986

Frederick CJ: Treatment of a tic by systematic desensitization and massed response evocation. J Behav Ther Exper Psychiatry 2:281–283, 1971

Fuchs A: Schwere Progressive Anankastische Entwicklung bei einen Falle von Genuiner Epilepsie. Arch Psychiatr Nervenkr 80:586–698, 1927

Gadelius B: Om Tvangstankar. Stockholm, Uppsalla, 1896, p. I. Cited in Skoog G. Acta Psychiatr Scand Suppl 134, 1959

Garmany G: Les etats obsessionales chez les epileptics (obsessional states in epileptics). Journal of Mental Science 93:639–643, 1947

Gaston A, Reda GC, Ciani N: Le obsessione nella patologia cerebrale. Neuro-psichiatria (Genova) 23:669–680, 1967

George MS, Trimble MR, Ring HA, et al: Obsessions in obsessive-compulsive disorder with and without Gilles de la Tourette's syndrome. Am J Psychiatry 150: 93–97, 1993

Glaser GH, Solitaire GE, Manuelidis EE: Limbic epilepsy in childhood. J Nerv Ment Dis 144:391–397, 1968

Goldflam S: Die Grosse Encephalitisepidemie des Jahres, 1920. Dtsch Z Nervenheilkd 73:1–7, 1922

Goldman S, Amrom D, Szliwowski HB: Reversible striatal hypermetabolism in a case of Sydenham's chorea. Mov Disord 8:365–368, 1993

Goldstein K: La Structure de l'Organism. Paris, Gallimard, 1951

Gonce M, Barbeau A: Seven cases of Gilles de la Tourette's syndrome: partial relief with clonazepam: a pilot study. Can J Neurol Sci 4:279–283, 1977

Gostling JVT: Herpetic encephalitis. Proc R Soc Med 60:693–696, 1967

Guinon: Sur la maladie des tics convulsifs. Revue de Medicine 1:50–80, 1886

Hammond WA: Myriachit, a newly described disease of the nervous system and its analogues. BMJ 2:758–759, 1884

Harris JS, Cooper HA: Late results of encephalitis lethargica. Med Press 194: 12–14, 1937

Hendricks I: Encephalitis lethargica and the interpretation of mental disease. Am J Psychiatry 7:989–1014, 1927

Hermann G: Zwangsmaessiges Denken u andere Zwangserscheinungen bie Erkrankungen des Striaren Systems. Monatschrift fur Psychiatrie and Neurologie 52:324–330, 1922

Hewlett WA: The use of benzodiazepines in obsessive compulsive disorder and Tourette's syndrome. Psychiatric Annals 23:309–316, 1993

Hill D: Psychiatric disorders of epilepsy. Med Press 229:473–475, 1953

Hillbom E: After-effects of brain injuries. Acta Psychiatr Neurol Scand Suppl 142: 1–195, 1960

Himmelhoch J, Pincus J, Tucker G, et al: Subacute encephalitis: behavioural and neurological aspects. Br J Psychiatry 116:531–538, 1970

Hohman L: Forced conjugate upward movements of the eyes in postencephalitic Parkinson's syndrome. JAMA 84:1489–1490, 1925

Hollander E, Liebowitz MR, DeCaria CM: Conceptual and methodological issues in studies of obsessive-compulsive and Tourette's disorders. Psychiatric Developments 7:267–296, 1989

Hollander E, Schiffman E, Cohen B, et al: Signs of central nervous system dysfunction in obsessive-compulsive disorder. Arch Gen Psychiatry 47:27–32, 1990

Hundert EM: Philosophy, Psychiatry and Neuroscience. Three Approaches to the Mind. New York, Oxford Press, 1990

Ingram IM: The EEG, obsessive illness and obsessive personality. Journal of Mental Science 106:686–691, 1960

Itard JMG: Memoire sur quelques fonctions involontaires des appareils de la locomotion, de la prehension et de la voix. Arch Gen Med 8:385–407, 1825

Jahrreiss W: Uber einen Fall von Chronischer Systematische Zwangserkrankung. Arch Psychiatr Nervenkr 77:596–612, 1926

Jelliffe ES: Psychopathology of forced movements in oculogyric crises. Journal of Nervous and Mental Disease Monograph Series 55:1–210, 1932

Kelman DH: Gilles de la Tourette's disease in children. A review of the literature. J Child Psychol Psychiatry 6:219–226, 1965

Kettl PA, Marks IM: Neurological factors in obsessive-compulsive disorder. Two case reports and a review of the literature. Br J Psychiatry 1–49, 315–319, 1986

Kienzle JD, Breger RK, Chun RW, et al: Sydenham's MR manifestations in two cases. American Journal of Neuroradiology 12:73–76, 1991

Kiloh LG, McComas AJ, Osselton JW: Clinical Electroencephalography, 3rd Edition. New York, Appleton, Century & Crofts, 1972

King RA, Riddle MA, Goodman WK: Psychopharmacology of obsessive-compulsive disorder. Adv Neurol 58:283–291, 1992

Kligman D, Goldberg DA: Temporal lobe epilepsy and aggression. J Nerv Ment Dis 160:324–341, 1975

Lambertet P, Midenet P, Midenet J, et al: Traitement par la thioproperazine a haute dose de manifestations pseudo-obsessived d'origine encephalitique. J Med Lyon 47:1219–1224, 1966

Leckman JF, Chittenden EH: Gilles de La Tourette's syndrome and some forms of obsessive-compulsive disorder may share a common genetic diathesis. Encephale 16:321–323, 1990

Leckman JF, Hardin MT, Riddle MA, et al: Clonidine treatment of Gilles de la Tourette's syndrome. Arch Gen Psychiatry 48:324–328, 1991

Lees AJ: The neurobehavioral abnormalities in Parkinson's disease and their relationship to psychomotor retardation and obsessive-compulsive disorders. Behavioral Neurology 2:1–11, 1989

Leonard HL, Lenane MC, Swedo SE, et al: Tics and Tourette's disorder: a 2–7 year follow-up of 54 obsessive-compulsive children. Am J Psychiatry 149:1244–1251, 1992

Levy BS, Ascher E: Phenothiazines in the treatment of Gilles de la Tourette's disease. J Nerv Ment Dis 146:36–40, 1968

Lishman WA: Brain damage in relation to psychiatric disability after head injury. Br J Psychiatry 114:373–410, 1968

Lucas AR: Gilles de la Tourette's disease in children: treatment with phenothiazine drugs. Am J Psychiatry 124:146–149, 1964

Lucas AR, Rodin EA: The EEG in Gilles de la Tourette's disease. Dis Nerv Syst 34:85–89, 1973

Majluf E: Síntomas obsesivos-compulsivos y epilepsia en la infancia. A próposito de un caso clínico. Rev Neuropsiquiatr 14:415–426, 1951

Malamud N, Haymaker W, Pinkerton H: Inclusion encephalitis with a clinicopathological report of three cases. Am J Pathol 26:133–144, 1950

Mapother E: Mental symptoms associated with head injury. The psychiatric aspect. BMJ 2:1055–1061, 1937

Mayer-Gross W, Steiner G: Encephalitis lethargica in der Selbstbeobachtung. Z Neurol 73:283–286, 1921

McKeon JP, McGuffin P, Robinson PH: Obsessive-compulsive neurosis following head injury: a report of four cases. Br J Psychiatry 144:190–192, 1984

Meige H, Feindel E: Tics and Their Treatment. Translated and edited by Wilson SAK. New York, William Wood, 1907

Mesnikoff AM: Three cases of Gilles de la Tourette's syndrome treated with psychotherapy and chlorpromazine. Archives of Neurology (Chicago) 81:710–716, 1959

Meyerhoff JL, Snyder SH: Gilles de la Tourette's disease and minimal brain dysfunction: amphetamine isomers reveal catecholamine correlates in an affected patient. Psychopharmocology 29:211–220, 1973

Miller E: Gilles de la Tourette's syndrome. Workshop presented by the Society for Biological Psychiatry, New York, October 1975

Milman D: Gilles de la Tourette's syndrome. NY State J Med 75:892–895, 1975

Minski L: The mental symptom associated with 58 cases of cerebral tumors. Journal of Neurology and Psychopathology 13, 1933

Moldofsky H, Tullis C, Lamon R: Multiple tic syndrome (GIT). Clinical, biological, and psychosocial variables and their influence with haloperidol. J Nerv Ment Dis 15:282–292, 1974

Morphew JA, Sim M: Gilles de la Tourette's syndrome: a clinical and psychopathological study. Br J Med Psychol 42:293–301, 1969

Mulder DW, Daly D: Psychiatric symptoms associated with lesions of temporal lobe. JAMA 150:173–176, 1952

Oesterreich TK: Possession and Exorcism. New York, Causeway Books, 1974

Osler W: On Chorea and Coreiform Affections. Philadelphia, PA, Blakiston, 1894

Pacella B: Clinical and electroencephalographic studies of obsessive-compulsive states. Am J Psychiatry 100:830–838, 1944

Paradis CM, Freidman S, Hatch M, et al: Obsessive-compulsive disorder onset after removal of a brain tumor. J Nerv Ment Dis 180:535–536, 1992

Parkinson J: An Essay on the Shaking Palsy. London, Sherwood, Neely & Jones, 1817

Parsons OA: Human neuropsychology: the new phrenology. Journal of Operational Psychiatry 8:47–56, 1977

Pauls DL: The genetics of obsessive compulsive disorder and Gilles de la Tourette's syndrome. Psychiatr Clin North Am 15:759–766, 1992

Pauls DL, Leckman JF: The inheritance of Gilles de la Tourette's syndrome and associated behaviors. Evidence for autosomal dominant transmission. N Engl J Med 315:993–997, 1986

Pauls DL, Towbin KE, Leckman JF, et al: Gilles de la Tourette's syndrome and obsessive-compulsive disorder. Arch Gen Psychiatry 43:1180–1182, 1986

Pauls DL, Raymond CL, Stevenson JM, et al: A family study of Gilles de la Tourette syndrome. Am J Hum Genet 48:154–163, 1991

Pitman RK, Green RC, Jenike MA, et al: Clinical comparison of Tourette's disorder and obsessive-compulsive disorder. Am J Psychiatry 144:1166–1171, 1987

Polites DJ, Kruger D, Stevenson I: Sequential treatment in a case of Gilles de la Tourette's syndrome. Br J Med Psychiat 38:43–52, 1965

Pond DA: Psychiatric aspects of epilepsy. J Indian Med Prof 3:1441–1451, 1957

Pushkov VV: Differential diagnostic criteria of childhood diseases accompanied by hyperkinesias (in Russian). Zh Nevropatol Psikhiatr Imi S S Korsakova 85: 409–415, 1985

Reda GC: Nosografia della psiconevrosi ossessiva. Lavoro Neuropsichiatrico 39: 213–220, 1966

Robertson MM, Trimble MR, Lees AJ: The psychopathology of the Gilles de la Tourette syndrome. A phenomenological analysis. Br J Psychiatry 152:383–390, 1988

Rockwell J, Simons DJ: The EEG and personality organization in the obsessive-compulsive reactions. Archives of Neurology and Psychiatry 57:71–77, 1947

Rojo Sierra M: El Tipo Clínico Obsesivo. Valencia, Spain, Apuntes de Catedra, 1970

Rosen M, Wesner C: A behavioral approach to Tourette's syndrome. J Consult Clin Psychol 41:308–312, 1973

Roubicek J: Laughter in epilepsy with some general introductory notes. Journal of Mental Science 92:734–755, 1946

Sacks O: Awakenings. Paper presented at the meeting of the American Psychiatric Association, Toronto, May 1977

Sanchez Planell L: Sindromes obsesivoides en neurología. In Patología Obsesiva. Edited by Monserrat-Esteve S, Costa Molinari JM, Ballús C. Málaga, Spain, Graficasa, 1971, pp 341–361

Sand PL, Carlson C: Failure to establish control over tics in the Gilles de la Tourette syndrome with behaviour therapy techniques. Br J Psychiatry 122:665–670, 1973

Sarro R: Recuerdos obsesivos durante las crisis oculogiras. Analogias con el onirismo. Mundo Medico 14:568–569, 1932

Schilder P: The organic background of obsessions and compulsions. Am J Psychiatry 94:1397–1416, 1938

Schwab RS, Fabing HD, Pritchard JS: Psychiatric symptoms and syndromes in Parkinson's disease. Am J Psychiatry 107:901–907, 1951

Seignot JN: Un cas de maladie des tics de Gilles de la Tourette queri par le R-1625. Ann Med Psychol (Paris) 119:578–579, 1961

Seva Diaz A: Investigaciones en torno al fenómeno obsesivo. Actas Luso Españolas neurobilogía y Psiquitría 23:260–271, 1964

Shapiro AK, Shapiro E: Evaluation of the reported association of obsessive-compulsive symptoms or disorder with Tourette's disorder. Compr Psychiatry 33: 152–165, 1992

Shapiro AK, Shapiro ES: Gilles de la Tourette's syndrome. Am Fam Physician 9: 94–96, 1974

Shapiro AK, Shapiro ES, Brunn RD, et al: Gilles de la Tourette's Syndrome. New York, Raven, 1978

Shapiro E, Shapiro AK, Fulop G, Hubbard M, Mandeli J, Nordile J, Phillips RA: Controlled study of haloperidol, pimozide and placebo for the treatment of Gilles de la Tourette's syndrome. Arch Gen Psychiatry 46:722–730, 1989

Shulze A, Stephan P: Psychopathologic symptoms in torticollis spasmodi. Psychiatr Neurol Med Psychol (Leipz) 12:735–743, 1987

Singer HS, Walkup JT: Tourette syndrome and other tic disorders: diagnosis, pathophysiology, and treatment. Medicine 70:15–32, 1991

Skoog G: The anancastic syndrome and its relation to personality attitudes. Acta Psychiatr Scand 134:205–207, 1959

Slater E, Roth M: Clinical Psychiatry. London, Bailliere, Tindall, & Cassell, 1972

Snyder SH, Taylor KM, Cayle JT, et al: The role of brain dopamine in behavioral regulation and the actions of psychotropic drugs. Am J Psychiatry 127:199–207, 1970

Sprenger J, Kramer H: Malleus Malleficarum, 1486. Spanish translation. Buenos Aires, Argentina, Ediciones Oriam, 1975

Steiner G: Von Zwangerscheunungen bei Organischen Nervenkrank. Zeitschrift der Gesellschaft der Neurologie und Psychiatrie 128:515–527, 1930

Steingard R, Dillon-Stout D: Tourette's syndrome and obsessive-compulsive disorder: clinical aspects. Psychiatr Clin North Am 15:849–860, 1992

Stengel E: Zur Kenntnis der Beziehungen zwischen Zwangsneur und Paranoia. Archiven fur Psychiatrie 95:8–23, 1931

Stern F: Ubur Psychische Zwangsvorgange und ihre Entstehung bei Encephalitischen. Blickkrampfen mit Bemerkungen uber die Genese der Encephalitischen Blickkrampfe. Arch Psychiatr Nervenkr 81:522–560, 1927

Storring GE: Uber Zwangsdeken Blickrampfen. Arch Psychiatr Nervenkr 89:836–840, 1930

Swedo SE, Rapoport JL, Cheslow DL, et al: High prevalence of obsessive-compulsive symptoms in patients with Sydenham's chorea. Am J Psychiatry 146:246–249, 1989

Swedo SE, Leonard HL, Schapiro MB, et al: Sydenham's chorea: physical and psychological symptoms of St Vidus dance. Pediatrics 91:706–713, 1993

Tabarka K, Ticha M: Prispevek K Psychopatologii Morbus Gilles de la Tourette (A contribution to the psychopathology of Morbus Gilles de la Tourette). Cesk Psychiatr 71:234–238, 1975

Tapia F: Haldol in the treatment of children with tics and stutters, and an incidental finding. Psychiat Q 43:647–649, 1969

Taylor LD, Krizman DB, Jankovic J, et al: 9p monosomy in a patient with Gilles de la Tourette's syndrome. Neurology 42:1513–1515, 1991

Thomas EJ, Abrams KS, Johnson JB: Self-monitoring and reciprocal inhibition in the modification of multiple tics of Gilles de la Tourette. Am J Dis Child 101:778–783, 1971

Trousseau A: Des diverses espèces de chorée. Clinique Medical de l'Hotel-Dieu. 2:264–271, 1873

Turner WA: Epilepsy—A Study of the Idiopathic Disease. London, Macmillan, 1907

Van Bogaert L: A case of subacute sclerotic leucoencephalitis. Journal of Neurology and Psychiatry 8:101–120, 1945

van de Wetering BJ, Heutink P: The genetics of the Gilles de la Tourette syndrome: a review. J Lab Clin Med 121:638–645, 1993

Van Woert MH, Jutowitz R, Rosenbaum D, et al: Gilles de la Tourette's syndrome: biochemical approaches, in The Basal Ganglia. Edited by Yahr MD. New York, Raven, 1976, pp 459–465

Van Woert MH, Yip LC, Balis ME: Purine phosphoribosyl-transferase in Gilles de la Tourette syndrome. N Engl J Med 296:210–212, 1977

von Economo C: Encephalitis Lethargica: Its Sequelae and Treatment. London, KO Newman, 1931

Walkup JT, Leckman JF, Price A, et al: The relationship between obsessive-compulsive disorder and Tourette's Syndrome: a twin study. Psychopharmacol Bull 24:375–379, 1988

Ward CD: Encephalitis lethargica and the development of neuropsychiatry. Psychiatr Clin North Am 9:215–224, 1986

Ward CD: Transient feelings of compulsion caused by hemispheric lesions: three cases. J Neurol Neurosurg Psychiatry 51:266–268, 1988

Waxman SG, Geschwind N: Hypergraphia in temporal lobe epilepsy. Neurology 24:629–636, 1974

Yaryura-Tobias JA: Chlorimipramine in Gilles de la Tourette's disease. Am J Psychiatry 132:1221–1225, 1975

Yaryura-Tobias JA: Clinical and laboratory data on Tourette syndrome. Paper presented at the First International Gilles de la Tourette Syndrome Symposium, New York, May 27–29, 1981

Yaryura-Tobias JA, Neziroglu F: Gilles de la Tourette syndrome: a new clinico-therapeutic approach. Prog Neuropsychopharmacol 1:335–338, 1977

Yaryura-Tobias JA, Neziroglu F: Obsessive Compulsive Disorders: Pathogenesis, Diagnosis, and Treatment. New York, Marcel Dekker, 1983

Yaryura-Tobias JA, Neziroglu FA: Organicity in obsessive-compulsive disorder, in Biological Psychiatry, Vol 29. Edited by Racagni G. Amsterdam, The Netherlands, Elsevier, 1991, pp 337S

Yaryura-Tobias JA, Diamond B, Merlis S: Psychiatric manifestations of levodopa. Can Psychiatr Assoc J 17:123–128, 1972

Yaryura-Tobias JA, Neziroglu F, Fuller B: An integral approach in the management of the obsessive-compulsive patient. Pharmaceutical Medicine 1:155–167, 1980

Yaryura-Tobias JA, Neziroglu F, Howard S, et al: Clinical aspects of Gilles de la Tourette syndrome. Journal of Orthomolecular Psychiatry 10:263–268, 1981

Yates AJ: The application of learning theory to the treatment of tics. Journal of Abnormal Social Psychology 56:175–182, 1958

Yates AJ: Tics, in Symptoms of Psychopathology. Edited by Costello C. New York, Wiley, 1970

Yde A, Edel L, Faurbye A: On relation between schizophrenia, epilepsy, and induced convulsions. Acta Psychiatr Scand (Kobenhavn) 16:325–388, 1941

Section III

Research Issues

Section III reviews theoretical concepts, models, and empirical findings pertaining to the current direction of the investigation of obsessive-compulsive disorder (OCD).

One fundamental aspect is to study OCD and its spectrum and its association with other disorders. This study will assist in investigating pathological mechanisms and treatment choices.

Another area to discuss is neurobiological development including neuron plasticity and brain anatomy. This approach becomes helpful in understanding the natural course of OCD. A new pathophysiological dimension surfaces with the discovery of novel receptors and subreceptors, the application of biological challenges, the observation of anatomical findings, and the evaluation of cerebral metabolism related to OCD.

Finally, neuroendocrine and nutritional studies introduce a new avenue of research to further integrate the entire OCD biopsychosocial spectrum.

Chapter 13
Clinical and Experimental Research

Current obsessive-compulsive disorder (OCD) research focuses on anatomical, behavioral, phenomenological, pharmacological, neuropsycho-surgical, and biochemical aspects of the disorder. This approach is constructed around atomistic or particular areas of OCD. Although certain questions have been answered, our knowledge of OCD as a whole remains limited.

Gradually, OCD research is moving toward an integrative approach that allows researchers working on the different aspects of OCD to share their knowledge. These researchers study the biological, psychological, and social parameters that theoretically influence OCD's pathophysiology as it is currently known.

Comorbidity and Related Disorders

OCD is an experiential activity of human thought and behavior. It encompasses thought, movement, affect, volition, and somatosensory activity. The presence of OCD is indicated by numerous symptoms constituting a large pathological mosaic. This protean symptomatology may have its seat in the brain, accepting a priori that OCD is primarily housed in the brain. Because the brain is a complex organ with billions of cells and nerve fibers, we doubt the existence of a well-defined OCD territory. There are three reasons for our doubt: 1) the presence of symptoms associated with different brain activities, 2) the brain's interconnectedness, and 3) the possibility that different illnesses, such as OCD, are the manifestation of just one master illness.

First, we will focus on the concept that OCD is really several diseases and then on the one-disease theory. It is more admissible to entertain the idea of physiological sharing through histochemical "highways" that distribute and associate stimuli and regions, respectively. This activity generates different diseases that might overlap clinically or pathologically. The cerebral territory becomes essential to interpret OCD mechanisms and the disorder's anatomical correlates. Therefore, it is feasible to admit the concomitant or sequential presence of other disorders that seem to share part of the same territory.

With the addition of new processes, novel pathology is introduced; this pathology is blended, interconnected, or imbricated at different neurobiological levels with OCD. This transnosological approach may show emerging symptoms with an innovative perspective. This new-old concept can be traced back to the work of various neuropsychiatric investigators interested in the OCD equation. This concept posited that OCD was a disturbance sometimes associated with other clinical conditions such as major depression or schizophrenia. According to Prat et al.'s review (1971), investigators researching OCD nosology used the terms *obsesoid, obsessive-form, obsessionality,* and *pseudo-obsessions* to indicate the presence of obsessions grafted onto other clinical entities. Others have looked into the association between OCD and neurological syndromes such as encephalitis, extrapyramidalism, injured brain, chorea, Tourette's syndrome, tics, and epilepsy. In conclusion, Sanchez Planell (1971) did a review of the work of several researchers who propose that OCD is a secondary neurological disorder.

We approach OCD as a protean syndrome with symptomatology that overlaps with other conditions. Awareness of symptom imbrication helps refine the diagnosis and improves treatment modalities and outcome. Consequently, we classify OCD from a nosological perspective as primary OCD and related disorders (Yaryura-Tobias and Neziroglu 1983).

When OCD includes only those symptoms that are pathognomonic for the disorder, we call it a primary illness (i.e., primary OCD). When OCD encompasses symptoms of other diseases intertwined with symptoms of the primary disorder, we speak of a clinical spectrum including comorbidity, a nosological continuum, and related disorders. When several illnesses appear at the same time, the patient is said to have comorbidity or "parallel emergents." When these illnesses share symptoms in different degrees of intensity and frequency, the patient is said to have related disorders. When these disorders surface in chronological order to graft themselves onto the primary illness, the condition is called a nosological continuum. Because of our inability to determine onset time, we use, indistinctly, the words spectrum and comorbidity in this chapter (see Figure 13–1).

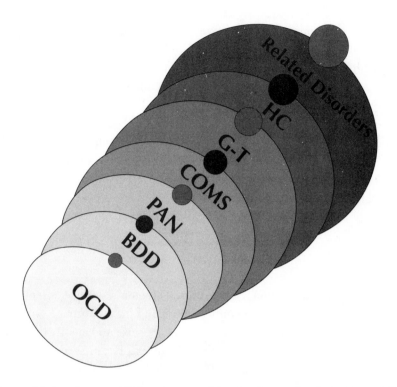

Figure 13–1. Spectrum of obsessive-compulsive disorder (ripple effect). *Note.*   OCD = obsessive-compulsive disorder. BDD = body dysmorphic disorder. PAN = panic disorder. COMS = compulsive-orectic-mutilative syndrome. HC = hypochondriasis. G-T =Gilles de la Tourette's syndrome.

Recent studies reported the presence of comorbidity in Axis I and Axis II disorders. Most studies reported at least a 50% rate of comorbid Axis I disorders (Hollander et al. 1992; Karno et al. 1988; Pigott et al. 1994; Rasmussen and Eisen 1992). Most patients with OCD meet the criteria for at least one Axis II personality disorder (Baer et al. 1992; Mavissakalian et al. 1990; McKay et al. 1996; Steketee 1990).

Comorbidity requires considerable epidemiological, semiological, and pathophysiological sameness, conducive to explaining why two or more conditions become comorbid.

Indirectly, comorbidity points toward the one-mental-illness theory of Griesinger (1867/1965). This theory postulates pathophysiological facts showing the brain as the seat of mental illness. Griesinger's concepts have a functional basis, stating cerebral ocular inspection is negative. This theory, advanced for its time, should be revisited in the light of new findings in cerebral pathology. We partially concur with Griesinger's one-mental-illness theory with our unified theory for OCD (Yaryura-Tobias 1990).

We accept a priori OCD as a pathological subsystem emerging from the brain. We acknowledge the presence of OCD and its spectrum, but we must still verify the existence of symptoms, behaviors, and pathology that must be connected. Therefore, in this chapter, the reader is introduced to an array of ideas, concepts, working hypotheses, and general material weaving the OCD mesh. To this end, we use three kinds of analysis: 1) conceptual, 2) epistemological, and 3) factual.

Philosophical Aspects

Based on Hume's dimensional theory, three elements—cause, effect, and necessity—are applied in the study of OCD and its spectrum. Kant's approach to human affairs states that thoughts organize and modify the outer world; thus, people can change both. In contrast, Hegel asserts that objects modify thoughts. Kant also affirmed the unity of consciousness as a nonfragmented body. Thus, the self remains intact, although we admit that it may become diseased without losing integrity. Patients with OCD adhere to Kantian thinking because it helps control the external world by modifying object perception and keeping them at peace with their consciousness.

Consciousness integration is achieved through four main processes: thought, emotionality, the somatosensory circuit, and motor activity.

Thought, as a complex function, controls analysis, decision, and execution. For these chores, four main cybernetic factors are required: 1) receptor, 2) operator, 3) moderator, and 4) effector. These functions are disorganized in OCD (see "Cybernetic model" in this chapter).

Emotionality interferes with or complements thinking. It derives from the term *emote* and is the process of elaborating feelings. This process is quick and has a minimal number of applied logic steps. Emotions are secondary to primary OCD symptoms, although these symptoms might be exacerbated by intense fear, anger, or depression. Intense emotions also are present in the OCD spectrum.

The somatosensory circuit, interconnected with thoughts and emotions, regulates the way we perceive the internal and external worlds. Kant proposed two main regulatory factors: sensorial and intellectual. These are subdivided according to their specific actions: shape, size, smell, color, touch, credences, expectations, planning, and normative codes. For example, distorted sensorial mechanisms may affect appetite (e.g., an eating disorder), body image (body dysmorphic disorder), the ability of OCD patients to make plans (loss of priorities, poor planning), or normative codes (moral hypertrophy).

The last factor is motor activity, that is, physical action to transport the body, perform physiological functions, express emotions through gestures, and talk. In addition, violent behavior is an extension of bodily movement. As part of the universe, motor activity blends with surrounding space and transcends skin boundaries as energy. Movement achieves orbital integration with the universe by means of the biosphere (Vernadsky 1930). The matter in the biosphere undergoes a constant transformation, represented by time and movement (Bergson 1944). A representative of universal motion in our bodily structure is the Brownian movement.

We posit thought as a nonvisual movement form specific to highly developed organisms and controlled by the neocortex and behavior as a movement form pertaining to the primitive brain. We may say that obsessionality is associated with the prefrontal region (e.g., moral hypertrophy, right or wrong), whereas compulsivity is associated with the primitive region (e.g., self-mutilation, hand-washing, picking). Thought and motion seem to work in a close relationship; both are frequently altered in neuropsychiatric pathology and are certainly altered in the pathogenesis of OCD and its spectrum. Motor activity in OCD may represent a behavioral response triggered by an urge to perform a physical act. This act does not require a mental reason to be done. A classical example is the behavior observed in patients with Tourette's syndrome (Yaryura-Tobias et al. 1981). This syndrome quite effectively integrates thought and motion pathology.

OCD and its spectrum pathology covers mental and somatosensorial functions that seriously affect the life of the patient (see Figure 13–1).

Three conclusions can be drawn: 1) not every compulsion requires previous reasoning, 2) some compulsions are mechanically programmed, and 3) an obsession does not always require the expression of a motor behavior.

Finally, people require perception, understanding, and knowledge to interact with, accept, and tolerate the views of the world outside themselves. A dysfunction of this triad affects our social projection (e.g., the family and social milieu of the patient with OCD).

Neurobiological Development

Following birth, neurobiological development continues in conjunction with developing psychological and social factors.

For earlier development stages, Freud proposed three phases: 1) oral, 2) anal, and 3) genital. These phases constitute the pillars of psychological growth; the anancastic personality results from phase 2.

Piaget's contribution to child development also consists of three primordial phases: 1) assimilation, 2) accommodation, and 3) acceptance or rejection. These phases seem altered in OCD; the inability of OCD patients to be flexible and less controlling is caused by not only rigid thinking, but also to a great degree by narcissism or "me-ness." These OCD traits incapacitate patients and prevent them from having positive relationships, eventually leading to periods of anger or depression and virtual isolation.

Awareness of these phases and their application may help patients and therapists modify false beliefs and maladaptive behaviors by using behavioral and cognitive techniques.

A Freudian approach to explaining OCD's dynamics involves unconscious or subconscious mechanisms; a Piagetian approach uses reasoning and emotion.

The Brain

The brain is responsible for bodily activities and coordinated functions. The brain's function is well demonstrated by neurobehavioral manifestations connecting the inner self to the outside world. The brain works mainly with acts, objects, and values, correlated to the dorsal-cortical sector (praxis responses), the ventral-cortical sector (pragmatic responses), the limbic ring (instinctual world), the cingulate gyrus (gross acts such as copulation), and the frontal region (values) (Goldar 1993).

Several schools have proposed outlines to subdivide the human brain's cortical surface (Brodman 1909; Economo 1929). The four cortical zones are: 1) idiotypic cortex, 2) homotypical isocortex, 3) paralimbic areas, and 4) limbic areas (allocortical structures) (see Figure 13–2).

This plain structural typology has far reaching implications for understanding the distribution of neural connectivity and behavioral specialization throughout the brain (Mesulam 1986). These concepts allow us to establish

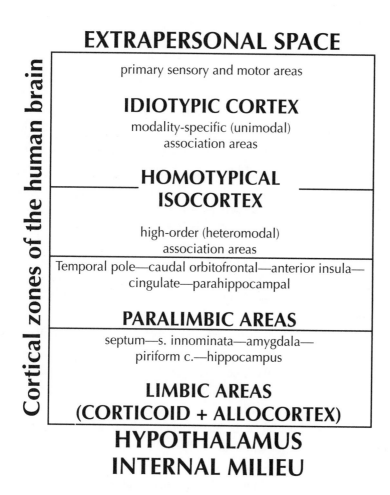

Figure 13–2. Subdivisions of the brain's cortical surface. *Note.* s. = substantia; c. = cortex. *Source.* M. Marsel Mesulam: *Principles of Behavioral Neurology.* Philadelphia, PA, FA Davis, 1986, p. 9. Reprinted with permission.

sound neurobiological OCD models and understand the organic basis of OCD symptoms.

The innermost (limbic) zone interconnects with the hypothalamus; regulates homeostasis, drive reduction, affect, and memory; and correlates well with OCD pathology. The outermost zone belongs to the outer world, receiving information and coordinating motor responses after starting the cybernetic operationality. Cybernetic operationality consists of the automatic control system formed by the nervous system and the brain and by mechanoelectrical communication systems and devices (e.g., computers, thermostats). It enables the exchange between the outer and the inner worlds. The two intermediate zones, containing the heteromodal and paralimbic areas, occupy most of the cortical surface. The process information, integrate, and set links with limbic input. Finally, the organization of the striatum, globus pallidus, and thalamus also is divided. The limbic system formed by the basal ganglia and parts of the thalamus regulates some aspects of memory, learning, and emotions.

The Neuron

The brain is composed of a neuron conglomerate ranging between 3 billion and 10 billion neurons. Each neuron seems to interconnect with 10,000 other neurons. In what region or regions of this multicellular organ is OCD placed? Will exploring the neuron result in an understanding of OCD pathology? Assuming that findings are gathered, what will be the benefits for the patient? We believe that any knowledge obtained about the neuron and the cerebral region's neural evolution might be applied to study OCD's evolution as a pathological construct.

The qualities of a neuron include 1) evolution, 2) preexistent diversity, 3) growth, 4) plasticity, 5) diversity of specific functions, 6) hierarchy, and 7) the right to die. Looking at the history of the cell, we wonder at its determination to become a neuron. So far, we know the cell's function and diversity are influenced by genetics and the environment. Neural connections are modulated by environmental factors such as postnatal development (Wiesel 1982) and by early childhood experiences of the surrounding environment. All contribute to perceptual competence in adulthood.

Hubel and Wiesel's experiments (1962), in which one of a kitten's eyelids was sewn shut during the critical growth period, demonstrated postnatal developmental changes. Sewing the kitten's eye shut modified ocular preference. As a result, the deprived eye's anatomy and physiology atrophied and, after reopening the closure, only unaffected cells responded to visual inputs (Hubel and Wiesel 1962). Furthermore, the anatomical brain counterpart atrophied (i.e., the lateral geniculate and the cortex), subsequently reshaping cortical anatomy. Similar results were observed by Blackmore and Mitchell (1973).

Myelinization is a crucial element in neurobiological development because myelin sheathing prevents electrical signals from fading out. Frontal myelinization continues until age 10 years, coinciding with Piaget formal operation, or at times until age 20 years. Others postulate myelinization as a constant life process (Yakovlev and LeCours 1964).

Some evidence indicates the presence of proteins critical for promotion of neural circuitry growth. These growth-associated proteins disappear after the critical growth period (e.g., the optical subsystem) and in mammals with defective or damaged nervous systems. The neuron can be selective and plastic but is always selective (Changeux and Danchin 1976; Edelman 1978). Now, however, the neuron is no longer accepted as the unit of brain function, but rather the unit of brain function is seen as a subsystem of neuron columns. These subsystems are selective. Knowing these subsystems' actions may facilitate symptom control through administration of psychotropic agents.

Ramon y Cajal (1933) described a neuron function known as plasticity that permits a diseased cell to remodulate and return to its primary function. Only when the allotted recovery time passes does chronicity set in. Along the same line, two researchers discovered the protein B-50, which permits neurons to change (Benowitz and Routtemberg 1987) and their synapses to undergo plastic changes (Lovinger et al. 1986). These current concepts in neuron growth and the renewed interest in neural plasticity (Changeux 1985) bring hope for patients with irreparably damaged neurons and chronicity. Loss of neuron plasticity in OCD's pathogenesis may indicate irreversible damage. This damage may be reflected in the treatment modalities' failure to reverse the OCD process. For example, an average of 50% to 70% improvement with drug and/or behavior therapy excludes a large group of nonresponders that should be accounted for. Perhaps loss of plasticity and damage to the cerebral structure are two of the factors responsible for treatment failure.

Two important neuron qualities are diversity of specific functions and hierarchy (Edelman 1978). When neurons become diseased, they lose hierarchy, as is observed in OCD patients, who can no longer effectively organize daily routines. Furthermore, diseased cells unable to continue executing their chores seem to become "unnecessary" and die.

OCD Correlates

Anatomical Aspects

Although neurology has primarily an anatomical foundation, psychiatry does not because it remains obscured in its own pathophysiology.

However, Kleist's clinical observations of wounded soldiers, Cannon's sham-rage phenomena, Moniz's psychosurgery, Papez's circuit, and Magoun's reticular activating system constitute a sufficient body of information to indicate neuropsychiatric involvement in OCD. Furthermore, current knowledge of neurohistochemistry and psychopharmacology and recent progress in cerebral imaging and determining cerebral metabolism add new information on OCD.

Crawford (1972) suggested that both the adrenergic and cholinergic divisions of the hypothalamus act down on the autonomic nervous system (ANS) and up on the cerebral cortex, where this activity is experienced as moods (Crow 1971). This associative concept—the interaction between the hypothalamus and the affect via an adrenocholinergic mechanism—calls for reflection because it suggests that a similar interaction may be involved in OCD pathology.

OCD patients have a gamut of symptoms involving thought, perception, mood, will, and motor activity. This symptom mosaic seems to emerge from an extensive cerebral territory comparable with the postencephalitic state, which is associated with some symptoms and behaviors identical to those associated with OCD. A wide range of cerebral lesions, with different size and shape changes, and cerebral circulatory insufficiency are related to OCD pathophysiology. The lesions include tumors, infarctions, gliosis, and atrophies. The areas affected are the frontal, parietal, and temporal lobes; the basal ganglia; and the insula (Alptekin et al. 1990; Daumezon et al. 1954; Laplane et al. 1988; Paunovic 1984; Yaryura-Tobias and Neziroglu 1991). Although these lesions are not located in a specific brain area, they all elicit obsessional thinking and compulsive behavior. This finding is explained by accepting the postulate that lesions in one area of the brain may indirectly affect other brain areas via neural connections.

Computed brain tomography shows changes in caudate nucleus volume (Luxemberg et al. 1988) and a higher ventricle-to-brain ratio in adolescents with OCD compared with healthy control subjects (Behar et al. 1984).

Magnetic resonance imaging of the brains of OCD patients registered T1 abnormalities, suggesting involvement of the orbitofrontal cortex, frontal white matter, cingulate gyrus, and lenticular nuclei (Garber et al. 1989).

Although the Papez circuit (1937) dominated subsequent development of the limbic system concept, its structures constitute only the medial half of that system as it is currently recognized (Livingston and Escobar 1971). In 1948 Yakovlev extended Papez's concept by including the orbitofrontal cortex and the insular and anterior temporal areas, together with their connections with the amygdala and dorsal medial nucleus in the thalamus. These cerebral regions seem related to OCD, as suggested by studies using magnetic resonance imaging and positron-emission scanning.

The reticular formation assumes the significance of an internal adjustment system of the brain (Nauta 1972). In the reticular formation, the raphe nuclei's role, representing the limbic system's midbrain extension, specifically relates to the homeostasis of affect (Hornykiewicz 1977). Furthermore, a disturbance in the serotonin metabolism of these nuclei might render this part of the reticular system vulnerable to external or internal stress, thus disturbing the homeostatic control of affect, resulting in excessive pathology (mood reactions).

The association between seizure disorders and OCD, the presence of abnormal electroencephalographic tracings in patients with OCD, and soft neurological signs favor an anatomical foundation for OCD pathophysiology.

Recent advances in understanding brain lateralization and hemispherical differences in cognitive specialization may assist in studying OCD. When surgically disconnected, the two cerebral hemispheres function like two separate minds as follows: the hemispheres specialize for different cognitive models (i.e., each hemisphere specializes for a different type of information processing). Such hemispheric specialization exists in the human brain.

To substantiate the organic theory of OCD, considerable data from neurosurgical procedures performed on the orbitofrontal, internal capsule, and cingulum regions have been reviewed (Mindus et al. 1994; Yaryura-Tobias and Neziroglu 1983). Neurosurgical interventions in OCD are considered when patients do not respond to noninvasive treatment procedures. It is unclear how these procedures affect the OCD process. Perhaps severing neural pathways interrupts the electrochemical transmissions related to OCD. As a result, clinical symptoms are abated. The surgical procedure suppresses obsessive-compulsive symptoms, reduces anxiety and depression, and blunts affect, with subsequent indifference to the obsessive-compulsive symptomatology. Although most studies were uncontrolled, it is safe to state that at least 30% of the patients improved and many patients remained improved during follow-up assessments (Baer et al 1995). Nonetheless, a relapse of OCD might be expected. The possibility of relapse after surgery suggests other mechanisms in the pathology of OCD. These mechanisms may have a functional foundation. On a strict anatomical basis, it might be argued that after the destruction of the anatomical site mediating the transmission of

OCD symptoms, a detour mechanism might be conceived. This theory could partially explain the recurrence of OCD symptoms.

Psychophysiological Parameters

Neurophysiological research helps explain the relation between anatomy and mental disorders. The responses to chronic electrical stimulation of the cingulum of persons with behavioral disorders about to undergo cingulotomy (Escobedo et al. 1973) were as follows: 1) vegetative responses, 2) motor responses, 3) psychological responses, and 4) behavioral responses.

Electrically stimulating the cingulum alters speech, producing dysphasia, perseveration, and rate or volume changes; modifies temporal lobe functions, resulting in picking at clothes, confusion, fixed gaze, lip smacking, rubbing the eyes and face, and akinetic mutism; modifies affective responses such as intense fear, pleasure, and agitation (Meyer et al. 1973); and results in compulsive motor phenomena (Talairach et al. 1973) and compulsory speech (Schaltenbrand 1965, 1975; Schaltenbrand et al. 1971). Summing up, some responses obtained via electrical stimulation are similar to OCD symptomatology. Some investigations clarifying the electrophysiological pathology of OCD were performed, including sleep, oculomotor activity, dysponesis, skin conductance, evoked potentials, and electroencephalography.

In 14 OCD patients, the sleep record disclosed a significant decrease of total sleep time with more awakenings, less stage 4 sleep, decreased REM efficiency, and shortened REM latency. These abnormalities evoke depression and might suggest a link between both disorders (Insel et al. 1982a). In another study, OCD patients' behavior during sleep deprivation remained unchanged (Joffe and Swinson 1988). In a comparative study of patients with schizophrenia and patients with OCD, patients with schizophrenia had insomnia (Gaillard et al. 1984).

Because disturbances in the neuronal circuitry of the basal ganglia and prefrontal cortex are linked to OCD, and because eye movements are often affected by lesions of these cerebral regions, oculomotor assessment of OCD patients was performed. OCD patients had more abnormal eye movements than a psychiatrically normal control group, including an increase in slow pursuit eye movements and an increased frequency of square-wave jerk intrusions (Sweeney et al. 1992). OCD patients made significantly more errors on a visual and goal-guided oculomotor task and had a significantly greater incorrect saccades rate on the goal-guided antisaccade task; this finding was most notable in male OCD patients. The authors claimed that these findings help diagnosis (Tien et al. 1992); however, they did not explain how. No correlation could be established among OCD, soft neurological signs, smooth pursuit eye movements, and saccadic eye movements (Nickoloff et al. 1991). Finally, OCD patients and psychiatrically normal control groups were different from patients with schizophrenia or depression who had abnormal eye movements (Kojima et al. 1992).

Dysponesis, an energy expenditure error interfering with the nervous system's function, relates, as a neurophysiological factor, to obsessive-compulsive states (Whatmore and Kohli 1968). Administering clomipramine reduces autonomic response to important or aversive stimuli that might predict clinical improvement (Zahn et al. 1984).

Investigating patients with OCD, other neurosis, schizophrenia, and major depression showed that the OCD group had a distinctive middle-latency pattern and somatosensory evoked potentials peak amplitude measurements compared with other groups (Shagass et al. 1984).

Flor-Henry (1973) presented the first electrophysiological OCD model. Using a heuristic approach, he found that predominantly lateral dominant temporal limbic neuronal disorganization was associated with schizophrenic syndrome, whereas predominantly unilateral nondominant temporal limbic dysfunction was associated with affective psychoses. Asymmetrical limbic system dysfunction explained the atypical depressions with paranoid symptomatology. Less dominant temporal limbic disturbance similarly led to psychopathology, whereas less nondominant disturbance led to types of neurotic depression. According to this model, disorganizing the central (anterior-thalamic-cingulate gyrus) limbic axis constitutes the neuronal basis underlying the obsessional syndrome (Flor-Henry et al. 1979).

Cybernetic Model

Cybernetics is the communication and control science. Its basis is transmitting information with a clean signal in a time unit and then codifying and decodifying it. Information is measured by Shannon's law (a law related to order); Boltzmann's law measures entropy (a law related to disorder). Because living organisms need information, they are ruled by Shannon's law (negative entropy), whereas inner matter is ruled by Boltzmann's law (positive entropy). Cybernetics interprets the individual mechanistically and unmodifiably, and physics in terms of cause and effect, producing efficacious action.

If we err, we need correction time, which may consist of a normal or—in the case of OCD patients—a delayed response. Through cybernetics, a continuous attempt is made to equilibrate the internal milieu with the outside world (von Bertalanffy 1968) using either a constant or a trend regulator. The latter usually manages disease. Cybernetics works by using a circuitry applicable to the brain's neuroanatomy and physiology. The pathology of OCD may affect the four main factors that control the cybernetic mechanisms of the brain.

The receptor presents two deficits: motor and auditory doubting (e.g., "Have I switched the lights off?" or "Did I hear the sound of broken glass?").

The operator displays continuous doubting and beliefs that occupy the "thinking time." This causes indecisiveness ("What decisions shall I make?") and the inability to shift from one task to another one. These impairments affect the ability to complete a given activity, either mental or motor. Slowness and inaccuracy are easily observable. Finally, a need to be iterative or redundant to be sure and certain is a hallmark of the OCD operator (see Table 13–1).

The motivator is affected by the inability to quantitatively or qualitatively move forward and execute the command. Three characteristics are part of this pathology: 1) repetition, 2) unfinished work, and 3) loss of the ability to shift from one task to another.

The major factor influencing the cybernetics of OCD is the tension level, which stimulates regulatory or compensatory mechanisms. We think the tension level in OCD benefits symptom control by distracting the patient from the main obsessional core. According to Piaget, psychasthenia lacks psychological tension; thus, the patient's coping ability falls considerably. This lack of tension might be compensated for by cybernetic mechanisms that minimize input or pick high-tension-provoking information. To illustrate, OCD decreased during World War II (Popov 1949) and in concentration camps (V. A. Kral 1951, quoted in Monserrat-Esteve 1971) because populations were exposed to situations (e.g., threats to survival) that provoked higher tension. Finally, dysponesis, as an error of energy expenditure, may alter the servomechanisms of OCD as tension does (see "Psychophysiological Parameters,"earlier in this chapter). Monserrat-Esteve (1971) wrote an excellent review of cybernetics and OCD.

The Organic Brain Model

One important etiopathogenic theory explaining OCD can be extracted from Goldstein (1924), later summarized by Rumke (1967). Goldstein extensively

Table 13–1. Cybernetic faulty mechanisms in obsessive-compulsive disorder

Region	Message	Response
Receptor	Lights off	Double-check
Operator	To act	Doubting
	To switch	Reverberation
Motivator	Forceful thought	Obsession
Effector	Execute	Onomatomania
		Arithmomania
		Tics
		Palikinesia
		Echolalia

contributed to the clinical description of the injured brain as well as the patient's response to the outside world and its demands on him or her. His ideas are fundamental to the modern view of the injured brain's problem and diagnosis and treatment considerations (Goldstein 1930, 1942; Goldstein and Katz 1937). Review of the literature for evidence outlining an organic OCD model showed that the brain-injured patient offered the best analogue.

Goldstein (1930, 1942) looked into three clinical areas that are important in OCD: 1) attitude toward the world, 2) thought processes, and 3) motor activity.

In the patient with brain injury, Goldstein (1930, 1942) described two attitude types: 1) relatively primitive and concrete, where thinking is determined by, and cannot proceed beyond, some immediate experience, object, or stimulus; and 2) relative detachment from experiences, where thoughts and actions are directed by general concepts embracing the immediate situation as one of a certain class of phenomena. The individual with a brain lesion cannot assume an abstract or categorical attitude and cannot shift from one to the other. Nevertheless, losing the capacity for abstraction may not be specific to brain damage (Zangwill 1964). The similarities subsection of the Wechsler Adult Intelligence Scale indicates normal abstract reasoning in OCD patients (F. A. Neziroglu, personal communication, July 1977).

Goldstein (1930, 1942) cited the following as characteristic of the abstract attitude: 1) assuming a mental set voluntarily (e.g., association and judgment); 2) shifting voluntarily from one aspect of a situation to another; 3) keeping in mind simultaneously various aspects of a situation; 4) grasping the essential of a whole, breaking up the given whole, and isolating the parts voluntarily; 5) abstracting common properties, ideally planning ahead, assuming an attitude to be merely possible (e.g., an event may or may not occur), and thinking of performing symbolically; and 6) detaching the ego from the outer world. The OCD patient has difficulties sorting out presenting problems, resolving conflicts, and making decisions.

One source of difficulty for patients with brain injury is their inability to perceive the difference between figure and background. As a result, while attempting to solve problems, even in everyday conditions, patients experience uncertainty and instability similar to psychiatrically normal persons when confronted with ambiguous figures. The figure-and-ground metaphor, widely used in Gestalt psychology, also may refer to brain-injured persons' difficulty in distinguishing essentials from nonessentials (Critchley 1953). OCD patients experience ambiguity as a result of doubting. Furthermore, they are unable to prioritize because they cannot differentiate essentials from nonessentials.

Speech defects observed in some cases of presenile dementia, such as logoclonia, aphasic perseveration, and palilalia, also may be present in certain forms of OCD (e.g. Tourette's syndrome).

Brain-injured patients appear normally susceptible to external stimuli; they are distractible rather than inattentive. Actually, their attention may be difficult to divert in some circumstances, and patients are often aware of this subjectively as an inability to shift attention voluntarily from one part of the environment to another. In some situations, this inability ties patients to the stimulus. This also is true in OCD patients, who show displeasure if interrupted while they perform a task. Furthermore, Vallejo Ruiloba (1978) showed in his psychophysiological studies that obsessive patients may have low attention and concentration levels, perhaps because of morbid thinking or adhering to previous stimuli.

Goldstein (1930, 1942) established the idea that a perseveration trend is a common point between neurological and obsessive alterations, and this tendency toward perseveration either lies in deeper subcortical regions or constitutes subcortical dominance. The mental difference between "neurologically" obsessive patients and "functionally" obsessive patients is that patients with neurological lesions present intense perseverative activity and report episodes appearing alien to the mind (e.g., ego dystonic). Perseveration and retracing are two OCD symptoms.

According to Goldstein (1930, 1942), brain-injured patients unconsciously try readjusting their lives to accommodate the demands of the environment.

However, brain-injured patients cannot cope with the world and have a catastrophic reaction characterized by mental, motor, and ANS symptoms. Patients become anxious, agitated, solemn, angry, and evasive. The neurological deficit worsens, and disturbances of the ANS showed by dyspnea, tachycardia, and tearfulness are present. The catastrophic OCD reaction is severe, irreversible OCD, also called the malignant form of OCD. This form might be accompanied by serious brain disorganization experienced during a severe panic attack.

To prevent the catastrophic reaction described in the previous paragraph, brain-injured patients avoid exposure to their environment and anxiety-provoking situations (similar to patients with OCD and phobic behaviors). Consequently, patients become loners, withdrawn, and indifferent to life events; this behavior brings a substantial decrease in anxiety. Patients may undertake all sorts of purposeless hyperactivity, known as occupational delirium, which is found in many dementia cases. This iterative activity is carried out because patients feel comfortable and safe performing activities with which they are familiar. Repetition and familiarity are almost automatic; this phenomenon gradually becomes obsessive (Burger and Mayer-Gross 1928).

Nine patients with organic OCD, confirmed by cerebral MRI, manifested concrete, rigid, and partially primitive thinking. Although all patients had insight about their illness, they could not adhere to the treatment, remained indifferent to their problem, and did not show anxiety (Yaryura-Tobias and Neziroglu 1991).

Some symptoms encountered in brain trauma and OCD patients appear to confirm the Jacksonian concept of positive symptoms equilibrating functional deficits from illness or injury. For example, the patients' possessions are frequently arranged in a stereotyped and meticulous manner, although there is no logical reason for the arrangement chosen. This orderliness also may show itself as a compulsive tendency to order others' property and make impossible demands on children's orderliness. This behavior is common among OCD patients wishing to impose their lifestyles on other family members. This behavior may be carried to extremes; for example, an OCD patient may force relatives to perform rituals on his or her behalf or hire employees for the same purpose.

Goldstein indicated that brain-injured persons tend to quell knowledge of their disability. This tendency is more easily achieved by patients with destroyed functions than by those whose disability is incomplete. This illness ignorance also can be seen in OCD patients who measure their behavioral responses using abnormal parameters. For example, in the housecleaning syndrome, the patient sees her activity as a virtue; other homemakers fall short of her expectations. The ignoring-a-disability rule holds for perceptual defects such as blindness and deafness, limb paralysis, and speech disturbances. The disability adjustment is often better for patients with a complete hemiplegia than for those with an incomplete hemiplegia; more emotional disturbance is commonly present in patients with severely impaired sight than in patients who are totally blind. A patient with organic OCD is more ready to accept the resulting disability than a patient affected by functional OCD. This concept might be useful when treating patients on a long-term basis for rehabilitation purposes. A new equilibrium based on adapting to a limited environment seems difficult to acquire when there is partial continuation of the impaired function.

In addition to the presence of structural or functional changes, an OCD patient displays robust evidence of higher intellectual and emotional injury. Sadness, anxiety, guilt, uncertainty, distrust, and incompleteness of daily life clearly illustrate pathology and personal and social handicaps. The question is whether we can put into perspective the anatomical, biochemical, and psychosocial aspects of OCD to make sense of what seems to be a chronic condition.

Biochemical Aspects

Neurotransmitter Research Applicable to OCD

Recently, new advances in understanding neurotransmitter function, anatomical locations of receptors and subreceptors, and their interconnection in the brain have received considerable attention from those interested in the OCD pathogenesis. As a result, the original serotonin OCD hypothesis now requires in-depth revision. The new view of neurotransmitters is that they are dynamic, rather than static, elements working flexibly with the anatomical and electrohistochemical environment. In this regard, some fundamentally important findings demand brief review.

A neurotransmitter fast chemical signal results from a neurotransmitter stimulating the opening-receptor controlled ion channels of the postsynaptic cell in a millisecond; this stimulation seems to mediate the passage of amino acids, notably glutamate and γ-aminobutyric acid.

A neurotransmitter slow chemical signal seems to operate in monoamines and neuropeptides in several seconds or even minutes (Iversen and Goodman

1986). Neurotransmitters operating with slow signals behave as modulators rather than excitatory or inhibitory substances and may act at a distance; this is called chemical addressing (Iversen 1984). If chemical addressing occurs between two specific neurons at one specific synapse, the neurotransmitter is anatomically addressed. Because of chemical addressing, the brain can influence other structures from a distance, causing symptoms unrelated to the original site of a lesion.

Programming chemical neurotransmission also is influenced by the rate of neurotransmitter release (Stahl and Wets 1988). Rate control comes from a pulsatile, not a continuous, manner of drug administration (Norstedt and Palmiter 1984; Stahl and Wets 1988); a pulsatile manner sensitizes the receptors, whereas a continuous manner desensitizes them or causes tolerance (Martin-Iversen et al. 1987; Stahl and Wets 1988). This fact should be considered when patients develop tolerance with long-term drug administration. To prevent tolerance, a twice-daily or three-times-daily dosage regimen should be chosen.

Some neurotransmitter variables to consider when choosing a drug therapy program are 1) a neurotransmitter's predominate chemical behavior over other neurotransmitters in one site of action; 2) biphasic action; 3) loss of neurotransmitter equilibrium; 4) the degree of sensitization or saturation (e.g., refractory response, paradoxical response); 5) tissue immaturity (e.g., ongoing myelinization in children); 6) tissue degeneration; and 7) loss of neural plasticity.

Paradigms favorable to understanding OCD are as follows:

1. Pavlovian mechanisms of excitation and inhibition
2. Repetitive neural activity, in other words reverberant circuits of Lorente de No, or referent circuits

These paradigms are observed in intellectual motoric symptoms such as iterativeness or inability to switch tasks. For example, OCD patients ask repetitive questions and they perform repetitive tasks. These tasks cannot be interrupted until completion. If interrupted, patients may become angry and disturbed.

Animal Experimentation

McKinney (1989) evaluated animal schizophrenia models that seem applicable to OCD. There are four general kinds of animal models:

1. Those simulating a specific human disorder sign or symptom (behavioral similarity models)
2. Those evaluating a specific etiological theory (theory-driven models)
3. Those studying underlying mechanisms (mechanistics models)
4. Those permitting preclinical drug evaluations (empirical validity models)

The biochemical mental disorder models in animal experiments are tested with substances that are either normally present in the brain or have psychotropic or psychotomimetic properties. These models usually target the aminergic or amino acid pathways. The results are measured on two behavioral levels: mental and motor. The animal OCD models are natural or induced. The natural model requires clinical observation of animals in their normal habitat or the laboratory; the induced model is commonly used.

The natural presence of obsessive and compulsive behavior was observed in the animal kingdom, similar to the perseveration observed in animals in captivity (Brion and Ey 1968). Attention to body surface (orofacial, hair, musculoskeletal, and other areas) as a substitute for the fight-or-flight response has been noted in the literature. In this regard, Mitchell (1968) emphasized several behaviors such as teeth grinding, lip biting, hair pulling, nail biting, and compulsive hand washing. Canine acral lick dermatitis consisting of compulsive licking of a patch of skin or a paw has been suggested as an animal model of OCD (Goldberger and Rapoport 1991; Rapoport et al. 1992).

Catecholamine System

Dopamine is a neurotransmitter present in the central nervous system and the peripheral nervous system. Dopamine is irregularly distributed in the brain. However, there are specific areas of higher concentration such as the striatum, limbic system, substantia nigra, and amygdala. Several neuropsychiatric pathologies seem associated to dopamine. These nosologies include conditions with prominence of movement disorders (e.g., Parkinson's disease, choreas, Tourette's syndrome, hyperkinetic syndromes) and conditions with prominence of thought pathology (e.g., schizophrenia). At times and under unclear circumstances, these conditions seem related to OCD. From these associations a new nosology emergent appears, indicating a distinct anatomical and chemical circuitry.

Pharmacotherapy acts on dopamine by modifying neurotransmitter receptor activity. Two main receptor families are related to dopamine: 1) excitatory (responsive to apomorphine stimulation) and 2) inhibitory. These receptors operate in the presence of the adenyl cyclase enzymatic system. They are further subdivided into subreceptors: the most studied ones are D_1, D_2, D_3, D_4, and D_5. These subreceptors have been studied with respect to their relationship with schizophrenia and the use of neuroleptic medication.

Administering amphetamines to study animal behavior produces stereotypy and repetitive behavior (Fog 1972; Randrup and Munkvad 1967), stereotypy with apomorphine (Randrup and Munkvad 1974) and then catatonia after administering mescaline (de Jong 1931), and endless motor activity, self-mutilation, presence of circular movements, cannibalism, and social disorganization (Carranza-Acevedo et al. 1970).

Amphetamine-like stereotypy can be produced by other agents, such as phenylethylamine, indolethylamine derivatives, cocaine, and monoamine oxidase inhibitors. With amphetamines and apomorphine, it is believed that stereotyped behavior absolutely depends on transmitting dopamine in the mammalian brain's basal ganglia (Randrup and Munkvad 1974); noradrenergic components also are an influence (Mogilnicka and Braestrup 1976). Furthermore, use of neuroleptics can potentiate and inhibit the amphetamine-induced stereotypy (Lal and Sourkes 1972).

The gnawing compulsion induced by apomorphine in mice results from stimulation of dopaminergic neurons in the corpus striatum and is not reduced by α-methyltyrosine (Ernst and Smelick 1966). Furthermore, high gnawing intensities were obtained with tricyclic antidepressants (Pedersen 1967), reduced by α-methyltyrosine, and reactivated by dopa (Pedersen 1968).

These results indicate that catecholamines, probably dopamine, are important to the mechanism of the gnawing compulsion syndrome produced by apomorphine and enhanced by administration of p-chlorophenylalanine or apomorphine combined with tricyclic antidepressants.

It seems that suppression of gnawing with large systemic morphine doses and related analgesics may be mediated by a serotonergic pathway. Bergmann et al. (1976) suggested that gnawing is stimulated via a catecholaminergic mechanism and the inhibition of gnawing via a serotonergic mechanism. This excitatory-inhibitory mechanism places the neurotransmitters dopamine and serotonin in a state of equilibrium. Loss of this balance may affect motoric activity.

Is there a relationship between obsessive-compulsive behavior and a disturbance of the dopaminergic system? The symptoms of amphetamine psychosis are manic, compulsive, and motor but not obsessive. However, patients with amphetamine psychosis have motor compulsive symptoms similar to those described in OCD. We assume that there is an interconnecting mechanism that requires an extensive neurotransmitter system to produce OCD pathology. Therefore, we presuppose the presence of several neurotransmitters forming the chemical skeleton of OCD pathology.

Although experimental animal and human models can reflect behaviors similar to OCD after the administration of drugs, these experiments are not conclusive. Years ago, an attempt to correlate animal and human behavior was made without success (Fog 1972; Randrup and Munkvad 1972), and the observation that there is no correlation remains valid.

In drug abusers, stereotyped, repetitive activities, teeth grinding, rubbing of the tongue, and compulsive behavior characterized by taking objects apart, sorting them, and on rare occasions, putting them back together have been observed (Ashcroft et al. 1965; Kramer et al. 1967; Mattson and Calverly 1968; Randrup and Munkvad 1967; Rylander 1966). In other studies OCD symptoms (Faillace et al. 1970), such as grimacing, constant combing of the hair, and iterative working have been observed (Schirring 1969).

However, Ellinwood (1967) only observed stereotyped compulsive behavior in addicted persons with amphetamine psychosis. Thus, amphetamine addicts may compulsively pluck their hair, pull their skin, play with clothes, and pick up lint.

The presence of obsessive-compulsive symptoms in patients with encephalitis, with postencephalitic parkinsonism, or after neuroleptic therapy (where a decreased level of dopamine in the basal ganglia has been suggested) makes questionable a clinical amphetamine hypothesis for OCD.

However, in Parkinson's disease and in extrapyramidal syndromes, different dopamine levels are found. For example, in striatal syndromes such as dystonia, Wilson's disease, Huntington's chorea, familiar tremor, torticollis, choreoathetosis, and Sydenham's chorea the levels of dopamine are high, whereas in postencephalitic and arteriosclerotic parkinsonian patients, the levels of dopamine are low (Barbeau and Sourkes 1961). Of note, reports indicating the presence of obsessive-compulsive symptoms in chorea suggest that dopamine levels are not the only variable that determines the presence or absence of OCD symptoms. Parkinsonism that may cause OCD symptoms often follows encephalitis or neuroleptic therapy. In fact, the administration of L-dopa (Anden et al. 1970) or its discontinuation (Sacks 1977) may cause obsessive-compulsive symptoms in parkinsonian patients.

On various grounds, the action of catecholamines has been questioned in the pathology of OCD. In this regard, several experiments were performed.

Plasma catecholamines and their metabolites did not differ between a control sample and 13 patients with OCD (Benkelfat et al. 1991). However, a sample of 61 patients with OCD had significantly lower levels of norepinephrine compared with patients with generalized anxiety disorder ($n = 34$) and significantly lower levels of dopamine compared with patients with major depression ($n = 22$).

At the 95% interval of confidence, 17% of a group of patients with OCD showed low levels and 7% showed high levels of serotonin, whereas 13% of the patients showed low levels and 7% showed high levels of 5-hydroxyindoleacetic acid (5-HIAA) in plasma (Yaryura-Tobias 1988).

The administration of the α_2-adrenergic agonist clonidine to patients with OCD has resulted in a transient reduction of OCD symptoms. This clinical observation may indicate the participation of a noradrenergic mechanism in the pathogenesis of OCD (Hollander et al. 1991). After a loading test with L-dopa, an impairment of adrenalin metabolism was reported in patients with obsessive fear neurosis (Russian classification) (Vasilev et al. 1988). There is some evidence that the anti–obsessive-compulsive agent clomipramine, a potent blocker of serotonin reuptake, exerted antidopaminergic activity in preclinical and clinical trials, indicating the presence of neuroleptic-like properties (Austin et al. 1991; Kim and Dysken 1991).

Two psychostimulants, dextroamphetamine and methylphenidate, were given to patients with OCD to study their effects on OCD symptomatology. Only dextroamphetamine had an antiobsessive effect (Joffe et al. 1991). In another study with patients with OCD ($n = 13$), an antiobsessive response to methylphenidate was observed in four patients (Joffe and Swinson 1987). However, administration of intravenous methylphenidate to a group of patients with OCD modified their behavior, resulting in dysphoria, mood elevation, worsening of OCD symptoms, and stereotypic movements. This finding highlights the need to investigate the role of the dopaminergic system in OCD (Lemus et al. 1991).

Cholinergic System

Acetylcholine has peripheral and central roles, acting as a mediator in neuromuscular transmission, autonomic ganglia, and the central nervous system, notably in the thalamic and limbic regions. Acetylation and hydrolysis are the two major steps in the metabolic cycle of acetylcholine, an activity mediated primarily by the enzyme acetylcholinesterase.

The main cholinergic receptors are nicotinic and muscarinic. The nicotinic receptors participate in skeletal muscle contraction, and the muscarinic receptors determine the activity of secretory glands and smooth muscles.

The cholinergic system is related to the pathology of mental disorders through two main syndromes: schizophreniform syndrome and confusional syndrome. These are characteristic results of administering, or excessively administering, psychopharmacological agents, causing an iatrogenic delirium or "atropinic madness." Perhaps the cholinergic system interacts with other neuronal systems to cause OCD by altering the brain's biochemical balance. Anticholinergic drugs potentiated stereotyped behavior, probably of dopaminergic origin (Fog 1967; Scheel-Kruger 1970). Also, anticholinergic drugs antagonized several behavioral effects considered highly characteristic of neuroleptic drugs (Morpurgo 1962; Morpurgo and Theobald 1964). In a study involving pseudocholinesterase levels in patients with anxiety-related disorders, the OCD group had significantly higher pseudocholinesterase serum activity. The meaning and implications of these results remain unknown (Aizenberg et al. 1989).

Serotonin System

Because of our limited knowledge, to gain direct insight into the mechanisms involved in the normal and abnormal function of serotonin (5-HT), we should proceed with caution. Recent advances in identifying receptors and messengers widen the possibilities to further explore serotonin's action and that of all other neurotransmitters and their involvement with OCD pathology.

Currently, OCD's serotonin hypothesis needs to be revised. Several questions have been raised:

1. Is serotonin the only neurotransmitter involved?
2. Do neurotransmitters operate in isolation or cooperation?
3. How do neurotransmitters' biphasic activities fit the OCD biochemical model?
4. Among the neurotransmitters, what is the percentage of each to trigger OCD?
5. What is the role of the subreceptors?

The various steps taken by serotonin in the indoleaminergic pathway may be affected by OCD pathology. These steps include synthesis, distribution, metabolism, and catabolism.

The amine serotonin is synthesized from L-tryptophan via 5-hydroxytryptophan in serotonergic neurons and then stored in electron-dense subcellular organelles in the nerve terminals. The rate-limiting step in serotonin's synthesis is tryptophan's hydroxylation (Lovenberg 1973). Therefore, tryptophan's hydroxylation becomes important because altering it disturbs serotonin synthesis. A decrease in cell body tryptophan hydroxylase can be caused by lithium (Knapp and Mandell 1973), amphetamine (Mandell et al. 1974), and LSD (Zivkovic et al. 1974).

Injecting 5-hydroxytryptophan induces an immediate, important, and long-lasting increase in serotonin release. In contrast, acute tryptophan injection leads to a transient and moderate elevation of serotonin release (Ternaux et al. 1976).

Serotonin is widely distributed in the brain. This multianatomical location seems to modulate several normal physiological and emotional behaviors. Serotonin modulates sleep and wakefulness, endocrine activity, appetite, bodily temperature, blood pressure, and pain regulation. Basically, serotonin is intimately bound to the limbic system to perform important activities. In addition, serotonin is associated with depression, OCD and its spectrum, self-mutilation, rage, and schizophrenia.

Distribution of serotonin in the brain may be influenced by changes in biosynthetic enzymes, tryptophan 5-hydroxylase, and aromatic L-amino acid decarboxylase. Most serotonin-containing nerve cell bodies are localized in the raphe nuclei, in the midline from the pyramidal decussation in the medulla through the pons and caudal mesencephalon. There also are important serotonin concentrations in the hypothalamus, thalamic region, and striatum.

A neurotransmitter may or may not respond to various drugs that act on it, depending on its anatomical location. Collard and Roberts (1974) showed that administration of L-tryptophan produced significant increases in the forebrain concentrations of serotonin and 5-HIAA, whereas coadministration of clomipramine had no effect on the elevation of serotonin by L-tryptophan but significantly increased the 5-HIAA concentration. These findings provide additional support for the hypothesis that elevation of the 5-HIAA concentration after raphe stimulation results from the extraneuronal release of serotonin, followed by uptake and catabolism.

The heterogenicity of serotonergic receptors results in a complex activity regulating neurotransmission. To this date, 10 subfamilies of serotonin receptors have been classified, many of them with neuropsychiatric activity. The serotonin receptor family belongs to two gene superfamilies:

1) G-protein coupled and 2) ligand-gated ion channel. It is important to identify the role of each subreceptor in the pathogenesis of brain disease. Finding the specific ligands for the respective subreceptors will assist in identifying these receptors. Eventually, therapeutic manipulation of these receptors may modify the course of OCD.

Human Research

Indolaminergic Hypothesis of OCD

Assuming that clomipramine, a potent serotonin reuptake blocker, has specific anti–obsessive-compulsive activity (Capstick 1975; Fernandez de Cordoba and López-Ibor 1967; Reynynghe de Voxurie 1968; Yaryura-Tobias and Neziroglu 1975) and that brain chemistry could be affected in OCD (Rack 1970), a serotonergic disturbance was proposed as a cause of OCD (Yaryura-Tobias 1977; Yaryura-Tobias et al. 1976). Later, evidence that blood serotonin levels in obsessive-compulsive patients were significantly lower than those in control subjects was reported (Yaryura-Tobias et al. 1977). Furthermore, patients with prominent motor compulsion symptoms seemed to have significantly lower serotonin levels than patients with ideational compulsions.

Central nervous system 5-HIAA (Thoren et al. 1980a, 1980b) and platelet serotonin (Flament et al. 1985) were inversely correlated to symptom severity and positively correlated to treatment response. However, Goodman (1989) was unable to replicate those findings.

Moreover, no differences in platelet serotonin levels between OCD patients and healthy control subjects were reported by Cottraux et al. (1987) and Flament et al. (1987). Nevertheless, in the latter study patients with higher serotonin concentrations responded better to clomipramine therapy. There was no difference in blood serotonin levels between juvenile patients with OCD and psychiatrically normal control subjects. However, those patients with a family history of OCD had significantly higher blood serotonin levels than the control subjects or patients without a family history of OCD (Hanna et al. 1991b).

Challenge studies with the serotonergic agonist m-chlorophenylpiperazine aggravated OCD symptoms (Zohar et al. 1988), whereas administration of the 5-hydroxytryptophan antagonist metergoline decreased OCD symptoms (Zohar et al. 1987).

Because the amino acid L-tryptophan is the precursor of serotonin, whole blood serotonin was measured before and after the administration of L-tryptophan. Results indicated an elevation of serotonin levels in blood without modification of urinary 5-HIAA (Yaryura-Tobias et al. 1979). Furthermore, it was reported in an uncontrolled study that the administration of L-tryptophan improved the clinical symptoms of obsessions and compulsions (Ciprian Ollivier et al. 1982; Yaryura-Tobias 1981; Yaryura-Tobias and Bhagavan 1977). These biochemical findings support the serotonergic hypothesis.

The available data to support the serotonergic hypothesis have been challenged. At this time we may speak of a dysregulation of the serotonergic system with coparticipation of coenzymatic factors (e.g., pyridoxal phosphate) and the chloride pump. Certainly, studies of the receptor subtypes and genetic codes will bring new questions that will require further studies in the pathogenesis of OCD.

Serotonin Receptors

One question recently addressed is the nature of 5-HT_{1A}'s response in OCD patients. To answer that question, 5-HT_{1A}-mediated thermoregulatory and neuroendocrine activity was measured in OCD patients and psychiatrically normal control subjects with the ligand ipsapirone (Lesh et al. 1991) and with buspirone (Lucey et al. 1992); both groups had the same response. In an experiment, chronic administration of fluoxetine after the administration of ipsapirone resulted in a decrease in receptor activity (Lesh et al. 1991).

Peripheral-type benzodiazepine receptors were analyzed in lymphocyte membranes from OCD patients by using specific [^{3}H]PK11195 binding; results indicated that the number of binding sites was significantly reduced (Rocca et al. 1991). In a study of hyperserotoninemia and antiserotonin antibodies in autism, OCD, Tourette's syndrome, and multiple sclerosis, binding inhibition by antibody-rich blood fractions was highest for multiple sclerosis and was not specific to the serotonin receptor as currently defined (Yuwiler et al. 1992). These trials are at a primary stage, and results are unclear.

Our understanding of the biochemical aspects related to the pathogenesis of OCD is still in an embryonic stage. Hypotheses involving neurotransmitters, coenzymes, hormones, or trace minerals are currently under investigation, and their preliminary results are inconclusive.

Biological Changes

Measuring biological variables requires considering various biopsychosocial factors that should meet good methodological protocol rules. These factors include, among others, age, gender, biological individuality, diagnosis, chronicity of condition, acute or subacute state, medication program, degree of adaptive behavior to the disorder, comorbidity, working and school records, and an acceptable laboratory technique.

Fulfilling these requisites is almost impossible; therefore, one may have to reduce expectations. With OCD, there is an extraordinary array of symptoms and behaviors, manifested by surging pathological states such as ANS dysregulation, anxiety connected to the ANS, or stress as a pivotal factor (Curtis and Glitz 1988). Anxiety is an OCD symptom, so extreme OCD is still classified as an anxiety disorder. Therefore, we wonder whether the biological variables measured in OCD include anxiety variables as well. The general consensus indicates the limitations outlined above.

Researchers measuring biological variables in OCD study the relationship between OCD and the neuroendocrine system. The neuroendocrine system is regulated by the hypothalamic-pituitary-adrenal axis and includes the production of cortisol, prolactin, growth hormone, thyroid-stimulating hormone, thyroid-releasing hormone, vasopressin, follicle-stimulating hormone, and luteinizing hormone.

Abnormal hormonal values may indicate participation of a specific hormone in OCD's pathogenesis, may reflect a disorder of neurotransmitters related to OCD, or may be the response to OCD electrohistochemical changes.

Imipramine Binding

[^{3}H]Imipramine binding is used to study platelet activity as a central neuron function. [^{3}H]Imipramine-binding sites in the platelet membranes of OCD patients might imply serotonin involvement or represent an adaptive response to a chronic disease.

Several studies of [^{3}H]imipramine binding in OCD patients have shown contradictory results; some indicated decreasing maximal binding (Bastani et al. 1991; Marazzitti et al. 1992; Weizman et al. 1986) or a reduction in binding that is not OCD related (Black et al. 1990). Other studies did not demonstrate changes (Insel et al. 1985; Kim and Dysken 1991; Pfohl et al. 1990; Vitiello et al. 1991), including one using ^{125}I-labeled LSD in 5-HT$_2$ receptors (Pandey et al. 1993). In a comorbidity study of Tourette's syndrome and OCD, decreased imipramine binding was shown (Weizman et al. 1992).

We have studied the effect of intensive behavior therapy on [³H]imipramine binding in drug-free OCD patients. Results indicated changes in [³H]imipramine binding without indications of a definite pattern and without clinical correlation (Neziroglu et al. 1990).

Dexamethasone Suppression Test

The dexamethasone suppression test measures cortisol's response to administration of dexamethasone. This test is designed to be a biological marker for major depression. Because OCD may have depressive symptomatology, the dexamethasone suppression test has been given to OCD patients (Cameron et al. 1986).

Results have been equivocal and might be explained by age and gender (Catapano et al. 1990), family psychiatric history for depression (Insel et al. 1982b), or the presence of OCD subsets (Cottraux et al. 1984). One study indicated that OCD patients are nonsuppressors (Lieberman et al. 1985).

Other Biological Challenges

D-Fenfluramine, an indirect serotonin agonist, induces prolactin release when given to OCD patients. However, no differences were noticed between patients and control subjects (McBride et al. 1992). Conversely, fenfluramine blunted prolactin's release in OCD patients but not in control subjects (Hewlett et al. 1992; Hollander et al. 1992). The cortisol and prolactin responses to D-fenfluramine in nondepressed OCD patients were unspecific (Lucey et al. 1992).

Hanna et al. (1991a) measured basal prolactin concentrations before clomipramine treatment in children with OCD. Prolactin levels were influenced by a history of chronic tic disorder, and increased duration and severity of the illness was associated with an increase in the basal prolactin levels, indirectly suggesting an adaptive serotonergic receptor response (Hanna et al. 1991a).

Negative results were observed in the response of desipramine-induced growth hormone to dexamethasone suppression test in OCD patients (Lucey et al. 1992). Nonetheless, an elevated growth hormone response to pyridostigmine in OCD patients indicated cholinergic supersensitivity (Lucey et al. 1993).

The level of somatostatin, a peptide stimulating serotonin release and inhibiting growth hormone release, was significantly higher in OCD patients' cerebrospinal fluid compared with that of psychiatrically normal volunteers. This finding's relevance is unclear (Altemus et al. 1993). In children with OCD, levels of somatostatin in cerebrospinal fluid were normal, in contrast to levels in a sample of children with disruptive behavior (Kruesi et al. 1990). Noteworthy is a report that children with OCD have shorter stature compared with a psychiatrically normal sample of children (Hamburger et al. 1989). The meaning of this finding in a neuroendocrine context is not known.

Another serotonin agonist, MK-212, blunted prolactin and cortisol secretion in OCD patients (Bastani et al. 1990). A cortisol increase was registered after administering behavior exposure to OCD patients (Kasvikis et al. 1988). A urinary cortisol increase, with a decrease after administering clomipramine, was observed in a sample of OCD patients (Gehris et al. 1990). It was suggested that the serotonin agonist m-chlorophenylpiperazine, by inducing prolactin and cortisol release, indicates that these responses are serotonin mediated (Kahn et al. 1990). The significant increase in anxiety and obsessive-compulsive symptoms in OCD patients after administration of m-chloro-phenylpiperazine was blocked by administering metergoline, further supporting the hypothesis that serotonin mediates m-chloro-phenylpiperazine effects (Pigott et al. 1991).

Tryptophan, serotonin's precursor, also was investigated. Administration of tryptophan and m-chlorophenylpiperazine to OCD patients and psychiatrically normal volunteers showed significantly higher responses in female patients and normal volunteers than in male patients. Interestingly, neither m-chlorophenylpiperazine nor tryptophan affected obsessive-compulsive symptoms (Charney et al. 1988). Plasma tryptophan was significantly lower in patients with major depression but not in patients with OCD compared with psychiatrically normal subjects (Lucca et al. 1992). Although prolactin had a blunting effect in depressed patients after intravenous tryptophan administration, this effect was not observed in OCD patients (Price et al. 1990).

In another experiment, decreasing immunoreactive β-endorphin, without cortisol or growth hormone changes, was observed in OCD patients (Weizman et al. 1990).

Levels of thyroid-stimulating hormone, prolactin, and growth hormone were measured after stimulation with thyroid-releasing hormone; results indicated that only thyroid-stimulating hormone was significantly blunted by thyroid-releasing hormone (Aizenberg et al. 1991). Hantouche et al. (1991) found that thyroid function in OCD patients was not depressed. Basal values for thyroid hormones and thyroid-stimulating hormones were normal; however, the authors reported a curious comorbidity between OCD and Grave's disease found in 3 of 50 (6%) OCD patients (Hantouche et al. 1991).

Menstrual Cycle and Pregnancy

A few reports indicated that the menstrual cycle and pregnancy might precipitate or modify OCD's evolution. Pregnancy and childbirth have been associated with OCD's onset (Ingram 1961; Lo 1967; Pollitt 1957; Sichel et al. 1993), and in one case an obsessional state was associated with depression (Brandt and MacKenzie 1987). This issue was specifically addressed by Neziroglu et al. (1992), who examined 106 female OCD patients. Of the women without children (n = 42), 28.6% experienced OCD onset between the ages of 13 and 15 years; those women with children (n = 59) had two onset peaks: at ages 22–24 and 29–32 years. Of the patients with children, 39% had onset of OCD symptoms during pregnancy. An additional five women experienced an onset of their symptoms while pregnant, but symptoms disappeared when they had a miscarriage or abortion.

One case of unusual cleaning during the luteal phase was reported. It is believed that this behavioral change was caused by progesterone disturbances (Dillon and Brooks 1992). Two cases of obsessional symptoms with depression in prepubertal girls were reported; a prominent regression to the pre-oedipal level was thought to explain this onset (Ushijima and Kobayashi 1988). Dysmenorrhea in adolescents with obsessive-phobic disorder was reported in Russian literature (Mikirtumov 1985).

A comparison study of lifetime psychiatric diagnosis in women with premenstrual syndrome (PMS) showed that the diagnosis of OCD was made in PMS clinics and overlapped the specific symptoms of PMS (Stout et al. 1986). A case of amenorrhea after OCD with depressive symptomatology in a drug-free patient was reported (Cipollina Mangiameli 1973). Finally, we should mention the association of dysmenorrhea with OCD, eating disorders, and self-harm, as described in the compulsive-orectic-mutilative syndrome (see Chapter 11) (Yaryura-Tobias and Neziroglu 1978; Yaryura-Tobias et al. 1995).

Hormonal Therapeutic Changes

In a study with 12 OCD patients, administering oxytocin intranasally did not confirm the hypothesis that oxytocin is a potential antiobsessive agent (de Boer and Westenberg 1992). A preliminary trial of oxytocin and vasopressin failed to improve OCD patients (Salzberg and Swedo 1992). It was hypothesized that melatonin mediates serotonin reuptake inhibitors' therapeutic action in OCD by activating the pineal gland and facilitating melatonin's action (Sandyk 1992). In seven OCD patients, low plasma melatonin levels and higher cortisol levels were measured, but no correlation was found between clinical parameters and hormone levels (Catapano et al. 1992).

Metabolic Changes

Water metabolism. Because 57% of body weight is water, we assume that water may play a role in OCD pathology, as it has been reported to do in schizophrenia, where polydipsia occurs frequently (Bremner and Regan 1987).

The importance of the hypothalamic-pituitary-adrenal axis and kidney participation in regulating water metabolism suggests that psychogenic polydipsia may have organic roots. Water balance is controlled by renin, vasopressin, potassium, chloride, sodium, calcium, and glucose. Two main water-related clinical illnesses are diabetes insipidus and diabetes mellitus.

Is it possible to establish a clinical coincidence point between OCD and water metabolism? First, let us look for clinical evidence:

1. Is compulsive water drinking accompanied by other obsessive-compulsive symptoms?
2. Does the administration of anti–obsessive-compulsive agents cause alterations in water consumption or elimination?
3. Do the chloride pump and the sodium pump participate in the pathogenesis of OCD?
4. Considering the hydrophilic properties of glucose, does a glucose imbalance in OCD patients alter water concentration?

In 1894 Kruse described a relationship between OCD and water consumption disturbance (quoted in Barton 1965). Subsequent literature is scarce; the diabetes insipidus–obsessional neurosis syndrome is not put forward until 1965 (Barton 1965). Barton collected nine cases from different sources; he had observed three of these cases. One patient had an additional delusional olfactory syndrome, four patients apparently had postencephalitic parkinsonism, one had a pinealoma, and another had a concomitant psychosis. Interestingly, some patients were treated with vasopressin.

Our observations in this area are limited to 14 patients. Our first report was on a group of compulsive-orectic-mutilative syndrome patients ($n = 10$) who manifested compulsive water drinking, polyuria, or polydipsia (Yaryura-Tobias and Neziroglu 1978). The other four cases were collected from our clinical and research practice over a 16-year period (1978–1994).

In a sample of 12 OCD patients compared with psychiatrically normal control subjects, patients had significantly increased arginine vasopressin levels in the cerebrospinal fluid and significantly increased arginine vaso-pressin secretion into the plasma in response to hypertonic saline adminis-tration (Altemus et al. 1992).

A case of neuroleptic malignant syndrome in an OCD patient with major depression was reported (Langlow and Alarcon 1989). The symptoms of neuro-leptic malignant syndrome were accompanied by a brief polydipsia episode.

An OCD patient with bulimia nervosa who developed psychogenic poly-dipsia was successfully treated with fluoxetine (Deas-Nesmith and Brewerton 1992). We prescribe hydrochlorothiazide for some of our OCD patients with polydipsia with equivocal results.

Glucose metabolism. In 1919 Kooy published the first report on carbo-hydrate metabolism and mental illness. Over the years, reports of associations of glucose pathology with ANS disorders and major psychiatric disorders, including OCD, appeared in the literature (Yaryura-Tobias and Neziroglu 1975).

In a sample of 100 OCD patients, 61% responded abnormally to a 5-hour oral glucose tolerance test (Yaryura-Tobias 1988); this result should be fur-ther investigated because glucose interacts with tryptophan to assist the regu-latory mechanism of cerebral physiology (Fernstrom et al. 1975). Positron-emission scanning corroborates that cerebral glucose metabolism plays a key role in brain physiology. Glucose metabolism increases in the whole cerebral hemisphere, caudate head, and orbital gyri in OCD patients (Baxter et al. 1987, 1988) as well as in patients with Tourette's syndrome (Baxter et al. 1990). Similar findings in OCD patients, but without involve-ment of the basal ganglia, also were reported (Nordahl et al. 1989). Com-pared with control subjects, children with OCD had increased cerebral glucose metabolism in the left orbital frontal, right sensorimotor, and bilateral pre-frontal and anterior cingulate regions (Swedo et al. 1989).

Interestingly, administration of drugs with a known anti–obsessive-compulsive action was associated with regional brain glucose metabo-lism returning to a more normal level in patients who responded favorably to drug therapy. This finding was true for clomipramine (Benkelfat et al. 1990), fluoxetine (Baxter et al. 1992), and trazodone, with and without use of a monoamine oxidase inhibitor (Baxter et al. 1987). It also was true in cases of childhood-onset OCD when patients were given clomipramine or fluoxetine (Swedo et al. 1992).

In patients with childhood-onset OCD, altered intercorrelations between regional glucose use rates were found in the left hemisphere superior pari-etal region and the left hemisphere anterior medial temporal area (which includes primarily the amygdala). Altered intercorrelations were also found in the anterior limbic and paralimbic regions (Horwitz et al. 1991).

Neuropsychological testing showed the cortical function modifying general activating systems of cortical function and a relationship between decreased glucose metabolism in the lateral prefrontal region and selective attention deficit (Martinot et al. 1990).

Regional cerebral glucose hypermetabolism was measured in women with trichotillomania. Patients had striking global cerebral glucose hypermetabolism in the right superior parietal region and the right and left cerebella (Swedo et al. 1991). Female patients with bulimia nervosa showed a correlation between lower left anterolateral prefrontal regional cerebral glucose hypermetabolism and greater depressive symptoms (Andreason et al. 1992).

The Unified Theory of OCD

The psychiatric history of hundreds of patients who have had more than one major psychiatric illness in their lives can be elicited by careful psychiatric examination. One sixth of a national probability sample (Karno et al 1988) in the United States had a history of three or more comorbid psychiatric disorders (see the section entitlted "Comorbidity and Related Disorders" earlier in this chapter); our personal clinical experience tends to support these findings. We have seen many OCD patients with more than one major mental illness. The mosaic of symptoms displayed by these patients validates the concept of the brain as one indivisible system, with a lesion in one area affecting many other cerebral functioning layers in due time.

As we see in this book, OCD has numerous parameters interwoven in a continuum. Therefore, we define OCD as an open-ended multivariate phenomenon affecting the individual's biopsychosocial architecture.

OCD appears to be related to, or associated with, several neuropsychiatric entities (see Figure 13–1). This cluster of associations makes us believe that OCD exists on a continuum of mental illness, rather than being one clinical entity (Yaryura-Tobias 1990).

The OCD continuum is like a Spanish fan; one condition leads to another, spreading like the unfolding of a Spanish fan from one subsystem to the other. Or the OCD continuum could be compared with a ripple effect, when a noxa intrudes and several resultant variables impinge on a subsystem causing a multiplicity of aftereffects on a range of subsystems (e.g., neurons, axons, neurotransmitters, cerebral regions). If multiple noxae impact the brain, they result in two or more waves overlapping, causing novel histochemical changes. Hence, we observe a surge in neurobehavioral responses or a clinical message (e.g., a symptom) to convey a new disorder's genesis.

Our nosological continuum is based on the concept of a chain reaction in physics; two subatomic particles collide, producing a ripple effect. Another example of the ripple effect is a small meteorological change resulting in an expansive phenomenon of great energy and destructive potential.

OCD has a large symptom spectrum that on observation may fall into predetermined compartments linked by a continuous energy flow in a framework of functions, structures, and fluctuations. With the unified theory of OCD, various nosologies are integrated into one consolidating pathophysiology. The energy flows in time and space, determining the illness's duration in a given anatomical and time trajectory (see Figure 13–1). If the trajectory follows a unidirectional path, the patient's condition deteriorates; if it fluctuates, the disorder waxes and wanes (e.g., Tourette's syndrome). If the trajectory is multidirectional, with back-and-forth displacements, there may be relapse or symptom recurrence.

However, OCD is an entity of gradual onset and growth that, if untreated, becomes chronic. When the illness trespasses on the neural plasticity frontiers (restitutio and integrum), regenerative healing ceases and the disorder becomes irreversible. Measurement of neural plasticity indicates the patient's capacity for adaptation (Bunge 1985), similar to Piaget's adaptation stage. Plasticity provides the ability to reverse the disease's ongoing mechanism (as Prigogine [1988] suggests in another context). We think reversibility is a function of the OCD phenomenon, unless the condition remains untreated or is treated at a later stage of its evolution. The OCD continuum holds together, in accordance with Bell's theorem rejecting the isolation of parts, or separateness, in the human system (Bell 1984).

The clinician must treat OCD and its spectrum. Generally, the prognosis seems to be guarded, and the pathology involved usually requires more than one medication as the therapeutic answer. However, introducing behavior therapy, with or without a cognitive approach, certainly betters the prognosis. As years go by and chronicity sets in, more unsolved therapeutic issues arise. Until we get answers, a multidisciplinary approach seems advisable; perhaps a biopsychosocial model should be applied.

References

Aizenberg G, Hermesh H, Karp L, et al: Pseudocholinesterase in obsessive-compulsive patients. Psychiatry Res 27:65–69, 1989

Aizenberg D, Hermesh H, Gil-ad I, et al: TRH stimulation test in obsessive-compulsive patients. Psychiatry Res 38:21–26, 1991

Alptekin K, Tunca Z, Pirnar T, et al: Magnetic Resonance Imaging of the Brain in Obsessive Compulsive Disorder. Izmir, Turkey, Dokuz Eylul University Faculty of Medicine, 1990

Altemus M, Pigott T, Kalugeras KT, et al: Abnormalities in the regulation of vasopressin and corticotropin releasing factor secretion in obsessive-compulsive disorder. Arch Gen Psychiatry 49:9–20, 1992

Altemus M, Pigott T, L'Heureux F, et al: CSF somatostatin in obsessive-compulsive disorder. Am J Psychiatry 150:460–464, 1993

Anden NE, Carlsson A, Kerstell J, et al: Oral L-dopa treatment of parkinsonism. Acta Med Scand 187:247–255, 1970

Andreason PJ, Altemus M, Zametkin AJ, et al: Regional cerebral glucose metabolism in bulimia nervosa. Am J Psychiatry 149:1506–1513, 1992

Ashcroft GW, Eccleston D, Waddell JL: Recognition of amphetamine addicts. BMJ 1:57–59, 1965

Austin LS, Lydiard RB, Ballenger JC, et al: Dopamine blocking activity of clomipramine in patients without obsessive-compulsive disorder. Biol Psychiatry 30:225–232, 1991

Baer L, Jenike M, Black DW, et al: Effect on Axis II diagnosis in treatment outcome with clomipramine in 55 patients with obsessive-compulsive disorder. J Arch Gen Psychiatry 49:862–866, 1992

Baer L, Rauch SL, Ballantine T, Martuza R, Cosgrove R, Cassem E, Giriunas I, Manza PA, Dimino C, Jenike M: Cingulotomy for intractable obsessive compulsive disorder. Arch Gen Psychiatry 52:384–392, 1995

Barbeau A, Sourkes TL: Some biochemical aspects of extrapyramidal diseases, in Extrapyramidal System and Neuroleptics. Edited by Bordeleau JM. Montreal, Canada, Editions Psychiatriques, 1961

Barton R: Diabetes insipidus and obsessional neurosis: a syndrome. Lancet 1:133–135, 1965

Bastani B, Nash JF, Meltzer HY: Prolactin and cortisol responses to MK-212, a serotonin agonist in obsessive-compulsive disorder. Arch Gen Psychiatry 47:833–839, 1990

Bastani B, Arora AC, Meltzer HY: Serotonin uptake and imipramine binding in the blood platelets of obsessive-compulsive disorder patients. Biol Psychiatry 30:131–139, 1991

Baxter LR Jr, Thompson JM, Schwartz JM: Trazodone treatment response in obsessive-compulsive disorder correlated with shifts in glucose metabolism in the caudate nuclei. Psychopathology 1:114–122, 1987

Baxter LR Jr, Schwartz JM, Mazziotta, et al: Cerebral glucose metabolic rates in nondepressed patients with obsessive-compulsive disorder. Am J Psychiatry 145:1560–1563, 1988

Baxter LR, Schwartz JM, Guze BH, et al: PET imaging in obsessive-compulsive disorder with and without depression. J Clin Psychiatry 51:61–69, 1990

Baxter LR, Schwartz JM, Bergman KS, et al: Caudate glucose metabolic rate changes with both drug and behavior therapy for obsessive-compulsive disorder. Arch Gen Psychiatry 49:681–689, 1992

Behar D, Rapoport JL, Berg CJ, et al: Computerized tomography and neuropsychological test measures in adolescents with obsessive-compulsive disorder. Am J Psychiatry 141:363–369, 1984

Bell JS: Physics, Vol 1. 1984

Benkelfat C, Nordahl TE, Semple WE, et al: Local cerebral glucose metabolic rates in obsessive-compulsive disorder patients treated with clomipramine. Arch Gen Psychiatry 47:840–848, 1990

Benkelfat C, Mefford IN, Masters CF, et al: Plasma catecholamines and their metabolites in obsessive-compulsive disorder. Psychiatry Res 37:321–331, 1991

Benowitz L, Routtemberg A: A membrane phosphoprotein associated with neural development, axonal regeneration, phospholipid metabolism and synaptic plasticity. Trends Neurosci 10:527–532, 1987

Bergmann F, Chaimovitz M, Pasternak V: Dual action of morphine and related drugs on compulsive gnawing of rats. Psychopharmacologia 46:87–91, 1976

Bergson H: Creative Evolution. Translated by Murray A. New York, Modern Library, 1944

Black DW, Kelly M, Myers C, et al: Tritiated imipramine binding in obsessive-compulsive disorder volunteers and psychiatrically normal controls. Biol Psychiatry 27:319–327, 1990

Blackmore C, Mitchell DE: Environmental modification of the visual cortex and the neural basis of learning and memory. Nature 241:467–468, 1973

Brandt KP, MacKenzie TB: Obsessive-compulsive disorder exacerbated during pregnancy: a case report. Int J Psychiatry Med 17:361–366, 1987

Bremner AJ, Regan A: Intoxicated by water: polydipsia and water intoxication in a mental handicap hospital. Br J Psychiatry 158:244–250, 1987

Brion A, Ey H: Psiquiatria Animal, Siglo XXI. Mexico City, Mexico, 1968

Brodman K: Vergleicmende Lokalisationlehre der Grosshirnrinde, in Ihren Prinzipien dargestelt auf Grund des Zellenbaues, Vol 6. Leipzig, Germany, JA Barth, 1909, p 324

Bunge M: El Problema Mente-Cerebro. Un Enfoque Psicobiológico. Madrid, Spain, Tecnos, 1985

Burger H, Mayer-Gross N: Uber Zwangssymptome Encephalitis Lethargica und uber die strukturd der zwangserscheinungen uberhaupt. Zeitschrift der Gesamte Zeitschrift der Neurologie und Psychiatrie 116:645–686, 1928

Cameron OG, Kerber K, Curtis TC: Obsessive-compulsive and DST. Psychiatry Res 19:329, 1986

Capstick N: Chlorimipramine in the treatment of true obsessional states: a report on four patients. Psychosomatics 16:21–25, 1975

Carranza-Acevedo J, Ortega-Corona BG, Ordonez S, et al: Cambios en la conducta producios por la Administracion Cronica de D-Anfetamina en Ratones. Arch Invest Med (Mex) 1:221–226, 1970

Catapano F, Moneleone P, Maj M, et al: Dexamethasone suppression test in patients with primary obsessive-compulsive disorder and in healthy controls. Neuropsychobiology 23:53–56, 1990

Catapano F, Monteleone P, Fuschino A, et al: Melatonin and cortisol secretion in patients with primary obsessive-compulsive disorder. Psychiatry Res 44: 217–225, 1992

Changeux JP: Neuronal Man-The Biology of Mind. Translated by Garey L. New York, Pantheon, 1985

Changeux JP, Danchin A: Selective stabilisation of developing synapses as a mechanism for the specification of neuronal networks. Nature 264:705–712, 1976

Charney DS, Goodman WK, Price LH, Woods SW, Rasmussen SA, Geninger GR: Serotonin function in obsessive compulsive disorder. A comparison of the effects of tryptophan and m-chlorophenylpiperazine in patients and healthy subjects. Arch Gen Psychiatry 45:177–185, 1988

Cipollina Mangiameli G: Amenorrea e disturbi comportamentali. Minerva Med 64:3765–3769, 1973

Ciprian Ollivier J, Gallardo F, Biganzdi B, et al: Desordenes obseso-compulsivos: tratamiento con clorimipramina. Daimon 6:33–37, 1982

Collard KJ, Roberts MHT: Effects of chlorimipramine on experimentally-induced changes in forebrain 5-hydroxyindoles. Eur J Pharmacol 29:154–160, 1974

Cottraux JH, Bouvard M, Claustrat B, et al: Abnormal dexamethasone suppression in agoraphobia with panic attacks. Psychiatry Res 15:301, 1984

Cottraux JH, Flachaire E, Renaud B: Dosage de la serotonin plaquettaire dans les obsessions compulsions. Presse Med 16:590–594, 1987

Crawford JP: Cerebral autonomic imbalance. Lancet 2:772–773, 1972

Critchley M: The Parietal Lobes. London, Arnold, 1953

Crow HJ: Cerebral Circulation and Stroke by KJ Zulch (book review). Neurol Sci 14:377, 1971

Curtis GC, Glitz DA: Neuroendocrine findings in anxiety disorders. Neurol Clin 6:131–148, 1988

Daumezon MG, Cor J, Moor L: Disparition de phénomènes obsessionnels graves après "autolobotomie" chez un grand déséquilibré. Ann Med Psychol 112: 93–97, 1954

Deas-Nesmith D, Brewerton TD: A case of fluoxetine-responsive psychogenic polydipsia: a variant of obsessive-compulsive disorder. J Nerv Ment Dis 180: 338–339, 1992

de Boer JA, Westenberg HG: Oxytocin in obsessive compulsive disorder. Peptides 13:1083–1085, 1992

De Jong H: Hormanale Experimentelle Katatonie. Proc R Acad Sci (Amsterdam) 34:576–587, 1931

Dillon KM, Brooks D: Unusual cleaning behavior in the luteal phase. Psychol Rep 70:35–39, 1992

Economo C: The Cytoarchitectonics of the Human Cerebral Cortex. London, Oxford University Press, 1929

Edelman GM: Group selection and phasic re-entrant signaling: a theory of higher brain function, in The Mindful Brain. Edited by Edelman GM, Mount Castle VB. Cambridge, MA, 1978, pp 51–100

Ellinwood E: Amphetamine psychosis. J Nerv Ment Dis 1:244–273, 1967

Ernst AM, Smelick P: Site of action of dopamine and apomorphine on compulsive gnawing behavior in rats. Experientia 22:837–838, 1966

Escobedo F, Fernandez-Guardiola A, Solis G: Chronic stimulation of the cingulum with behavior disorders, in Surgical Approaches in Psychiatry. Edited by Lattinen LV, Livingston KE. Baltimore, MD, University Park Press, 1973, pp 65–68

Faillace LA, Snyder SH, Weingartner H: 5-dimethoxy-4-methylamphetamine: clinical evaluation of a new hallucinogenic drug. J Pharm Pharmacol 22:337–379, 1970

Fernandez de Cordoba CE, Lopez-Ibor JJ: Monochlorimipramine in the treatment of psychiatric patients resistant to other therapies. Act Luso-Española Neurologia 26:119–147, 1967

Fernstrom JD, Jacoby JH, Milinview A: The interaction of diet and drug in modifying brain serotonin metabolism. Gen Pharmacol 6:253–258, 1975

Flament MF, Rapoport JL, Berg CJ, et al: Clomipramine treatment of childhood obsessive-compulsive disorder: a double-blind controlled study. Arch Gen Psychiatry 42:977–983, 1985

Flament MF, Rapoport JL, Murphy DL, et al: Clomipramine treatment of childhood obsessive-compulsive disorder. Arch Gen Psychiatry 44:219–225, 1987

Flor-Henry P: Psychiatric syndromes considered as manifestations of lateralized temporal-limbic dysfunction, in Surgical Approaches in Psychiatry. Edited by Laitinen LV, Livingston KE. Baltimore, MD, University Park Press, 1973, pp 22–26

Flor-Henry P, Yeudall L, Koles Z, et al: Neuropsychological and power-spectral EEG investigations in the obsessive-compulsive syndrome. Biol Psychiatry 14:119–130, 1979

Fog R: On stereotypy and catalepsy: studies on the effect of amphetamines and neuroleptics in rats. Acta Neurol Scand 48:1–64, 1967

Fog R: Role of the carpus striatum in typical behavioral effects in rats produced by both amphetamine and neuroleptic drugs. Acta Pharmacol Toxicol (Copenh) 25:49–59, 1972

Gaillard JM, Iorio G, Campajola P, et al: Temporal organization of sleep in schizophrenics and patients with obsessive-compulsive disorder. Recent Advances in Biological Psychiatry 15:76–83, 1984

Garber HJ, Ananth JV, Chiu LC, et al: Nuclear magnetic resonance study of obsessive compulsive disorder. Am J Psychiatry 146:1001–1005, 1989

Gehris TL, Kathol RG, Black DW, et al: Urinary free cortisol levels in obsessive-compulsive disorder. Psychiatry Res 32:151–158, 1990

Goldar JC: Anatomia de la Mente. Buenos Aires, Argentina, Editorial Salerno, 1993

Goldberger E, Rapoport J: Canine acral dermatitis: response to the anti-obsessional drug clomipramine. J Am Anim Hosp Assoc 22:179–182,1991

Goldstein K: Zur Frage der Restitution nach umschriebenem Hirndefekt. Schweizer Archiven fur Psychiatrie 13:283–296, 1924

Goldstein K: The Organism. New York, American Books, 1930, pp 485–489

Goldstein K: After Effects of Brain Injuries in War: Their Evaluation and Treatment. New York, Grune & Stratton, 1942, pp 485–489

Goldstein K, Katz SE: The psychopathology of Pick's disease. Archives of Neurological Psychiatry 38:473–485, 1937

Goodman W: Drug response and obsessive-compulsive disorder subtypes. Paper presented at the annual meeting of the American Psychiatric Association, Montreal, Canada, May 1989

Griesinger W: Mental Pathology and Therapeutics (1867). Translated by Ackerknecht EH. New York, Hafner Publishing, 1965

Hamburger SD, Swedo S, Whitake A, et al: Growth rate in adolescents without obsessive-compulsive disorder. Am J Psychiatry 146:652–655, 1989

Hanna GL, McCracken JT, Cantwell DP: Prolactin in childhood obsessive-compulsive disorder: clinical correlates and response to clomipramine. J Am Acad Child Adolesc Psychiatry 30:173–178, 1991a

Hanna GL, Yuwiler A, Cantwell DP: Whole blood serotonin in juvenile obsessive-compulsive disorder. Biol Psychiatry 29:738–744, 1991b

Hantouche E, Piketty ML, Poirier MF, et al: Obsessive-compulsive disorder and the study of thyroid function. Encephale 17:493–496, 1991

Hewlett WG, Vinogradov S, Martin K, et al: Fenfluramine stimulation of prolactin in obsessive-compulsive disorder. Psychiatry Res 42:81–92, 1992

Hollander E, McCarley A: Yohimbine treatment of sexual side effects induced by serotonin reuptake blockers. J Clin Psychiatry 53:207–209, 1992

Hollander E, DeCaria L, Nitescu A, et al: Noradrenergic function in obsessive-compulsive disorder: behavioral and endocrine response to clonidine and comparison to healthy controls. Psychiatry Res 37:161–177, 1991

Hollander E, DeCaria C, Nitescu A, et al: Serotonergic function in obsessive-compulsive disorder: behavioral and neuroendocrine responses to oral *m*-chlorophenylpiperazine and fenfluramine in patients and healthy volunteers. Arch Gen Psychiatry 49:21–28, 1992

Hornykiewicz O: The subcortical monoaminergic systems, in Neurosurgical Treatment in Psychiatry, Pain and Epilepsy. Edited by Sweet WH, Obrader S, Martin-Rodriquez JG. Baltimore, MD, University Park Press, 1977, pp 293–302

Horwitz B, Swedo SE, Grady CL, et al: Cerebral metabolic pattern in obsessive-compulsive disorder: altered intercorrelations between regional rates of glucose utilization. Psychiatry Res 40:221–237, 1991

Hubel DH, Wiesel TN: Receptive fields, binocular interaction and functional architecture in the cat's visual cortex. J Physiol (Lond) 160:106–154, 1962

Ingram IM: Obsessional illness in mental hospital patients. J Ment Sci 107: 382–402, 1961

Insel TR, Gillin JC, Moore A, et al: The sleep of patients with obsessive-compulsive disorder. Arch Gen Psychiatry 39:1372–1377, 1982a

Insel TR, Kalin NH, Guttmacher LB, et al: The dexamethasone suppression test in patients with primary obsessive-compulsive disorder. Psychiatry Res 6: 153–160, 1982b

Insel TR, Mueller EA, Alterman I, et al: Obsessive-compulsive disorder and serotonin: is there a connection? Biol Psychiatry 20:1174–1189, 1985

Iversen LL: Amino acids and peptides-fast and slow chemical signals in the nervous system? Proc R Soc Lond B Biol Sci 221:245–260, 1984

Iversen LL, Goodman E: Fast and Slow Chemical Signalling in the Nervous System. Oxford, England, University Park Press, 1986

Joffe RT, Swinson RP: Methylphenidate in primary obsessive-compulsive disorder. J Clin Psychopharmacol 7:420–422, 1987

Joffe RT, Swinson RP: Total sleep deprivation in patients with obsessive-compulsive disorder. Acta Psychiatr Scand 77:483–487, 1988

Joffe RT, Swinson RP, Levitt AJ: Acute psychostimulant challenge in primary obsessive-compulsive disorder. J Clin Psychopharmacol 11:237–241, 1991

Kahn RS, Kalus D, Wetzler S, et al: Effects of serotonin antagonists on M-chlorophenylpiperazine-mediated responses in normal subjects. Psychiatry Res 33:189–198, 1990

Karno M, Goldin JM, Sorenson SB: The epidemiology of obsessive-compulsive disorder in five US communities. Arch Gen Psychiatry 45:1094–1099, 1988

Kasvikis G, Basoglu M, Monteiro W, et al: Urinary cortisol during exposure in obsessive-compulsive ritualizers. Psychiatry Res 23:131–135, 1988

Kim SW, Dysken MW: Test of dopamine-blocking potential of clomipramine (letter). Am J Psychiatry 148:690, 1991

Knapp S, Mandell A: Some drug effects on the functions of the two measurable forms of tryptophan-s-hydroxylase: influence on hydroxylation and uptake of substrate, in Serotonin and Behavior. Edited by Barchas J, Usdin E. New York, Academic Press, 1973, pp 61–71

Kojima T, Matsushima E, Ando K, et al: Exploratory eye movements and neuropsychological tests in schizophrenic patients. Schizophr Bull 18:85–94, 1992

Kooy FH: Hyperglycemia in mental disorder. Brain 17:214–217, 1919

Kramer JC, Fishman VS, Littlefield DC: Amphetamine abuse. JAMA 305–309, 1967

Kruesi MJ, Swedo L, Leonard H, et al: CSF somatostatin in childhood psychiatric disorders: a preliminary investigation. Psychiatry Res 33:277–284, 1990

Lal S, Sourkes TL: Potentiation and inhibition of the amphetamine stereotypy and hypermotility. Arch Immunol Ther Exp 24:829–836, 1972

Langlow JR, Alarcon RD: Trimipramine-induced neuroleptic malignant syndrome after transient psychogenic polydipsia in one patient. J Clin Psychiatry 50: 144–145, 1989

Laplane D, Boulliat J, Baron JC, et al: Obsessive-compulsive behavior caused by bilateral lesions of the lenticular nuclei. Encephale 14:27–32, 1988

Lemus CZ, Robinson DG, Kronig M, et al: Behavioral responses to a dopaminergic challenge in obsessive-compulsive disorder. Journal of Anxiety Disorders 5: 369–373, 1991

Lesh KP, Hoh A, Schulte HM, et al: Long-term fluoxetine treatment decreases 5-HT1A receptor responsivity in obsessive-compulsive disorder. Psychopharmacology 105:415–420, 1991

Lieberman JA, Kane JM, Sarantakos S, et al: Dexamethasone suppression tests in patients with obsessive-compulsive disorder. Am J Psychiatry 142:747–751, 1985

Livingston KE, Escobar A: The anatomical bias of the limbic system concepts: a proposed reorientation. Arch Neurol 24:17–21, 1971

Lo WH: A follow-up study of obsessional neurotics in Hong Kong Chinese. Br J Psychiatry 113:823–832, 1967

Lovenberg W: Tryptophan hydroxylase and serotonin synthesis in the brain, in Pharmacology and the Future of Man: Proceedings of the 5th International Congress on Pharmacology, Basel, Vol 4. San Francisco, CA, Karger, 1973, pp 232–244

Lovinger DM, Colley PA, Akers RF, et al: Direct relation of long-term synaptic potentiation to phosphorylation of membrane protein F1, a substrate of membrane protein kinase C. Brain Res 399:205–211, 1986

Lucca A, Lucini V, Piatti E: Plasma tryptophan levels and plasma tryptophan/neutral amino acids ratio in patients with mood disorder, patients with obsessive-compulsive disorder, and normal subjects. Psychiatry Res 44:85–91, 1992

Lucey JV, Barry S, Webb MG, et al: The desipramine-induced growth hormone response and the dexamethasone suppression test in obsessive-compulsive disorder. Acta Psychiatr Scand 86:367–370, 1992

Lucey JV, Butcher G, Clare AW, et al: Elevated growth hormone responses to pyridostigmine in obsessive-compulsive disorder: evidence of cholinergic supersensitivity. Am J Psychiatry 150:961–962, 1993

Luxemberg JS, Swedo SE, Flament MF, et al: Neuroanatomical abnormalities in obsessive-compulsive disorder detected with quantitative X-ray computed tomography. Am J Psychiatry 145:1089–1093, 1988

Mandell A, Knapp S, Hsu LL: Some factors in the regulation of central serotonergic synapses. Life Sci 14:1–17, 1974

Marazzitti D, Hollander E, Lensi P, et al: Peripheral markers of serotonin and dopamine function in obsessive-compulsive disorder. Psychiatry Res 42:41–51, 1992

Martin-Iversen MT, Stahl SM, Iversen SD: Factors determining the behavioral consequences of continuous treatment with 4-propyl 9-hydroxynaphthoxazine, a selective dopamine D2 agonist, in Parkinson's Disease: Clinical and Experimental Advances. Edited by Rose FC. London, John Libbey, 1987, pp 169–177

Martinot JL, Allilaire JF, Mazoyer BM, et al: Obsessive-compulsive disorder: a clinical, neuropsychological and positron emission tomography study. Acta Psychiatr Scand 82:233–242, 1990

Mattson RH, Calverly JR: Dextroamphetamine-sulphate induced dyskinesias. JAMA 204:108–110, 1968

Mavissakalian M, Hamann MS, Jones B: Correlates of DSM-III personality disorders in obsessive-compulsive disorder. Compr Psychiatry 31:481–489, 1990

McBride P, DeMeo MD, Seeney JA, et al: Neuroendocrine and behavioral responses to challenge with the indirect serotonin agonist difenfluramine in adults with obsessive-compulsive disorder. Biol Psychiatry 31:19–34, 1992

McKay D, Neziroglu F, Todaro J: Changes in personality disorders following behavior therapy for obsessive compulsive disorder. Journal of Anxiety Disorders 10:47–57, 1996

McKinney WT: Animal model of schizophrenic disorder in schizophrenia. Sci Prog 15:141–154, 1989

Mesulam MM: Patterns in behavioral neuro-anatomy: association areas, the limbic system and hemispheric specialization, in Principles of Behavioral Neurology, Vol 1. Edited by Mesulam MM. Philadelphia, PA, FA Davis, 1986, pp 1–70

Meyer G, McElhaney M, Martin W, et al: Stereotactic cingulotomy with results of acute stimulation and serial psychological testing, in Surgical Approaches in Psychiatry. Edited by Laitinen LV, Livingston KE. Baltimore, MD, University Park Press, 1973, pp 39–58

Mikirtumov BE: Neuropsychiatric disorders in adolescent disorders of menstrual function. Zh Nevropatol Psikhiatr Im S S Korsakova 85:747–751, 1985

Mindus P, Rauch SL, Nyman H, et al: Capsulotomy and cingulotomy as treatments for malignant obsessive-compulsive disorder: an update, in Obsessive-Compulsive Disorder. Edited by Hollander E, Zohar J, Marazziti D, et al. England, John Wiley & Sons, 1994, pp 245–276

Mitchell JC: Dermatological aspects of displacement activity: attention to the body surface as a substitute for "fight or flight." Can Med Assoc J 98:962–964, 1968

Mogilnicka E, Braestrup C: Noradrenergic influence on the stereotyped behavior induced by amphetamine, phenylethylamine, and apomorphine combinations. J Pharm Pharmacol 28:253–255, 1976

Monserrat-Esteve S: Introduction, in Patologia Obsesiva. Edited by Monserrat-Esteve S, Costa Molinari JM, Ballús C. Málaga, Spain, XI Congreso Nacional de Neuropsiquiatria, Graficasa, 1971, pp 13–29

Morpurgo C: Effects of antiparkinson drugs on phenothiazine induced catatonic reaction. Arch Int Pharmacodyn Ther 137:84–90, 1962

Morpurgo C, Theobald W: Influence of antiparkinson drugs and amphetamine on some pharmacological effects of phenothiazine derivatives used as neuroleptics. Psychopharmacologia 6:178–191, 1964

Nauta WJH: The central nisceromotor system: a general survey, in Limbic System Mechanisms and Autonomic Function. Edited by Hockman CH. Springfield IL, Charles C Thomas, 1972, pp 21–33

Neziroglu F, Steele J, Yaryura-Tobias JA, et al: Effect of behavior therapy on serotonin level in obsessive compulsive disorder, in Psychiatry: A World Perspective, Vol 1. Edited by Stefanis CN, Rabavilas AD, Soldatos CR, Amsterdam, The Netherlands, Elsevier, 1990

Neziroglu FA, Anemone R, Yaryura-Tobias JA: Onset of obsessive-compulsive disorder in pregnancy. Am J Psychiatry 149:947–950, 1992

Nickoloff SE, Radant AD, Reichler R, et al: Smooth pursuit and saccadic eye movements and neurological soft signs in obsessive-compulsive disorder. Psychiatric Research 38:173–185, 1991

Nordahl TE, Benkelfat C, Semple WE, et al: Cerebral glucose metabolic rates in obsessive-compulsive disorder. Neuropsychopharmacology 2:23–28, 1989

Norstedt G, Palmiter R: Secretory rhythm of growth hormone regulates sexual differentiation of mouse liver. Cell 36:805–812, 1984

Pandey SC, Kim SW, Davis JM, et al: Platelet serotonin-2 receptors in obsessive-compulsive disorder. Biol Psychiatry 33:367–372, 1993

Papez JW: A proposed mechanism of emotion. Archives of Neurological Psychiatry 38:725–743, 1937

Paunovic VR: Syndrome obsessionnel au decours d'une atteinte cerebrale organique. Ann Med Psychol (Paris) 142:379–382, 1984

Pedersen V: Potentiation of apomorphine effect (compulsive gnawing behavior in mice). Acta Pharmacol Toxicol (Copenh) 25 (suppl 4):63–67, 1967

Pedersen V: Role of catecholamines in compulsive gnawing behavior in mice. Br J Pharmacol 34:219–220, 1968

Pfohl B, Black D, Noyes R Jr, et al: A test of the tridimensional personality theory: association with diagnosis and platelet imipramine binding in obsessive-compulsive disorder. Biol Psychiatry 28:41–46, 1990

Pigott TA, Pato MT, L'Heureux F, et al: A controlled comparison of adjuvant lithium carbonate or thyroid hormone in clomipramine treated patients with obsessive-compulsive disorder. J Clin Psychopharmacol 11:242–248, 1991

Pigott TA, L'Heureux F, Dubbert B, et al: Obsessive-compulsive disorder: comorbid conditions. J Clin Psychiatry 55:15–27, 1994

Pollitt J: Natural history of obsessional states: a study of 150 cases. BMJ 1:149–198, 1957

Popov EA: Von Einen Akuten Fall von Zwangneurose. Z BL Neur 87:539–547, 1949

Prat J, Porta A, Vallejo J: Sindromes obsesivoides en psiquiatria, in Patologia Obsesiva. Edited by Monserrat-Esteve S, Costa-Molinari JM, Ballus C. Malaga, Spain, XI Congreso Nacional de Neuropsiquiatria, Graficasa, 1971, pp 313–337

Price LH, Charney DS, Delgado PL, et al: Clinical studies of 5-HT function using i.v. L-tryptophan. Prog Neuropsychopharmacol Biol Psychiatry 14:459–472, 1990

Prigogine I: Tan Solo Una Ilusión? 2nd Edition. Barcelona, Spain, Tusquets, 1988

Rack PH: Experience with intravenous clomipramine, in Obsessional States and Their Treatment with Anafranil. Manchester, England, Geigy, 1970, pp 10–13

Ramon y Cajal S: Neuronismo o reticularismo? Las Pruebas objetivas de la unidad anatomica de las celulas neruiosas. Arch Neurobiol (Madr) 13:217–291, 1933

Randrup A, Munkvad I: Stereotyped activities produced by amphetamine in several animal species and man. Psychopharmacologia 11:300–310, 1967

Randrup A, Munkvad I: Influence of amphetamines on animal behavior: stereotypy, functional impairment and possible animal-human correlations. Psychiatr Neurol Neurochir 75:193–202, 1972

Randrup A, Munkvad I: Pharmacology and physiology of stereotyped behavior. J Psychiatr Res 11:1–10, 1974

Rapoport JL, Ryland DH, Kriet M: Drug treatment of canine acral lick: an animal model of obsessive-compulsive disorder. Arch Gen Psychiatry 49:517–521, 1992

Rasmussen SA, Eisen JL: The epidemiology and clinical features of obsessive compulsive disorder. Psychiatr Clin North Am 15:744–758, 1992

Reynynghe de Voxurie VG: Anafranil (G.34586) in obsessive neurosis. Acta Neurol Belg 68:787–792, 1968

Rocca P, Ferrero P, Gualerzi A, et al: Peripheral-type benzodiazepine receptors in anxiety disorders. Acta Psychiatr Scand 84:537–544, 1991

Rumke HC: Uber die Klinik und Psychopathologie der Zwangserscheinungen, in Eine Bluhende: Psychiatrie in Gefahr. Edited by Ritter W, Selbach OC. Berlin, Germany, Springer, 1967, pp 76–100

Rylander G: Addiction to preludin intravenously injected, in Proceedings of the IVth World Congress on Psychiatry. Edited by Lopez JT. Amsterdam, The Netherlands, Elsevier North-Holland, 1966, pp 1363–1365

Sacks O: Awakenings. Paper presented at the annual meeting of the American Psychiatric Association, Toronto, Canada, May 1977

Salzberg AD, Swedo SE: Oxytocin and vasopressin in obsessive-compulsive disorder. Am J Psychiatry 149:713–714, 1992

Sanchez Planell L: Sindromes obsesivoides en neurologia, in Patologia Obsesiva. Edited by Monserrat-Esteve S, Costa-Molinari JM, Ballus C. Málaga, Spain, XI Congreso Nacional de Neuropsiquiatria, Graficasa, 1971, pp 341–361

Sandyk R: Does melatonin mediate the therapeutic effects of 5-HT reuptake inhibitors in obsessive-compulsive disorder? Int J Neurol Sci 64:221–223, 1992

Schaltenbrand G: The effects of stereotactical stimulation in the depth of the brain. Brain 88:835–840, 1965

Schaltenbrand G: The effects on speech and language of stereotactical stimulation in thalamus and corpus callosum. Brain Lang 2:70–77, 1975

Schaltenbrand G, Spuler H, Wahren W, et al: Electroanatomy of the thalamic ventro-oral nucleus based on stereotactic stimulation in man. Z Neurol 199:259–276, 1971

Scheel-Kruger J: Central effects of anti-cholinergic drugs measured by the apomorphine gnawing test in mice. Acta Pharmacol Toxicol (Copenh) 28:1–16, 1970

Schirring E: Amfetamin-I focus for forsking og misburg. Ment Hyg 22:13–20, 1969

Shagass C, Roemer RA, Straumanis JJ, et al: Distinctive somatosensory evoked potential features in obsessive-compulsive disorder. Biol Psychiatry 19:1507–1524, 1984

Sichel DA, Cohen LS, Dimmock JA: Postpartum obsessive-compulsive disorder: a case series. J Clin Psychiatry 54:156–159, 1993

Stahl SM, Wets KM: Recent advances in drug delivery technology for neurology. Clin Neuropharmacol 11:1–17, 1988

Steketee G: Personality traits and disorders in obsessive-compulsives. Journal of Anxiety Disorders 4:351–364, 1990

Stout AL, Steege JF, Blazer DG, et al: Comparison of lifetime psychiatric diagnosis in premenstrual syndrome clinic and community samples. J Nerv Ment Dis 174:517–522, 1986

Swedo SE, Kruesi MJ, Leonard HL, et al: Lack of seasonal variation in pediatric lumbar cerebrospinal fluid neurotransmitter metabolite concentrations. Acta Psychiatr Scand 80:644–649, 1989

Swedo SE, Rapoport JL, Leonard HL, et al: Regional cerebral glucose metabolism of women with trichotillomania. Arch Gen Psychiatry 48:828–833, 1991

Swedo SE, Pietrini P, Leonard HL, et al: Cerebral glucose metabolism in childhood-onset obsessive-compulsive disorder: revisualization during pharmacotherapy. Arch Gen Psychiatry 49:690–694, 1992

Sweeney JA, Palumbo DR, Halper JP, et al: Pursuit eye movement dysfunction in obsessive-compulsive disorder. Psychiatry Research 42:1–11, 1992

Talairach J, Banland J, Geier S, et al: The cingulate gyrus and human behavior. Electroencephalogr Clin Neurophysiol 34:45–52, 1973

Ternaux JP, Boireau A, Bourgoin S, et al: In vivo release of 5-HT in the lateral ventricle of the rat: effects of 5-hydroxytryptophan and tryptophan. Brain Res 101:533–548, 1976

Thoren P, Asberg M, Bertilsson L, et al: Clomipramine treatment of obsessive-compulsive disorder, II: biochemical aspects. Arch Gen Psychiatry 37:1286–1294, 1980a

Thoren P, Asberg M, Cronholm B, et al: Clomipramine treatment of obsessive-compulsive disorder, I: a controlled clinical trial. Arch Gen Psychiatry 37:1281–1285, 1980b

Tien AY, Pearlson GD, Machlin SR, et al: Regional cerebral glucose metabolism of women with trichotillomania. Arch Gen Psychiatry 48:828–833, 1992

Ushijima S, Kobayashi R: The perimenarche syndrome (a proposal). Japanese Journal of Psychiatry 149:641–646, 1988

Vallejo Ruiloba J: Estudio psicofisiológico de la enfermedad obsesiva. Rev Depart Psiquiatría Facult Med Barcelona 5:221–238, 1978

Vasilev VN, Chugunov VS, Derbeneva LM, et al: The L-DOPA test in patients with obsessive fear neurosis. Vopr Med Khim 34:115–120,1988

Vernadsky VI: La Biosphere. Paris, Felix Alcan, 1930

Vitiello B, Shimon H, Behar D, et al: High affinity imipramine binding and serotonin uptake in obsessive-compulsive patients. Acta Psychiatr Scand 84:29–32, 1991

von Bertalanfly L: General System Theory. New York, George Brazillier, 1968

Weizman A, Carmi M, Haggai H, et al: High affinity imipramine binding and serotonin uptake in platelets of eight adolescent and ten adult obsessive-compulsive patients. Am J Psychiatry 143:335–339, 1986

Weizman R, Gil-ad I, Hermesh H, et al: Immunoreactive beta-endorphin, cortisol, and growth hormone plasma levels in obsessive-compulsive disorder. Clin Neuropharmacol 13:297–302, 1990

Weizman A, Mandel A, Barber Y, et al: Decreased platelet imipramine binding in Tourette syndrome children with obsessive-compulsive disorder. Biol Psychiatry 31:705–711, 1992

Whatmore GB, Kohli DR: Dysponesis: a neurophysiological factor in functional disorders. Behav Sci 13:102–124, 1968

Wiesel TN: The post-natal development of the visual cortex and the influence of environment (Nobel lecture). Biosci Rep 2:351–377, 1982

Yakovlev PL: Pathoarchitechtonic studies of cerebral malformations, III: arrhinencephalies (holotelencephalies). Neuropath Exp Neurol 18:22–55, 1948

Yakovlev PI, LeCours AR: The myelogenetic cycles of regional maturation of the brain, in Regional Development of the Brain in Early Life. Edited by Minkowski A. Boston, Blackwell Scientific Publications, 1964, pp 3–60

Yaryura-Tobias JA: Obsessive-compulsive disorder: a serotonergic hypothesis. Journal of Orthomolecular Psychiatry 6:317–326, 1977

Yaryura-Tobias JA: Clinical observations on L-tryptophan in the treatment of obsessive-compulsive disorders, in Abstracts of the III World Congress of Biological Psychiatry. Stockholm, Sweden, G Struve, 1981

Yaryura-Tobias JA: Desorden obseso-compulsivo primario: aspectos bioquímicos, in Psiquiatría Biológica, Vol 12. Edited by Ciprian-Ollivier J. Buenos Aires, Argentina, Cientifíca Inter Americana, 1988, pp 120–127

Yaryura-Tobias JA: A unified theory of obsessive-compulsive disorder, in A World Perspective, Vol 1. Edited by Stefanis CN, Rabavilas AD, Soldatos CR, et al. Amsterdam, the Netherlands, Elsevier Science Publishers, 1990, pp 568–571

Yaryura-Tobias JA, Bhagavan HN: L-tryptophan in obsessive-compulsive disorders. Am J Psychiatry 134:1298–1299, 1977

Yaryura-Tobias JA, Neziroglu FA: Psychosis and disturbance of glucose metabolism. Journal of the International Academy of Preventive Medicine 2:38–45, 1975

Yaryura-Tobias JA, Neziroglu F: Compulsions, aggression, and self-mutilation: a hypothalamic disorder? Journal of Orthomolecular Psychiatry 10:263–268, 1978

Yaryura-Tobias JA, Neziroglu F: Obsessive-Compulsive Disorder: Pathogenesis, Diagnosis and Treatment. New York, Marcel Dekker, 1983

Yaryura-Tobias JA, Neziroglu F: Organicity in obsessive compulsive disorder. Biol Psychiatry 29:335, 1991

Yaryura-Tobias JA, Neziroglu FA, Bergman L: Chlorimipramine for obsessive-compulsive neurosis: an organic approach. 20:541–548, 1976

Yaryura-Tobias JA, Bebirian RJ, Neziroglu F, et al: Obsessive-compulsive disorders as a serotonergic defect. Res Commun Psychol Psychiatr Behav 2:279–286, 1977

Yaryura-Tobias JA, Neziroglu FA, Fuller B: An integral approach in the management of the obsessive-compulsive patient. Pharmm Med 1:155–167, 1979

Yaryura-Tobias JA, Neziroglu F, Howard S, et al: Clinical aspects of Gilles de la Tourette Syndrome. Journal of Orthomolecular Psychiatry 4:263–268, 1981

Yaryura-Tobias JA, Neziroglu FA, Kaplan S: Self-mutilation, anorexia, and dysmenorrhea in obsessive compulsive disorder. International Journal of Eating Disorders 17:33–38, 1995

Yuwiler A, Shih JC, Chen C, et al: Hyperserotoninemia and antiserotonin antibodies in autism and other disorder. J Autism Dev Disord 22:33–45, 1992

Zahn TP, Insel TR, Murphy DL: Psychophysiological changes during pharmacological treatment of patients with obsessive-compulsive disorder. Br J Psychiatry 145:39–44, 1984

Zangwill OL: Neurological studies and human behavior. Br Med Bull 20:488–490, 1964

Zivkovic B, Guidoti A, Costa E: On the regulation of tryptophan hydroxylase in brain. Adv Biochem Psychopharmacol 11:19–30, 1974

Zohar J, Mueller EA, Insel TR, et al: Serotonergic responsivity in obsessive-compulsive disorder. Arch Gen Psychiatry 44:946–951, 1987

Zohar J, Insel TR, Zohar-Kadouch RC, et al: Serotonergic responsivity in obsessive-compulsive disorder. Arch Gen Psychiatry 45:167–172, 1988

Index

*Page numbers that appear in **boldface** refer to tables or figures.*